Modern Medicine and International Aid

New Perspectives in South Asian History 29

The **New Perspectives in South Asian History** series publishes monographs and other writings on early modern, modern and contemporary history. The volumes in the series cover new ground across a broad spectrum of subjects such as cultural, environmental, medical, military and political history, and the histories of 'marginalised' groups. It includes fresh perspectives on more familiar fields as well as interdisciplinary and original work from all parts of South Asia. It welcomes historical contributions from sociology, anthropology and cultural studies.

Modern Medicine and International Aid
Khunde Hospital, Nepal (1966–1998)

SUSAN HEYDON
University of Otago
New Zealand

Orient BlackSwan

ORIENT BLACKSWAN PRIVATE LIMITED

Registered Office
3-6-752 Himayatnagar, Hyderabad 500 029 (A.P.), India
E-mail: centraloffice@orientblackswan.com

Other Offices
Bangalore, Bhopal, Bhubaneshwar, Chennai,
Ernakulam, Guwahati, Hyderabad, Jaipur, Kolkata,
Lucknow, Mumbai, New Delhi, Patna

First Published 2009

ISBN 978 81 250 3697 5

Typeset by
OSDATA, Hyderabad 500 029
in Bembo (Aldine) 10.5/12.5

Printed at
De Unique
New Delhi 110 018

Published by
Orient Blackswan Private Limited
1/24 Asaf Ali Road
Email: delhi@orientblackswan.com

The external boundary of India as depicted in the map in this book is neither correct nor authentic

The publishers gratefully acknowledge the financial support received for this volume from the Wellcome Trust Centre for the History of Medicine at University College London

For all those for whom Khunde Hospital
has been a part of their life

Contents

Illustrations and Maps

Acknowledgements

I would not have been able to complete this book without the considerable support of many individuals and organisations. In New Zealand I would particularly like to thank Sir Edmund (who, sadly, died in January 2008) and June Lady Hillary, members, associates and friends of the Himalayan Trust and Khunde Hospital volunteers for their time in sharing with me their knowledge and memories and for the considerable hospitality I have received. I would also like to thank the Trust for giving our family the chance to go to Khunde Hospital in 1996 and to return for a couple of months at the end of 2001.

Altogether, we spent almost two-and-a-half years living in the Sherpa area of Khumbu. People made us feel welcome, gave us enormous hospitality and above all friendship. My interest in the history of the hospital began almost from the start, and I would particularly like to thank Mingma Temba and Kami Temba (now Dr Kami Temba and in charge of Khunde Hospital) for their guidance and patience with our endless questions about the hospital, the area and practising medicine in a Sherpa community.

This interest in Khunde Hospital became my doctoral project a few years later. During the course of my research I was able to return to Nepal for six weeks in May 2003. I would like to thank June Lady Hillary for including me in the "Hillary party" during the Everest fiftieth anniversary celebrations in Kathmandu, Dr Kami Temba for inviting me back to stay at Khunde Hospital and Ang Rita, the Himalayan Trust's Chief Administrative Officer, for inviting me to stay at his home in Kathmandu. I returned for a further six weeks in March 2004 and again would like to thank Dr Kami Temba for having me to stay at the hospital and Ang Rita for enabling me to stay in the Trust flat in Kathmandu. Both Ang Rita and

Dr Kami Temba have given me considerable support, assistance and advice throughout my research.

Nepal and New Zealand, however, are a long way from one another. I would particularly like to acknowledge the financial assistance, first of the Historical Research Advisory Group of New Zealand's Ministry of Foreign Affairs and Trade, that helped in 2002 with travel and expenses in New Zealand, and in 2003 funded my trip to Nepal. I would also like to thank the Ministry in Wellington and the High Commission staff in India for permission in 2004 to consult files held in New Delhi. I am also very grateful to the Asia 2000 Foundation and NZASIA for their funding of my visit to Nepal in 2004 and to the Asian Studies Research Centre at the University of Otago for help with funding my research in New Zealand in 2002. A three-year University of Otago Postgraduate Scholarship supported my doctoral research.

An important part in the development of this project has been the opportunity to participate in conferences. I would like to thank the University of Otago and the New Zealand Federation of Graduate Women (Otago Branch) for funding to enable me to present a paper at the 10th Seminar of the International Association for Tibetan Studies held at the University of Oxford, England, in September 2003. I am also very grateful to Alex McKay and Sanjoy Bhattacharya of the Wellcome Trust Centre for the History of Medicine at University College London for their invitation, and the British Academy for its financial support, to participate in the conference on "frontier medicine" in November 2004. I have benefited very much from the advice and encouragement of both. During the visit to London I was able to stop on the way over and carry out research at the New Zealand High Commission in New Delhi, and on the return to stop in Toronto and carry out research at the office of the Sir Edmund Hillary Foundation. I am very grateful to Zeke O'Connor and the Foundation for their support of my visit while in Toronto. I would like to thank Jorge Lossio and the Wellcome Unit for the History of Medicine at the University of Manchester, England, for the invitation and funding to participate in the first conference on the history of high-altitude medicine in Manchester in December 2005 and Mona Schrempf who organized the panel and obtained funding from the Fritz Thyssen Foundation to present a paper at the 11th Seminar of the International Association for Tibetan Studies in Bonn, Germany in August/September 2006.

This exploration of the histories of Khunde Hospital has been an enjoyable and exciting project. I would like to thank my doctoral supervisors Barbara Brookes, Brian Moloughney and Tony Ballantyne for their guidance and encouragement. Each had something particular to contribute—Barbara for first supporting the project and then for not letting me forget my Western world, Brian for his careful reading and sound advice about many issues and Tony for letting me run with my ideas but always being willing to help me work through when I was stuck. To Natalie Smith, thank you for your companionship along this journey. I would also like to thank Ruth Fitzgerald of the Anthropology Department for her enthusiasm, friendship and for letting me regularly present a seminar on Khunde Hospital and Sherpa beliefs and practices to her Anthropology of Health course. Whether I have been in Dunedin or travelling in a challenging environment, I remain very grateful to Simon Høgh for his advice and practical computer assistance. I would also like to thank Bill Mooney in the Geography Department for the map of Khumbu and staff in the University library for their help in locating material from around the world. During the writing, valuable help in reading chapters and answering questions was provided by Alex McKay, Ang Rita, Mike and Linda Gill, John and Diane McKinnon, Jim and Ann Wilson and my husband, John. From early on in our time in the mountains of Nepal, I wanted to write a book about Khunde Hospital. I owe a special thank you to Sanjoy Bhattacharya for his enthusiastic support that has enabled it to happen, to the Wellcome Trust Centre for the History of Medicine at University College London for their financial assistance and to Veenu Luthria and Padmaja Anant at Orient BlackSwan for their considerable and patient help during the latter stages of the book's production.

Finally, I thank my husband John and children Emma, Edward and Christopher, for their support, forbearance and patience throughout the whole period whether I was at home, about to go away, was somewhere else or planning the next trip. They have been part of my Khunde Hospital experience from the beginning, and continue so as we remain involved with the hospital. We are all grateful to Sir Edmund Hillary and the Himalayan Trust and to the Sherpas of Khumbu for the wonderful opportunity we were given and to whom I offer this book.

Notes on Orthography and Terminology

The Sherpa language is one of many dialects of spoken Tibetan. Written Tibetan, which is used in religious texts, is unfamiliar to almost all lay Sherpas and I have not used it in this book. Although a considerable volume of literature exists about Sherpas, almost all of which is written by overseas scholars from a variety of disciplines, there is no agreed convention for writing the Sherpa language. I have, therefore, adopted the same method as other authors of phonetically rendering Sherpa words and checking these with indigenous Sherpa speakers. The meaning of the word is also considered important. Nevertheless, for a variety of reasons that may be inconsistent, authors then also make their own decisions. I am no different. Pronunciation has also changed since the 1960s, particularly of place and people names.

In this book I use Khunde, which has more local meaning, rather than the common alternative of Kunde that is used on the sign at the hospital and in the Agreement with the Nepalese government. On the other hand I use the more widely understood *gompa* for a temple or monastery rather than *gomba* or the Sherpa *gonda.* In terms of historical changes in name pronunciation, I use a common version in current use, unless it is in a quotation or more appropriate to do otherwise. As a result I use, for example, Ang Rita rather than Ang Hrita and Phortse rather than Phorche.

Regarding terminology, in this book the words Sherpa or Sherpas only denote the ethnic group and do not refer to an occupational category within expeditions.

Sherpas have dual names, one of which is often the day of the week on which they were born. The number of names is quite small. Where confusion may arise, such as more than one person in this book having the name of Ang Rita, further clarification is given. When Sherpas live outside the area, travel overseas or write a publication, "Sherpa" becomes the surname.

Village names, particularly in the lower adjacent area of Pharak, present further difficulties as many are now more commonly known by their Nepali names. In Khumbu the significant place name change is in the area's administrative centre where Namche Bazar replaces Nauche. *Sagarmatha* is Nepali for Everest and appears in the name of the Sagarmatha National Park in which Khumbu is now situated.

Lastly, I use Nepalese to describe nationality and Nepali to denote the language.

Abbreviations

ANZ	Archives New Zealand/Te Rua Mahara o te Kawanatanga, Head Office, Wellington
BBC	British Broadcasting Corporation
BCG	Bacille Calmette-Guérin (vaccine against tuberculosis)
CIDA	Canadian International Development Agency
EPI	Expanded Programme on Immunisation
ESCAP	Economic and Social Commission for Asia and the Pacific
HAC	Hospital Advisory Committee (see also HACB and MHAC)
HACB	Hospital Advisory Committee Book
HMG	His Majesty's Government. Also, HMG/N – His Majesty's Government of Nepal. Government of Nepal now replaces both
HT	Himalayan Trust (see also HTK)
HTK	Himalayan Trust office, Kathmandu
IDD	Iodine Deficiency Disorders
INGO	International Non-Governmental Organisation
IUCD	Intra-Uterine Contraceptive Device
KH	Khunde Hospital
MHAC	Minutes of the Hospital Advisory Committee
NGO	Non-Governmental Organisation
NZ	New Zealand
OIDP	Ontario International Development Program
OIOC	Oriental and India Office Collection and Records, British Library, London
PHC	Primary Health Care
SEHF	Sir Edmund Hillary Foundation
SNP	Sagarmatha National Park

SPCC	Sagarmatha Pollution Control Committee
TB	Tuberculosis
UMN	United Mission to Nepal
UNHCR	United Nations High Commissioner for Refugees
UNICEF	United Nations Children's Fund
USAID	United States Agency for International Development
VDC	Village Development Committee
VSA	Volunteer Service Abroad
WHO	World Health Organization

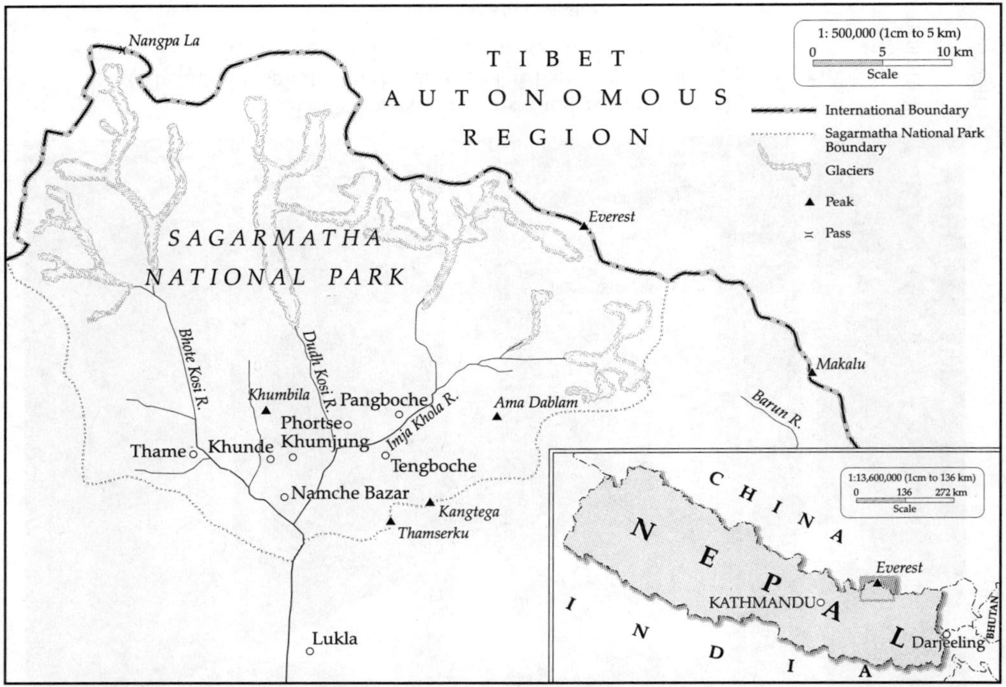
1: 500,000 (1cm to 5 km)
0
5
10 km
Scale
TIBET
AUTONOMOUS
REGION
International Boundary
Sagarmatha National Park Boundary
Glaciers
Peak
Pass
Nangpa La
SAGARMATHA
NATIONAL PARK
Everest
Makalu
Barun R.
Bhote Kosi R.
Dudh Kosi R.
Imja Khola R.
Khumbila
Pangboche
Phortse
Khumjung
Khunde
Thame
Tengboche
Ama Dablam
Namche Bazar
Kangtega
Thamserku
Lukla
1:13,600,000 (1cm to 136 km)
0
136
272 km
Scale
CHINA
NEPAL
INDIA
Everest
KATHMANDU
Darjeeling
BHUTAN

Khumbu

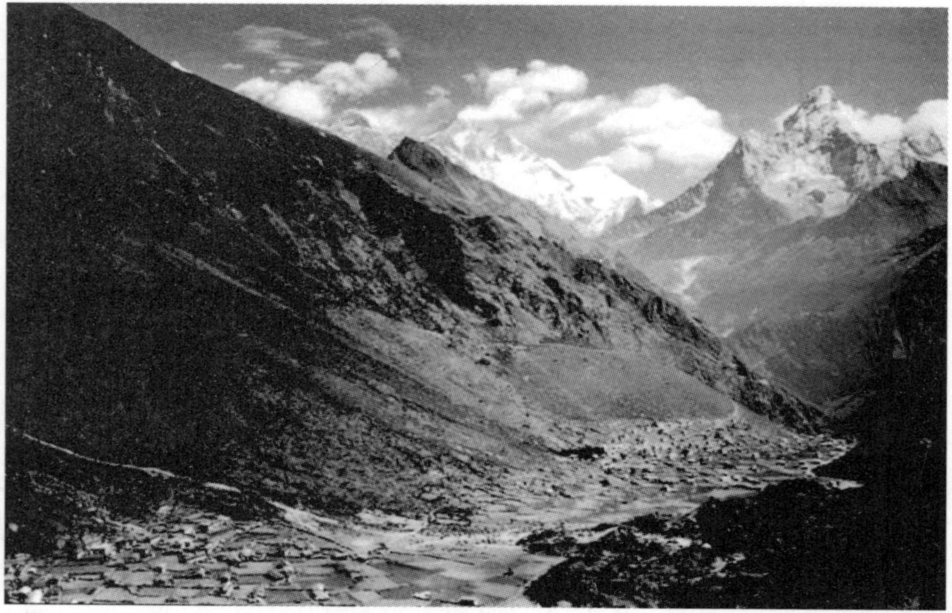

The villages of Khunde and Khumjung
(Khunde Hospital is in the bottom left hand corner of the photograph.
Mt Everest is the peak in the distance, left of centre.)

Source: Heydon family

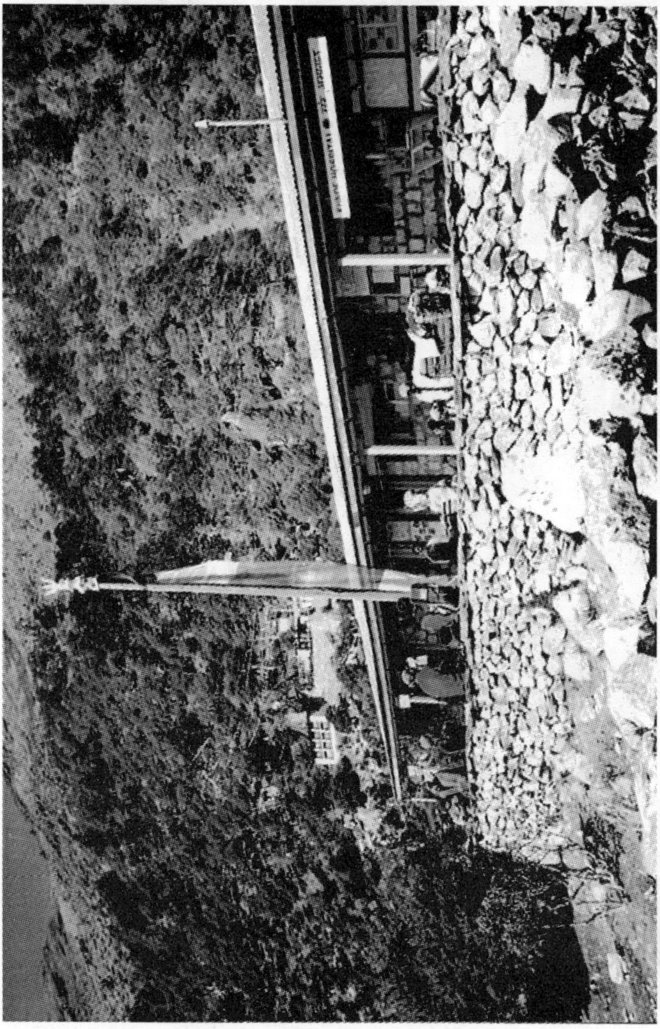

Khunde Hospital

Source: Heydon family

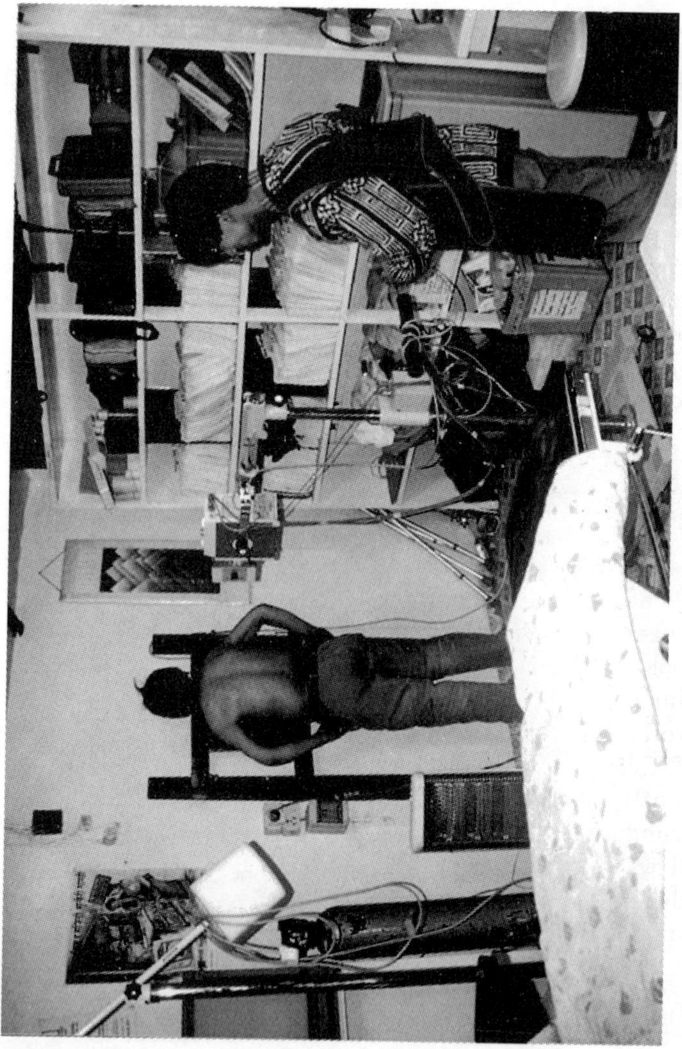

Inside the Clinic

Source: Heydon family

Introduction

In December 1966 a small hospital opened in a remote, mountainous and high-altitude region of Nepal to provide medical services for the approximately three thousand people who lived in a series of villages in the surrounding four valleys. Although little more than a one-roomed, if well stocked, clinic with facilities for patients to stay, the hospital offered a range of outpatient and inpatient, curative and preventive services. It soon became the main provider of biomedical services for the area, a position that it continues to occupy today.[1]

Why Read a History About a Small Hospital in the Mountains of Nepal?

At this point the reader could be forgiven for wondering why anyone from outside the region would be interested in the handful of buildings and staff that provide medical services for this small group of people, but three things make Khunde Hospital a very distinctive institution. It is situated near Mt Everest, the highest mountain in the world; the local inhabitants are Sherpa who became internationally renowned during the twentieth century through their role in Himalayan mountaineering; and the hospital was built and is still administered through the Himalayan Trust which was established by New Zealander Sir Edmund Hillary, who became famous worldwide when he and Tenzing Norgay were the first to step on to the summit of Mt Everest on 29 May 1953.[2]

[1] For how I approach the term "biomedical", see note 12.

[2] My discussion of Sherpas in this book and use of the expression "the Sherpa" is in no way intended to homogenise the considerable variation that exists within and between different groups of Sherpas. See chapter two of this book.

The Everest area is one of Nepal's most popular tourist destinations and Khunde Hospital enjoys a high international profile, receiving hundreds of visitors each year. Hillary's aid work is well known around the world and much has been written about his life, but a study of his work in Nepal is lacking. While a book about the hospital is of interest to those who would like to know more about the people involved and the place, this book is a detailed institutional study that also adds to the extensive and diverse scholarly literature about Sherpas and change and development in the Everest region. Its focus is on an agent of the modernising process instead of those being modernised, and its analysis, although drawing on work from other disciplines, is historical. This study of Khunde Hospital is grounded in a discussion of Hillary's particular form of aid, the shifting discourse of international medical aid between the 1960s and the 1990s and the unique world of the Sherpa of Khumbu (the Sherpa name for this area). It reveals the complexities and interconnectedness of the dual processes of the implementation and ongoing management of a foreign aid project and the introduction and continuing provision of biomedical services.

Yet, to be of more than local interest a book needs to address and make a contribution to wider debates. This history of Khunde Hospital starts from a position of considerable disadvantage: histories of hospitals, and about medical institutions in general, are unfashionable topics for current historians; the case study method faces an inherent weakness of whether general inferences can be drawn from a study of a particular example; and additional to this concern, Khunde Hospital is very small and very unusual.[3] It is neither a representative "Third World" hospital nor a representative "Third World" aid project.

Nevertheless, anyone who goes into a hospital knows that medical institutions are too important to be ignored. More investigation is needed—not less, but this research needs to shift from the antiquarianism of many institutional histories.[4] The case study approach is

[3] I would like to thank my anonymous reviewer for the insightful and helpful comments.

[4] Many hospital histories are commissioned and it may be difficult to avoid such an approach.

a positive strategy in this book, because its focus on a single project allows the possibility of being able to undertake detailed analysis of the institution, its work and the wider society in which it is situated. The small size of Khunde Hospital becomes an advantage. The project of analysing the hospital as a whole becomes manageable and in so doing reveals the multiple complexities involved in providing health care—about which we need to know much more. All medical institutions and health systems, regardless of their size or location have both unique and common features, and we can learn from their similarities and differences. We can also learn from their histories. "Path dependency", the idea that historical developments can significantly influence current policy arrangements and the capacity for change, is a key notion in the study of policy.[5] Similarly in institutional theory, history shapes institutions.[6]

This history of Khunde Hospital provides a case study for examining one of the most important issues concerning international health today—the implementation of aid.[7] For most of the sixty years since the end of the Second World War a conceptual framework of "development" has underpinned relations between the world's "developed" and "un-" or "underdeveloped" states. This book, however, is not the place to explore at an international or even national level the complexities of these relationships, the political and economic self-interest of Western intervention, the use made by leaders of emerging nations of the rhetoric of "development" and "modernisation" or the underlying continuities between colonial

5 For example, Robin Gauld uses it as one of the themes in Robin Gauld, ed., *Comparative Health Policy in the Asia-Pacific* (Maidenhead: Open University Press, 2005).

6 Robert D. Putnam, *Making Democracy Work: Civic Traditions in Modern Italy* (Princeton: Princeton University Press, 1993), 8.

7 The literature on aid and development is vast. For a recent comprehensive analysis of aid, see John Degnbol-Martinussen and Poul Engberg-Pedersen, *Aid: Understanding International Development Cooperation,* translated by Marie Bille (London: Zed Books/Copenhagen: Mellemfolkeligt Samvirke Danish Association for International Cooperation, 2003). Despite the many problems with aid and the authors' belief in the need for improvement, Degnbol-Martinussen and Engberg-Pedersen argue for the retention of aid as the main mechanism for promoting greater equality between and within countries.

and post-colonial ideas and practices that Randall Packard argues have "played a significant role in undermining the effectiveness of efforts to improve the health of developing nations".[8]

In developing countries, foreign aid and health care are deeply entwined because a large proportion of the limited funds in a country's budget for health services may come from outside sources.[9] Despite all the reports and the literature about aid and development we know remarkably little about the practical implementation of policies and, as Frederick Cooper and Packard note, how institutions, whether a small non-government organisation (NGO) such as Khunde Hospital or at the other end of the scale, the World Bank, actually operate.[10] Similarly, emphasis on universal models and policies or "the West" or "the state", as David Mosse writes "conceals the contingent networks of practice" overlooking the diversity of those involved and their particular interests and perspectives.[11] It is such concerns that this book addresses. What happens in the

[8] Randall Packard, "Visions of Postwar Health and Development and Their Impact on Public Health Interventions in the Developing World", in *International Development and the Social Sciences: Essays on the History and Politics of Knowledge,* ed. Frederick Cooper and Randall Packard (Berkeley: University of California Press, 1997), 93. For a wider discussion see the excellent introduction by Packard and Cooper in the same volume. Also see Sunil Amrith's significant recent study of international health policies, ideas and practices which focuses on India but includes the wider region (although with few mentions of Nepal). Sunil S. Amrith, *Decolonizing International Health: India and Southeast Asia, 1930–65* (Houndmills: Palgrave Macmillan, 2006). In talking of "Western" I acknowledge interpretations vary, but in general I mean the countries of Europe and North America, Australia and New Zealand.

[9] In Nepal aid as a percentage of the government's total budget reached its highest level in 1958/59 at an estimated 76.8 per cent. This has since declined and fluctuated annually. In 1997/98 the figure was 29.33 per cent. Sudhindra Sharma, "Half a Century of Foreign Aid", introductory chapter in *Foreign Aid and Politics in Nepal: A Case Study,* Eugene Bramer Mihaly, 2nd ed. (Lalitpur: Himal Books, 2002 [1965]), liii–lvi.

[10] Frederick Cooper and Randall Packard, "Introduction", in Cooper and Packard, *International Development and the Social Sciences,* 28.

[11] David Mosse, "Global Governance and the Ethnography of International Aid", in *The Aid Effect: Giving and Governing in International Development,* ed. David Mosse and David Lewis (London: Pluto Press, 2005), 14.

various stages of a process that begins with an idea, to its becoming policy and then being implemented? Even more importantly, what occurs afterwards—both in the short and the longer term? What is the relationship between those who give aid and those who receive it? How does this work in practice? Very often we read about what appear to be very worthwhile policies and projects that are not working as intended.

In aid for health projects, a central issue is the "medicine" itself.[12] The Western medicine system is the paradigm of international health programmes, but it is well documented that many people use other medical systems and continue to hold other beliefs about sickness and its treatment. It is easy to write about non-compliance, low uptake of services, lack of knowledge and so on and then exhort people to do better, to provide more information, to involve the community and set targets to be achieved with the assumption that if all of this is done a one-dimensional line of progress will be the result. Yet does the practice follow the rhetoric of the theory?

By considering Khunde Hospital as a whole and by focused analysis of what happened at the hospital and what was important for the hospital and those working in it, such broader issues can be addressed. In so doing the study moves from being one of purely local interest to one that has much wider relevance. That this history is grounded in the specific location of the spectacular Mt Everest area of Nepal, is about Sherpa beliefs and practices and Sherpa desires for modernisation in their mountain home of Khumbu and involves international mountaineering hero Sir Edmund Hillary, is a bonus.

[12] Khunde Hospital provides what is variously referred to in the literature as Western medicine, modern medicine, cosmopolitan medicine, scientific medicine, biomedicine or allopathic medicine. Multiple names reflect multiple views and unease over terminology. In this book different terms will be used. "Western" best describes the practice of medicine at Khunde, both in terms of medical services and of the establishment and ongoing management of the hospital through Western aid organisations. In line with other literature "biomedicine" is used in a more general and neutral way to denote this type of medical system, even though it is less familiar in medical practice. Sherpas talk about this type of medicine as "modern" medicine. In Nepal the term "allopathic" is also often used.

People and Place

When flying into Kathmandu, the capital city of Nepal, the skyline in clear weather conditions is dominated by the distant, soaring, snow-capped peaks of the high Himalaya. The triangular shape of the top of Everest is just visible behind other mountains and acts as a magnet for the thousands of visitors who now arrive each year. The lure of Everest is a frequent theme in the literature, especially the many articles in popular magazines and newspapers, guidebooks, books about climbing or the accounts of mountaineering expeditions and travellers. While a few visitors hope to fulfil their dreams and climb to the summit (8,850 metres), most people are content to reach Everest Base Camp, more than three thousand metres lower, or the small peak across the valley of Kala Patthar (5,643 metres) from where one may access unobstructed views of the South Col and the summit.

From Kathmandu, the journey to Everest continues for the majority of today's visitors with a flight of just under one hour on a small plane to the busy mountain airport at Lukla, and then on foot for several days as there are no roads in the rugged Everest region. Khunde Hospital (3,840 metres) is a thousand metres higher than Lukla and is reached by walking along the narrow, steep-sided river valley of the fast-flowing Dudh Kosi till its confluence with the Bhote Kosi. Here the track heads steeply upwards to the natural amphitheatre that contains Namche Bazar (3,440 metres), the main settlement of the area, and higher still, and slightly detouring off the main Everest trail, to the small horseshoe-shaped valley that contains the villages of Khumjung and Khunde.

Until 1950, this area of Nepal was unknown territory for people from Western countries (who make up the majority of today's visitors to these mountains and valleys) as the Nepalese government allowed few to visit Nepal and none to travel to the Everest region.[13] Access to Everest was via Tibet to the north, but in 1950 the Chinese intensified their presence in this large and remote land.

[13] The mapping of the Himalaya in the nineteenth and early twentieth centuries went around Nepal. See Kenneth Mason, *Abode of Snow: A History of Himalayan Exploration and Mountaineering* (London: Rupert Hart-Davis, 1955).

The door was shut to Western mountaineering expeditions in Tibet, but political change was occurring to the south of Everest in Nepal. Edmund Hillary, a beekeeper from Auckland in New Zealand who enjoyed climbing in his free time, first visited the Nepalese side of the mountain in 1951. Despite the splendour of New Zealand's mountains, he described in awe the landscape around him. It took him three days from Namche Bazar to reach the foot of Everest:

> but in many ways they were the most exciting and dramatic days I had ever spent. The rivers foamed through great gorges; the hillsides were clothed in dense forest, broken only here and there by a sheer rock face or a sharp crag. And then, high above the early autumn tints, towered the unbelievable peaks of the Khumba region—mighty ice-fluted faces, terrific rock buttresses, and razor-sharp jagged ice ridges soaring up to impossible summits.[14]

The valleys of the Dudh Kosi and the Bhote Kosi form a triangular-shaped area of ascending height, in which Namche Bazar is the apex, Khunde and Khumjung the centre and the base is Everest and the other mountains along Nepal's northern border.

If the physical landscape is spectacular, it is also harsh. The temperature is cold, being regularly below freezing in winter at Khunde Hospital, and the altitude high. Human beings require oxygen for survival, but as American climber Charles Houston, who was in the first party of Westerners to visit the Khumbu region in 1950, later wrote, "on the top of Everest man is at his utmost limits".[15] When Hillary and Tenzing set off to climb the final few hundred metres in 1953, they carried supplemental oxygen both to assist their endeavour and because they did not know for certain if human beings could survive even a short while at such heights. The body deteriorates, both mentally and physically. Judgement is impaired. Sleep is difficult, food unappealing and the "physical effort of raising one foot above the other requires half a dozen breaths before

[14] Edmund Hillary, *High Adventure* (London: Readers Book Club, 1957 [1955]), 44.

[15] Charles S. Houston, *Going High: The Story of Man and Altitude* (Burlington, Vermont: Charles S. Houston and The American Alpine Club, 1980), 1.

the climber has enough energy to take the next step".[16] At Base Camp there is more oxygen for the body to use, but effectively only half the amount that exists at sea level. At Khunde Hospital, there is two-thirds that of sea level, but still not enough for the body to function as it does at sea level.

Everest straddles the border between the small independent state of Nepal and the Tibet Autonomous Region of China. While visitors struggle in this environment the local inhabitants are acclimatised, or to be more accurate, adapted, to living at high altitude.[17] The human body makes adjustments to cope with the challenges of the physical environment. The Sherpa of Khumbu are ethnically Tibetan people who came over the mountain passes of the Himalaya in the early sixteenth century into what was then an uninhabited area.[18] The Sherpa language is a dialect of Tibetan. While this book primarily is about Sherpas in Khumbu, people who consider themselves to be, or are recognised by others to be Sherpa, inhabit a large part of the area between the Sun Kosi and Arun rivers in eastern Nepal, with the largest concentration of Sherpas being found in Solukhumbu District.[19] Sherpas constitute less than one per cent of the population of Nepal.[20] The name Sherpa, or *sharwa*

[16] L. V. Bryant, *New Zealanders and Everest* (Wellington: A. H. & A. W. Reed, 1953), 15. Bryant, a New Zealander, was a member of the 1935 British Mt Everest Expedition.

[17] The term "acclimatisation" has a physiological explanation in high-altitude medicine, unlike earlier discussions about race and climate where it often reflected moral judgements of the "other".

[18] The broad definition of an ethnic group that I have used is that of people sharing a cultural heritage who are viewed by themselves and others as distinctive: Frank N. Magill, ed., *Survey of Social Science* (Pasadena: Salem Press, 1994), Sociology Series 2: 689. Self-definition is particularly relevant in terms of a population census on which assessments of the Sherpa population are based.

[19] Stanley Stevens, *Claiming the High Ground: Sherpas, Subsistence and Environmental Change in the Highest Himalaya* (Delhi: Motilal Banarsidass, 1996 [1993]), 35–37.

[20] Central Bureau of Statistics, *Statistical Year Book of Nepal 2001* (Kathmandu: Central Bureau of Statistics, 2001), 12 and 52. These figures are taken from the 1991 population census that recorded 110,358 Sherpas and a total Nepalese population of 18,491,097.

as Sherpas call themselves, means "Easterner" and comes from two words, *shar* meaning east and *wa* or *pa* meaning people.[21] In the eighteenth century the area became incorporated into the Gorkha kingdom that became the modern state of Nepal. The new rulers were Hindu while the Sherpa, like a number of small groups living along the Himalaya, were Buddhist. Both their geographically remote and (for most other people) undesirable location, as well as their marginal social and political position in Nepal, meant that apart from the payment of taxes Sherpas were largely left alone.[22] Few government officials visited.

Khumbu Sherpas live in a series of permanent villages and temporary settlements and in the past largely managed their own affairs.[23] The six main villages of Namche Bazar, Khumjung, Khunde, Thame, Phortse and Pangboche occupy some of the few reasonably flat areas of ground between the heights of 3,400 and 4,000 metres. Before the 1950s, Sherpa livelihood was based on a mixture of agriculture and pastoralism.[24] In the twentieth century the potato became their staple food, while yaks supplied many other needs.[25] They provided meat, nak milk for butter and cheese, manure for fertiliser and fuel, hair for weaving into blankets and hide for boots.[26] Yaks were also used as pack animals. Trade supplement-

[21] It is uncertain as to what is meant by "east" in this context.

[22] Stevens, *Claiming the High Ground,* 53–54.

[23] Christoph von Fürer-Haimendorf, *The Sherpas of Nepal: Buddhist Highlanders* (London: John Murray, 1964), 100. There are many academic and popular studies about Sherpas from the 1950s onwards. *The Sherpas of Nepal* is the earliest academic work and remains the broadest account, but has been criticised by other anthropologists for its "rosy" view of Sherpas. See also chapter two of this book.

[24] See Barbara Brower, *Sherpa of Khumbu: People, Livestock and Landscape* (Delhi: Oxford University Press, 1992 [1991]); and Stevens, *Claiming the High Ground*.

[25] It is commonly thought that the potato was introduced into Khumbu during the second half of the nineteenth century and quickly became established. Stanley Stevens provides the most considered discussion and suggests that the initial diffusion was still taking place in the 1920s. Stevens, *Claiming the High Ground*, 225.

[26] A nak is a female yak.

ed the Sherpa subsistence economy, since the area was located on a long-distance route between northern India and Tibet.[27]

The fame of the Sherpa, however, was not built upon this way of life that they shared with other mountain peoples living along the border.[28] Their international reputation was earned outside both Khumbu and Nepal. Like many other people who make up Nepal's diverse ethnic mix, an alternative to this way of life for Sherpas was to leave Khumbu, on either a temporary or permanent basis.[29] A popular destination in the nineteenth century was Darjeeling, a hill station in British India, where the first district census in 1901 recorded 3,450 Sherpas.[30] They found employment in a variety of occupations, but in the first half of the twentieth century Darjeeling became an important recruitment centre for Sherpas accompanying mountaineering expeditions in the Himalaya.[31] During this period Sherpas became renowned for their key role as high-altitude support personnel for these expeditions, a reputation that was built both on their ability and personal attributes.[32] They could,

[27] For Sherpa trading before and after 1950, see Stevens, *Claiming the High Ground,* 335–55. For a broader discussion, see Wim van Spengen, *Tibetan Border Worlds: A Geohistorical Analysis of Trade and Traders* (London: Kegan Paul International, 2000).

[28] For a description of the different groups in Nepal, see the work of prominent Nepalese anthropologist Dor Bahadur Bista, *People of Nepal* (Kathmandu: Ratna Pustak Bhandar, 1972 [1967]). Use of "*People*" in the title is significant as Nepalese government policy promoted the idea of unity (one Nepalese people) rather than the ethnic diversity that was popular with the increasing number of foreign anthropologists in the region. Also see James F. Fisher, "The Historical Development of Himalayan Anthropology", *Mountain Research and Development* 5, no. 1, 1985, 99–111; and Don Funnell and Romola Parish, *Mountain Environments and Communities* (London: Routledge, 2001).

[29] See Mark Poffenberger, *Patterns of Change in the Nepal Himalaya* (Boulder: Westview Press, 1980), 57–66.

[30] Arthur Jules Dash, *Darjeeling* (Alipore: Bengal District Gazetteers, 1947), 72. This total would have included Sherpas from various areas.

[31] Sherpas in Khumbu also crossed directly into Tibet and joined the 1922 British Everest expedition.

[32] The role of Sherpas in expeditions is described in many accounts, but for a Sherpa-centred analysis, see Sherry B. Ortner, *Life and Death on Mt. Everest:*

and would, work in the difficult high-altitude conditions and were commonly considered cheerful companions.[33] The name Sherpa became synonymous with their occupation on the expeditions.[34] Success on Everest in 1953, however, resulted in Sherpas becoming famous beyond mountaineering circles. Other Western outsiders became fascinated by the Sherpa and often idealised them.[35]

Like many climbers, Edmund Hillary in the early 1950s respected and liked Sherpas, but it is wrong to assume an automatic and unilinear progression from the triumph on Everest to the aid programme that he subsequently developed.[36] He was involved in other adventures; furthermore, as a result of the nationalistic fervour that the climb generated in Nepal and India, he was not overly happy that Tenzing was adulated and his achievement belittled.[37] Fame after 1953 may have placed Hillary in a position to help the

---

Sherpas and Himalayan Mountaineering (New Delhi: Oxford University Press, 2000 [1999]). For a comparison of Sherpas with guides in the European Alps, see Peter H. Hansen, "Partners: Guides and Sherpas in the Alps and Himalayas, 1850s–1950s", in *Voyages and Visions: Towards a Cultural History of Travel,* ed. Jás Elsner and Joan-Pau Rubiés (London: Reaktion Books, 1999), 210–31.

33 Although Sherpas are adapted to living at high altitude, this does not mean that they could not get altitude sickness. Mountaineering accounts contain many examples where they did.

34 This has led to confusion. In this book Sherpa only refers to the ethnic group and not to the occupational category.

35 See Vincanne Adams, *Tigers of the Snow and Other Virtual Sherpas: An Ethnography of Himalayan Encounters* (Princeton: Princeton University Press, 1996). Hillary did not idealise Sherpas. The Gurkhas of the British and Indian armies are another group from Nepal with a positive, high international profile, but unlike Sherpas come from a number of different ethnic groups from a wide area of the hill region. See Lionel Caplan, *Warrior Gentlemen: "Gurkhas" in the Western Imagination* (Providence: Berghahn Books, 1995).

36 This in hindsight is a popular perception and was very evident in the tributes following Hillary's death in January 2008.

37 Sir Edmund Hillary, *View from the Summit* (London: Doubleday, 1999), 25. For different nationalist narratives about the first ascent of Mt Everest, see Peter H. Hansen, "Confetti of Empire: The Conquest of Everest in Nepal, India, Britain and New Zealand", *Comparative Studies in Society and History* 42, 2000, 307–32.

Sherpa, but it was eight years later, in June 1961, that he built a school in the village of Khumjung. Further projects followed in 1963 and 1964, and in 1966 he built the small hospital at Khunde. Hillary's determination and ability took him to the top of Everest, while determination and the means to assist led to the implementation of an aid programme in the Solukhumbu district of Nepal. What was unusual about Hillary's work was that it occurred at all. Although some mountaineers do give generously, most go to Everest, climb and leave. Hillary's aid to the Sherpa was wide-ranging and continuous.

In 1953 Hillary had coped well with the physical challenges of the Everest environment, and like others he appreciated the contribution of Sherpas to the triumph of the expedition. A successful climbing team, such as that of Hillary and Tenzing, required the two to work together and trust one another.[38] Only Hillary had a non-Western climbing partner. The friendship and respect that developed between Hillary and Sherpas continued to grow after the successful climb and provides the key to their relationship—a relationship that was also sustained by Hillary's personal feelings of a moral obligation to help others if he was able to. For more than forty years later, Hillary continued to help Sherpas with a broad range of assistance. On 29 May 2003, the fiftieth anniversary of the first ascent, King Gyanendra Bir Bikram Shah Dev bestowed honorary citizenship of Nepal on Sir Edmund Hillary.[39] Permitted under the 1990 Constitution, Hillary was the first foreign recipient of this honour that was awarded for both his success on Everest and his valuable contribution to the health and social sectors in Nepal.[40] For Hillary and the Sherpa, the fiftieth anniversary celebrations were, therefore, about much more than climbing Everest. Mountaineering had made Sherpas famous, but Hillary played a

[38] Although Tenzing's achievement on Everest made the Nepalese Sherpas famous around the world, he was born in Tibet around 1914. As a young child he was brought to live in Khumbu. In 1932 he moved to Darjeeling.

[39] Tenzing died in 1986.

[40] I am grateful to Ang Rita Sherpa, Chief Administrative Officer of the Himalayan Trust in Nepal, for a copy of the citation's English translation from the Home Ministry of the Government of Nepal.

major role in the changes that subsequently occurred in their home of Khumbu.

To Western visitors, Nepal in the 1950s provided a journey into the past, although British journalist Ralph Izzard provided a rare description of a Kathmandu that was beginning to modernise before the restoration of the monarchy in 1951 which brought with it the promise of modernisation throughout the country.[41] Foreign aid that began to trickle and then pour into the country mostly went into the small and fertile Kathmandu Valley that contained in the 1952/54 census two-thirds of the country's small urban population.[42] Nepal was, and remains, a predominantly rural country that in the 1950s and 1960s lacked the infrastructure that fostered development.[43]

In Nepal, development was associated with the government.[44] Influenced by Khumbu's situation near the border, government activity began to increase slowly with the establishment of a small school and medical clinic, but Hillary's support provided the impetus to hasten the process. An increasing number of Hillary schools

41 Ralph Izzard, *The Innocent on Everest* (London: Hodder and Stoughton, 1954), 47–49. Izzard visited in 1947 and noted that the city centre had electricity since 1911, an "abundant" water supply, some "modern plumbing" and "X-ray apparatus for the clinics". He also commented on the presence of "two or three hundred" cars and a "thousand or so" bicycles in the Kathmandu Valley. For Nepal in this period pre-1951, see Ludwig F. Stiller, *Nepal: Growth of a Nation* ([Kathmandu], Nepal: Human Resources Development Research Centre, 1999 [1993]).

42 Harka Gurung, *Nepal: Social Demography and Expressions* (Kathmandu: New Era, 2001), 10. The population of the Valley was 181,082. The total population of Nepal recorded in the 1952/54 census (regarded as the first modern census for Nepal) was 8,256,625.

43 See Satish Despande, "Modernization", in *The Oxford India Companion to Sociology and Social Anthropology,* ed. Veena Das (New Delhi: Oxford University Press, 2003), 63–98. Although the essay is specifically about India, many of the ideas can also be applied to Nepal.

44 See particularly the work of Stacy Leigh Pigg, "Unintended Consequences: The Ideological Impact of Development in Nepal", *South Asia Bulletin* 18, nos. 1 and 2, 1993, 45–58, and "Inventing Social Categories Through Place: Social Representations and Development in Nepal", *Comparative Studies in Society and History* 34, 1992, 491–513.

introduced secular education throughout the district while Khunde Hospital brought modern, Western style medical services.[45] The construction of an airstrip at Lukla in 1964, with the aim of providing more direct access for getting supplies to build the hospital, became, as anthropologist James Fisher describes it, an unintended "major conduit" for tourists that would "spark a burgeoning, radically new industry in Khumbu".[46] The number of visitors rose from 20 in 1964 to 5,310 in 1980/81 and to 17,412 in 1996/97.[47] Sherpas built lodges and shops and a variety of other services developed to supply the needs of the visitors. By 1998 visitors could eat pizza and access the internet. Visitor numbers have increased further, although they have also fluctuated in response to ongoing political uncertainties within Nepal.

On 29 May 2003, Sherpas and their foreign friends gathered from Khumbu, Kathmandu and around the world for an evening of celebration in Kathmandu. The event highlighted the considerable changes of the previous fifty years. Although it took place in the heat and humidity of a pre-monsoon bustling city and was far removed from the cold, high-altitude mountains of Khumbu, the worlds of Sir Edmund Hillary of New Zealand and the Sherpa of Nepal met. It was primarily a gathering of friends, who at times over the years came together, but on other occasions went their separate ways. Hillary had led expeditions to different places, was involved with other organisations and lived with his family in New Zealand, while Sherpas took advantage of the developing tourism industry in the Everest area and sought to improve their own social and economic position.[48] An increasing number travelled overseas

[45] The small government school and clinic were in Namche Bazar.

[46] James F. Fisher, *Sherpas: Reflections on Change in Himalayan Nepal* (Delhi: Oxford University Press, 1997 [1990]), xxiv. Fisher was a member of Hillary's expedition in 1964 and helped to build schools and the airstrip. In this study he examines the effects of the schools and tourism on Sherpas. I am grateful for copies of documents about the expedition and an email interview in February 2003.

[47] See Appendix 5.

[48] Also see Kurt Luger, *Kids of Khumbu: Sherpa Youth on the Modernity Trail* (Kathmandu: Mandala Book Point, 2000).

for training and employment. Among the event's organisers and guests were many Sherpas and foreigners associated with Khunde Hospital, making the hospital an integral part of this large, colourful and international occasion.

Khunde Hospital

Despite its small size, Khunde Hospital has always been called a hospital.[49] The main building has a single storey and contains a one-room clinic in which most examinations, investigations and treatments are carried out. An adjacent room provides inpatient facilities for acutely ill patients. A separate building initially provided eight beds for tuberculosis patients, but was later used more generally for patients requiring a long-term stay at the hospital. Although it underwent some changes—an extra room was added as a classroom at one end of the main building and a bedroom at the other, the long-stay accommodation rebuilt and internal reorganisation carried out—Khunde Hospital in 1998 looked remarkably similar to what it did in 1966.

In the 1960s Nepal had few doctors or other trained health workers, and so the Nepalese government gave Hillary permission to bring in foreign medical staff.[50] These were volunteers who went to work and live at Khunde for around two years. Initially all such volunteers were New Zealanders; in the early 1980s, however, vol-

[49] In colonial South Asia dispensaries were the main institutions providing medical servies to the general population, especially in rural areas. They were under the control of a doctor and provided curative and preventive services particularly on an outpatient basis. They could also have inpatients. See, for example, Mark Harrison, *Public Health in British India: Anglo-Indian Preventive Medicine, 1859–1914* (Cambridge: Cambridge University Press, 1994).

[50] For a very useful overview and discussion of the development of Nepal's health services, see Hemang Dixit, *The Quest for Health: The Health Services of Nepal* (Kathmandu: Educational Enterprise, 1995). A second edition was published in 1999. The brief reference to the Himalayan Trust (p. 207), however, still confuses Khunde Hospital with Phaphlu Hospital, which was the second hospital Hillary built and which became the district hospital for Solukhumbu.

unteer appointments began to alternate between New Zealand and Canada from where much of the hospital's funding now came. For most of the period the volunteers were the only foreigners living in Khumbu on a year-round basis, with their home being a small flat at one end of the main hospital building. They were supported by a small number of local staff, some of whom lived at the hospital and shared the kitchen with the volunteers. Close bonds often developed between them, with local Sherpa staff guiding the volunteers about living and working in a Sherpa community.

Most people were seen and treated as outpatients for a wide range of curative and preventive health services. Between 1967 and 1997 the number of outpatients increased from an annual total of 1,924 to 7,294.[51] While the most commonly presented conditions were respiratory, gastro-intestinal and skin problems, on any one day the medical staff might have to respond to minor coughs and colds, major problems such as tuberculosis, serious trauma or an obstetric complication, acute and chronic illness, common and rare conditions, or novel cases such as a sick or injured yak. The main preventive health programmes were immunisation, family planning and controlling the effects of the region's iodine deficiency. Antenatal care was encouraged and health education activities were also carried out. Most patients came from the resident and predominantly Sherpa population, but, as tourism and government services developed, the hospital also began to treat an increasing number of patients from other Nepalese groups and visitors from overseas. Treating altitude sickness, particularly during the two trekking seasons in the spring and autumn, became a significant component of the hospital's work.

As Khumbu has no roads, both staff and patients had to walk everywhere. While most people came to the hospital, hospital staff also made home visits and travelled out to the villages. Seriously ill patients were carried to the hospital, usually by another person. From the beginning, the volunteers began to train health workers and de-

[51] See Appendix 3. These totals convey overall trends, but caution should be exercised in interpreting the hospital's statistics because of the patchiness of data collected and inconsistencies such as different criteria used in reporting and varying time periods of reports.

velop village-based services so that people could receive basic health care, both curative and preventive, closer to where they lived.

In the 1960s Khumbu was isolated within Nepal. While part of the history of Khunde Hospital concerns the slow expansion of Nepalese government health services and the hospital's gradual integration into its programmes, throughout the period the hospital operated independently as a private aid project. Khunde Hospital was supported and administered primarily from New Zealand, by Hillary's Himalayan Trust under a renewable Agreement with the Nepalese government. Funds for Hillary's aid work came from a variety of private and official sources. In the mid-1970s Khunde Hospital became a Canadian as well as a New Zealand aid project when it attracted (what developed into very substantial but often inadequately recognised) assistance from the Sir Edmund Hillary Foundation (SEHF) and the Canadian International Development Agency (CIDA).

"Worlds"

Khunde Hospital, therefore, was a foreign institution and it contributed to the changes that were occurring in Khumbu by providing medical services and employment. At the same time, it was also affected by what was happening around it. The hospital was both distinct from and a part of the changing lives of the local inhabitants. This separation and connection raised questions of how to approach research and writing about the history of Khunde Hospital. Existing historiography was both unhelpful, and for this period, lacking.[52] Furthermore, unlike much of the South Asian region, Nepal was not colonised. We know much more about the introduction of biomedical services in the earlier context of colonialism than we do in the post-colonial world of foreign aid and development.

[52] Despite an active medical historical scholarship for the South Asian region, this interest has only recently extended to the Himalaya. For the first major study of the introduction and spread of biomedicine in the Himalayan region (although Nepal is not included), see Alex McKay, *Their Footprints Remain: Biomedical Beginnings Across the Indo-Tibetan Frontier* (Amsterdam: University of Amsterdam Press, 2007).

Should this study of Khunde Hospital be a narrative of a dominant discourse about the introduction and spread of medicine and international aid? Should it adopt a more "subaltern" approach of retrieving a Sherpa perspective?[53]

The problem was that neither of these binary methods that polarised people and ideas adequately reflected medical encounters at Khunde Hospital or the wider role of the hospital in the community.[54] If those providing health care initially anticipated a meeting with the spirit-suffused beliefs and practices of the Sherpa that would result in displacement of the latter, then the implementation was far less oppositional in practice than in theory. Hillary considered Sherpas his friends and respected their wishes and their way of life. He worked with them and responded to their requests for help, rather than seeking to impose what as an outsider he thought was best for them. If that meant doing something differently or not at all, Hillary was receptive and if change occurred slowly, then Hillary was patient. The relationship was very different from the standard top-down approach still current in the 1960s.

In this book I approach the history of Khunde Hospital through the conceptual device of distinct but overlapping "worlds" in order to explain and understand what occurred at the hospital, and to explore and analyse issues from different perspectives (with their varying relationships) to show the complex, interrelated yet fractured and porous nature of medical encounters. I argue that the hospital existed and operated simultaneously within multiple worlds that, while separate, were also interconnected. These worlds were physical, social and intellectual spaces within which there were rules and norms of behaviour that structured action. This does not, however,

53 Peter Hansen examines the lack of subaltern studies in Tibet in comparison to their considerable influence in South Asia, in Peter H. Hansen, "Why is There No Subaltern Studies for Tibet?" *Tibet Journal* 28, no. 4, winter 2003, 7–22.

54 Sherry Ortner in *Life and Death on Mt. Everest* raises similar issues about how to accommodate different perspectives in a single work. She discusses further her ongoing "tinkering" with practice theory in "Introduction: Updating Practice Theory", in Sherry B. Ortner, *Anthropology and Social Theory: Culture, Power, and the Acting Subject* (Durham: Duke University Press, 2006), 3.

imply rigidity and uniformity. Each world was important and influenced what happened at the hospital in different ways. At times these worlds engaged with one another, but in other circumstances their interests diverged. These worlds were not one-dimensional. They could meet, articulate, overlap or collide. Their boundaries could be fixed, fluid or porous, a line or a zone, yet the worlds they encompassed retained a certain coherence and discreteness of their own.

Use of the word "world" is common in today's historiography but is an idea derived from an understanding of an underlying common set of assumptions in a "world view".[55] In 1964 James Fisher was an American Peace Corps volunteer teacher who became a member of Hillary's Himalayan Schoolhouse Expedition, and subsequently became an anthropologist; he wrote later:

> I left Khumbu older and, I hope, wiser, but the longer I had stayed there, the more I had realized how little I understood of the Sherpa world. Although Sherpa culture seemed transparent and the people open, straightforward, and down-to-earth in a way easily grasped by a young American, I increasingly sensed vast differences between us in world-view.[56]

My "worlds" in this book are broader. They go beyond culture, encompassing institutions, political structures and knowledge communities. They allow culture to be embedded in place and for different geographical spaces to be linked. Different worlds can be considered consistently without privileging one discourse over another. Such a device, therefore, also provides an alternative to binary discussions of cross-cultural encounters.

This pragmatic concern to find a way of examining the hospital's history that more adequately reflected what took place, the different groups of people involved and their relationships, also developed as a response to my own experiences of living and working as a volunteer at Khunde Hospital between 1996 and 1998 and subsequent visits in 2001, 2003 and 2004. Furthermore, it ad-

55 See, for example, Robert H. Winthrop, *Dictionary of Concepts in Cultural Anthropology* (New York: Greenwood Press, 1991), 324–27.

56 Fisher, *Sherpas,* 53.

dressed questions being raised in the wider literature about ways to approach and research health services, their problems and cross-cultural situations.[57] In her valuable and insightful study of foreign aid and health development in Nepal, anthropologist Judith Justice considered the value of taking into account the multiple views and interests of participants and argued for the importance of cultural information to assist in planning appropriate programmes.[58] Linda Stone went further and asked "Primary Health Care for Whom?"[59] She concluded that the major international health policy of Primary Health Care (PHC) would not achieve its objective of "Health for All by the Year 2000" "until the perspectives of the people themselves, and not just their scientifically defined health problems, are both considered and respected".[60] Sjaak van der Geest, Johan Speckmann and Pieter Streefland also referred to studies from Nepal and suggested the need for multi-level research, both vertically and horizontally, to explore different perspectives and so overcome what they saw as the one-sided interest of much research.[61] Using

[57] For example, Paul Unschuld questions how to approach the long-term development of diverse health care concepts in China, in Paul U. Unschuld, *Medicine in China: A History of Ideas* (Berkeley: University of California Press, 1985).

[58] Judith Justice, *Policies, Plans, & People: Foreign Aid and Health Development* (Kathmandu: Mandala in association with University of California Press, 1986). For a major historical case study of the control and eradication of smallpox from India that similarly emphasises multiple and multi-level complexities, see Sanjoy Bhattacharya, Mark Harrison and Michael Worboys, *Fractured States: Smallpox, Public Health and Vaccination Policy in British India, 1800–1947* (New Delhi: Orient Longman, 2005); and Sanjoy Bhattacharya, *Expunging Variola: The Control and Eradication of Smallpox in India 1947–1977* (New Delhi: Orient Longman, 2006).

[59] Linda Stone, "Primary Health Care for Whom? Village Perspectives from Nepal", *Social Science & Medicine* 22, no. 3, 1986, 293–302.

[60] Stone, "Primary Health Care for Whom?" 302.

[61] Sjaak van der Geest, Johan D. Speckmann and Pieter H. Streefland, "Primary Health Care in a Multi-Level Perspective: Towards a Research Agenda", *Social Science & Medicine* 30, no. 9, 1990, 1025–34. They sought to explore why, despite the unanimous approval of the policy of Primary Health Care (PHC) on its adoption at the Alma Ata conference in 1978, criticism began almost immediately.

the conceptual device of worlds, however, enables a mapping of the multiple and different perspectives of those involved to take place in a non-oppositional structure that allows each to be considered and, hopefully, respected.

The "worlds" of Khunde Hospital

Searches of the literature and the internet uncover many references to Khunde Hospital, but no single account or critical study of the hospital exists. The hospital is popularly perceived to be "doing a good job" and provides good publicity for Hillary's programme as a whole.[62] Modern medicine and modernisation are also how the few Sherpa written accounts have contextualised Khunde Hospital.[63] Sherpas were and remain aware of their changing world, but do not wish to return to the harshness of their previous way of life. Health care from the hospital is a positive factor.

Ethnographic discussions of Khunde Hospital are less favourable. The most substantial references and discussion are contained in the works of Vincanne Adams and John Draper and are based primarily on research in different areas of Khumbu in the 1980s.[64] Both Adams and Draper found fault with Khunde Hospital, although they acknowledged that the hospital did valuable medical work. In Draper's view the hospital "remains a highly centralized and somewhat alien institution for most Sherpas".[65] Both Adams and Draper located their descriptions and discussions in a broader

62 See chapter one.

63 See chapter two.

64 Vincanne Adams, "Modes of Production and Medicine: An Examination of the Theory in Light of Sherpa Medical Traditionalism", *Social Science & Medicine* 27, no. 5, 1988, 505–13; Adams, "Healing Buddhas and Mountain Guides: The Production of Self Within Society Through Medication" (Ph.D. thesis, University of California, Berkeley, 1989); Adams, *Tigers of the Snow and Other Virtual Sherpas;* John Draper, "Beyond Medicine: Sickness, Healing, and Order in Sherpa Society" (Ph.D. thesis, University of Sydney, [1995]).

65 Draper, "Beyond Medicine", 164. By the early 1990s Draper had become involved in development activities and the last chapter reflects his changing career path.

thesis in which the actual issues of Sherpa ill health were not their primary interest. Just as medicine has been used as an avenue to explore colonialism in other places and periods of history, so among Sherpas sickness became a lens through which to explore issues of continuity and change, identity, knowledge and power in Sherpa society. Sadly, Draper died in 1994; and the extensive material about sickness beliefs and practices that is contained in the thesis (which was submitted shortly after his death) has been ignored by other scholars. Draper's published articles about knowledge and power deal much more with religion than sickness.[66]

In this book I have placed Khunde Hospital at the centre and make it the primary site for debate. I use the criteria of what happened at the hospital, or what was of relevance for the hospital, as the focus for analysis. Discussion about the implementation of aid therefore shifts from ideas and policies to practice, from the international arena to a small community in the mountains of Nepal, and from a linear view to one of ongoing interaction between different people with different ideas and with different needs and considerations. In order to explore the history of Khunde Hospital I set it within four distinct but overlapping worlds: that of Sir Edmund Hillary, the Sherpa, Western medicine and international aid. These are worlds that I have identified as being important for the questions I am looking at and each is the subject of a chapter in the book since each world also has its own literature and debates. Chapter one focuses on the role of Sir Edmund Hillary as the donor for the project, chapter two considers the hospital and the recipients of modern medicine and international aid, chapter three discusses practising medicine at Khunde Hospital and chapter four places the hospital in the wider international aid process. The important point is that all of these worlds influenced the provision of health care at and from Khunde Hospital in different ways, sometimes separately but often simultaneously, and at some times and for some issues more than others.

[66] Draper considered the control of knowledge "the primary axis of inequality" in Sherpa society. Draper, "Beyond Medicine", 398. For an obituary, see Elizabeth Stutchbury, "Remembering John Norman Draper, 1955–1994", *Himalayan Research Bulletin* 17, no. 2, 1997, 4–5.

That Hillary had money and could exercise power places the hospital within a discourse of a dominant representation, particularly when coupled with another discourse of a dominant representation—that of biomedicine's superiority. Yet, as Sherry Ortner has shown in respect of Himalayan mountaineering, which was an activity controlled by the outsider climbers, Sherpas had lives both on and off the mountain.[67] They had their own agendas, their own desires, sometimes engaging with outsider others and sometimes not. Khunde Hospital was part of both that Sherpa world and Hillary's world—worlds that articulated sometimes around the hospital and at other times did not. What went on within each affected events, ideas and practices at the hospital. The way Hillary ran his aid projects and how Sherpas viewed modern medicine contributed to the outcome.

Other influences also had an impact. The role of the hospital was to provide medical services. The medical world had its own culture, with its specialist practitioners and distinctive ideas about health and disease. Health workers were trained (whether in New Zealand, Canada or Nepal) to provide medical services that reflected specific views about ill health and its treatment. Nepal, however, was not a wealthy developed country. The post Second World War period saw the rise of international medical aid programmes and Nepal was offered and received assistance from many countries, international aid agencies and individual people and organisations. As the Nepalese government relaxed its isolation policy, international medical aid agencies and governments were ready to step in. Biomedicine was the main paradigm. These aid programmes operated within a framework that contained specific ideas and practices about what was appropriate for countries such as Nepal and rural areas such as Khumbu.[68] Khunde Hospital should offer basic medical services

[67] Ortner, *Life and Death on Mt. Everest.*

[68] See Draper, "Beyond Medicine", chapter 12, for how this could apply to Khumbu. Focusing on primary health care in general, Draper believed that a large percentage of health programmes continued to focus on biomedical curative services and that not enough resources and energy had been directed towards "community-based, socioculturally appropriate, prevention-oriented, self-care activities" (p. 390). He applied this approach to Khumbu

and emphasise preventive programmes that achieved gains at the level of community rather than at an individual patient level.

Hillary, the Sherpa community, staff at the hospital and international aid organisations all had their own ideas about health services and levels of involvement, and their own expectations about what could or should be done. Sometimes they coincided, such as in the belief about the need to provide services in rural areas. Sometimes they differed. Patients wanted access to curative services rather than talk about prevention. In the 1970s international aid discourse shifted away from a hospital-based model of care towards primary health care and community health services. Each participant in the aid process could influence those at the hospital trying to deal with an issue. Decisions about staffing the hospital and its village clinics, for example, had to take into account Hillary's and the Himalayan Trust's ideas, those of the local community, the lack of trained health workers in the area, medical views on the type and training of staff and aid priorities for the type and gender of health workers. Medical programmes similarly had to take into account a range of perspectives.

While researchers rightly concentrate on specific health problems or broader issues such as poverty, the need nevertheless exists to also look at people, organisations and institutions. In practice, the outcomes of policies and programmes to a large extent depend on these. The history of Khunde Hospital between 1966 and 1998 provides a detailed example of the implementation of an overseas aid project that continued to operate as an aid project more than thirty years later.[69] What happened, and how and why it happened is the subject of this book.

---

and was highly critical of Khunde Hospital and Hillary's Himalayan Trust for not moving further towards a community and prevention model.

69 For practical reasons my analysis closes at 1998 when we left Khunde. An epilogue continues the narrative of the hospital to the present, identifying significant features of both continuity and change.

Sources

A wide range of written primary and secondary sources exists to allow such an analysis, including books and articles by Sir Edmund Hillary, members of his family and the Himalayan Trust, and the volunteers at Khunde Hospital. One of the features of the primary sources is their diversity and scattered location in New Zealand, Nepal, Canada, England and India.

The book draws heavily on the written records held at Khunde Hospital. These range from the hospital's annual reports, inpatient and outpatient registers, files and ledgers about other hospital activity, and assorted but incomplete files of correspondence to and from the overseas volunteers. The sources cover a wide variety of issues, but the content is diverse, gaps exist and criteria for recording differ.[70] One of the features of the post-1950 period in Nepal has been the need to provide information for people to write reports, but difficulties remain in gathering data and ensuring its reliability.[71] Khunde Hospital occupied a mostly independent situation on the fringe of Nepal's health services and was unimportant in terms of the government's plans.[72]

Whether in unpublished archival sources or published literature, easily identifiable personal medical information can often be found. Often the person's name is given. Academic researchers have usually tried to find another way to use examples. With the small pool of Sherpa names and a small subject population, a different problem may occur when the person being written about is given a pseudonym. Mistaken identity can result. Privacy becomes an issue of even greater concern since many of the sources are recent, even contem-

[70] Hospital statistics reflect the work of the hospital and how people used the hospital. I do not use them as a measure of the community's health problems.

[71] This is frequently discussed in the literature. Also, compulsory registration of births and deaths does not occur.

[72] I also needed to keep in mind that Khunde Hospital and other Himalayan Trust projects were ongoing. The difficulties of obtaining access to Health Department files for foreign researchers precluded use from this source, but extensive statistical and other information about health issues exists in other available sources.

porary. Sickness is a personal matter and confidentiality is important. Although I am concerned with examining medical encounters I have avoided using identifiable information from archival sources unless it is public knowledge within the community and acceptable to those most involved.[73]

While multiple languages can be heard at Khunde Hospital, the working language of the hospital and its documentation is English. The Sherpa world is primarily an oral one. While Khumbu Sherpas speak Sherpa amongst themselves, the national language is Nepali, which is written in Devanagari script. Some patients speak Tibetan, while foreign visitors to the hospital arrive speaking a range of other tongues. Although I wanted to be able to speak the local language, I did not. I started learning Nepali in Kathmandu, but throughout my time at Khunde I remained unsure as to whether I should have learned Sherpa or Nepali. Only the very young children of the Canadian doctors at Khunde in the mid-1990s ever learned to speak like a Sherpa.[74] In the end I spoke English, as did most of the staff and an increasing number of hospital patients and people in the community. I also became aware that my inability to speak Sherpa gave people in the close environment of the hospital and the community their own space.[75] Sherpa was their language and gave them control.

As well as using the considerable volume and range of documents, a large part of the material for this study was gained orally and by participant observation.[76] I talked with people who had a variety of links with Khunde Hospital, both to Sherpas and to those from other countries. Many people have been involved for long periods and some since inception. Khunde Hospital is an ongoing project. I used a multi-pronged strategy for gaining oral information. Some interviews were conducted formally taking notes at the time, while

[73] Unfortunately, not all previously published examples meet this criteria and I have not referred to these.

[74] This comment was often made to us by Sherpa staff at the hospital and people in the community.

[75] This probably occurs in similar situations elsewhere.

[76] This study received ethical approval from the University of Otago in 2002. See the bibliography for a list of people with whom I talked.

others have been more informal and written up as soon afterwards as was possible. Some of the most useful material came from casual conversations, which I always wrote up afterwards. Often this occurred as a result of something happening in the clinic or community. While I could have used a tape recorder on some occasions, much of the time this would have been inhibitory or inappropriate for the social context. While some of the people I spoke to I met only once, most people I saw I met on several occasions throughout my stay. I could then talk further, clarify a point from a previous conversation that I was unsure about or ask a specific question. I used this approach with both Sherpa and Trust informants who were informed throughout about my project. My Sherpa sources knew that my project was primarily about Khunde Hospital and was not an ethnography about them. Similarly Sir Edmund Hillary understood that my interest was in his work rather than himself.

I used English and most of my conversations with Sherpas from the local community were in English. I used an interpreter when the other person did not speak English, whether I was at the hospital or in the community. Local staff at the hospital translated for the overseas volunteers both inside and outside the clinic, and therefore people were very used to having someone act as interpreter and to conversations being conducted in multiple languages.[77] When people did not want to talk about something they ignored the question and changed the subject.

My time at Khunde Hospital, and continued involvement with the hospital and the Himalayan Trust, gave me an entry into the local community and people's lives that was more difficult for an outside researcher. I was invited into many people's homes and participated in a wide variety of community events. I did not wish, however, to abuse this privilege and people's hospitality by asking questions that I knew people would not want to answer. Sickness was not something Sherpas liked other people to know about.[78] I also knew that there were people with whom it would have been

[77] For an informative discussion of how a good interpreter can overcome many problems during fieldwork, see van Spengen, *Tibetan Border Worlds*, 240–44.

[78] People usually knew because they visited one another, and along the trail people always ask where you are going or where you have come from.

useful to talk, especially those more ambivalent towards the hospital, but because I was associated with the hospital they would have been reluctant to criticise it. They would have found other ways to express this, as they did with using the hospital. They might not have been there when I went to call or would have said "I don't know". I am fortunate, however, that ethnographic accounts assist in filling some of these gaps.

I spent over two years living and working at Khunde Hospital before I began my doctoral research. I was always amazed by the diversity of events and activities that occurred each day, each being an integral part of what life at Khunde Hospital was all about, but each often very different from one another. "Multiple worlds" was indeed the term I would use to describe the world I encountered. My involvement with Khunde Hospital began in 1995 when my husband, John, a medical doctor, and I were appointed by the Himalayan Trust to be the next volunteers to run Khunde Hospital. We left Dunedin, New Zealand with our three children, Emma, Edward and Christopher, in May 1996, just as an Everest tragedy was unfolding in which New Zealand climbers Rob Hall and Andrew Harris and nine other people died. During the intervening time our world in Dunedin of family, university and hospital had begun engaging with the world of Sir Edmund Hillary, the Himalayan Trust and the Everest area. For over three weeks in the Nepalese capital of Kathmandu we were still part of Hillary's world. We learned a little Nepali, met people and began to discover how things did and did not work in Nepal. We then flew by small plane to Lukla. We were met by hospital staff and began our walk up to Khunde along the trail that was a two-way highway for people, animals and goods. It was June and the early monsoon. The temperature was mild, although cooler than Kathmandu, but everywhere was green, the crops were growing and flowers were blooming.

Then began our introduction to the Sherpa world of Khunde Hospital. Just before we reached the village where we were to stay on our second night John, the new "Khunde doctor", was called to assist a woman who was in labour in a house further back along the trail. She was upstairs, alone in a smoky loft, but first he was given something to eat and drink downstairs in the main room of the house. Here his Western medical beliefs of first seeing the patient met the obligations of Sherpa hospitality. Only then could he begin his work. As night approached the only light came from his headlight. The doctor, the woman and her mother were all on the floor with a layer of smoke filling the space above them. He had no equipment or medicines with him, but fortunately all went smoothly and mother and baby were well. Afterwards, the family gave him a beer to celebrate the birth.[79] Then, as it was now very late, he stayed the night and rejoined us the following morning.

Onwards and upwards we made our way in the mist and drizzle to the hospital, to the tiny flat at the end of the building that was to be our home and our personal space, to the kitchen that was the focal point of much of hospital life, to meeting the Canadian family we were succeeding and the Sherpa staff. The next week was a whirl—the hospital handover, participating in *Dumje* which was the major religious festival on the Sherpa calendar, parties and struggling to adjust to the altitude. Then Khunde Hospital was "ours" for the next two years.[80]

The damp, cloudy weather continued, but one morning a month later we awoke to find sunshine streaming into the flat. Beyond our valley and upwards soared the magnificent snow-capped peaks of Thamserku, Kangtega and Ama Dablam.[81] Outside our window the village of Khunde was waking up to a new day. A haze of juniper smoke hung over the houses, people made their way to the fields that surrounded the houses and some came to the hospital. By nine o'clock in the morning the mist had returned, but we had had our first glimpse of the mountain world of the Sherpa of Khumbu.

[79] This is common practice. The use of bottled beer rather than the local drinks reflects increasing affluence in the area and people wanting to display that they have the money. Bottled drinks are expensive because of the high transport costs of bringing such items into the area. Nevertheless, pressures are also created for those who have less money.

[80] Or so we thought initially. We soon learned that Khunde Hospital was a space we shared with other hospital staff and the community.

[81] All three peaks had New Zealanders who were associated with Hillary in the first ascents in the early 1960s.

The following chapters are my attempt as a historian to explore the multiple worlds and histories of Khunde Hospital. I began the research because I wanted to find out more and I began writing thinking that I should not be part of the stories. I soon found that I was. As one of the volunteers brought in by Sir Edmund Hillary to run the hospital between 1996 and 1998, I was both an observer and a participant. Khunde Hospital was my home and my world.

1

Khunde Hospital, Sir Edmund Hillary and Giving Aid

> It is commonly accepted that the isolated mountain valleys of the Himalayas are Shangri-Las where there is no sickness and people live on forever. Such, alas, is not the case—or certainly not in the various Himalayan regions I have visited.
>
> Sir Edmund Hillary, *Schoolhouse in the Clouds* [1]

> The Himalayan Trust is a diverse band of firm and sometimes fiery friends bonded together by experience of and fascination by Nepal, and by strong affection for and loyalty to Ed.
>
> Jim Wilson, Himalayan Trust Newsletter [2]

High childhood mortality, mothers dying in childbirth and cases of tuberculosis were not images that fitted in with the world's perceptions of the exotic mountain environments of the remote Himalaya. In 1964 Sir Edmund Hillary outlined in *Schoolhouse in the Clouds,* his book about the first Himalayan Schoolhouse Expedition (of 1963), his views about the ill health of the local people that he had encountered in his travels. Lack of modern medicines and scientific medical knowledge meant that people either recovered or died in "A Land Without Convalescents". [3] Himalayan expeditions had built up a tradition of treating the sick, but such actions were a short-term response. Hillary believed that there was a long-term need to meet

[1] Sir Edmund Hillary, *Schoolhouse in the Clouds* (London: Hodder and Stoughton, 1964), 100.

[2] [Dr] Jim Wilson, Himalayan Trust Newsletter 1988, 13 [Wilson papers]. Wilson was a lecturer in philosophy and comparative religion at Canterbury University (Christchurch, New Zealand), a climber and a long-time friend of Hillary.

[3] Hillary, *Schoolhouse in the Clouds,* 100 and 107.

the lack of medical facilities in Khumbu and so in his characteristic practical fashion planned to do something about the problem. Two years later, at the end of 1966, he built a small hospital on the edge of the Sherpa village of Khunde.

Nepal had assumed an increasing and important place in Hillary's life during the five years since establishing a school in the adjacent village of Khumjung in 1961. He spent several months each year in the country planning and organising, meeting officials, undertaking new projects, supporting and supervising his aid programme. The involvement continued outside these visits with preparation, fund-raising in New Zealand and overseas, public engagements and writing. His capacity for hard work was enormous, but others gave considerable time to help. Although Hillary and his team became incorporated as the Sherpa Trust Board in 1966 (becoming the Himalayan Trust Board in 1971), it continued to function as an informal group of friends, family and associates with its "office" at Hillary's home in Auckland. Throughout, the principal influence in the Trust was Hillary. As a result, his particular version of helping others suffused the whole programme.[4]

This chapter looks at Hillary's relationship with Khunde Hospital and uses it to highlight the role and the wide-ranging influence of the aid donor. Motives for giving assistance to others have varied and continue to vary, whether one is discussing different countries, organisations or individuals. The most important reasons relate to moral and humanitarian ideas, political and national security issues, and economic and trade interests.[5] Ideas have also changed over time and in today's international development framework of "global governance" the agency of the donor is increasingly hidden. Identifying the reasons behind the giving of aid, however, remains important because of the considerable influence these have had on the type of aid given and the process of implementing that aid.[6] That Hillary was a private individual and his organisation small, in

[4] The broader international aid context in which Khunde Hospital operated is discussed in chapter four.

[5] Degnbol-Martinussen and Engberg-Pedersen, *Aid,* 9.

[6] Mosse, "Global Governance and the Ethnography of International Aid", 12, and Degnbol-Martinussen and Engberg-Pedersen, *Aid,* 7.

no way lessens the significant impact of his role and influence as an aid donor.

Hillary was responsible for the hospital's establishment and subsequent management, but his personal philosophy of friendship and working with Sherpas in carrying out a broad aid programme had a defining role on how the hospital functioned. The overseas staff were expected to live and work as part of the local community, respecting their mostly Sherpa neighbours and the Sherpa and Nepalese way of life. The hospital was not an autonomous institution. Although its location was remote, it was run as an integral part of Hillary's programme. Despite the distance between Nepal and New Zealand, Hillary and the Trust's practical and personal support ensured the hospital's continuing ability to provide medical services in a country where most rural health work suffered from a lack of infrastructure, personnel and medicines. The overseas staff at the hospital would have found their life and work at Khunde very difficult; indeed they would not have been there without the organisational and financial support from Hillary through the Himalayan Trust and later also the Canadian Sir Edmund Hillary Foundation (SEHF). Khunde Hospital needed to be part of Hillary's world to continue to exist and function.

The first part of the chapter discusses why Hillary built the hospital at Khunde. Much of it is narrative. While this provides context for Hillary's involvement, its description demonstrates the crucial way in which Khunde Hospital was conceived, built and administered within Hillary's programme as a whole. It looks at his life, how and why he became involved in assisting the Sherpa and the events that led to building the hospital. The second section examines the ongoing role that Hillary and the Himalayan Trust played in the development of the hospital. On a day-to-day basis the hospital was run from Khunde with overseas volunteers in charge, but for Hillary it remained an integral part of his expanding assistance programme for which he took personal responsibility. Much of the initial organisational framework established by Hillary in the 1960s continued, but was adapted as circumstances changed within Nepal and overseas. The final part of the chapter reverses the focus and looks at the hospital's significant contribution to the wider Hillary/

Trust programme. Both the overseas volunteers and local Sherpa staff were involved with Hillary's other projects in the area. The hospital also gained positive international publicity, which helped to keep Hillary and the Trust's work in the public eye and so secure the donations that enabled these activities to continue.

Why Did Sir Edmund Hillary Build a Hospital at Khunde?

When Hillary descended from the summit of Everest on 29 May 1953, he had no idea of how quickly his successful first ascent of the world's highest mountain was to transform him into a very public person. Ed Hillary, the lanky New Zealand beekeeper became Sir Edmund Hillary, Everest hero. Awareness of the British expedition's success was heightened by its news being announced in England the day of the coronation of the new young Queen Elizabeth II. Yet Hillary was surprised that the public welcomes the expedition received around the world were repeated when he and George Lowe—also from New Zealand—returned to Auckland in August and were met with "handshakes, hugs, cheers and even a few tears—and all because we'd climbed a mountain!"[7] When a few weeks later the newly married Hillary flew into Sydney with his young bride, Louise, "there was another big crowd to see us with flashing cameras and inquisitive press men".[8]

Sir Edmund Hillary remained newsworthy. He was interviewed and written about regularly, and continued to be perceived in New Zealand as a legend and was to a surprising degree free from criticism. Yet for someone whose fame stretched back for over fifty years and who held such an iconic status within contemporary New Zealand society, his presence until recently was almost absent from New Zealand's general history books.[9] At the beginning of the twenty-first century, however, historian Michael King considered that Hillary had "earned the uncontested title of 'greatest New

[7] Edmund Hillary, *Nothing Venture, Nothing Win* (London: Hodder and Stoughton, 1975), 168. Also see Hansen, "Confetti of Empire," 307–32.

[8] Hillary, *Nothing Venture, Nothing Win,* 168. They had married the previous day on 3 September 1953, Louise's twenty-third birthday.

[9] Hillary's image is on the NZ$5 note.

Zealander'".[10] King believed that Hillary would have been famous throughout his life if the only thing he had done was the first ascent of Everest, but Hillary used the "almost accidental fame" that Everest brought him to do practical good both at home and overseas for more than forty years. For King, Hillary's status was not just about what he did, but was more importantly about how he conducted himself:

> Through all this he remained reticent, strong, dependable, unboastful, good-humoured, a man who accepted with patience and grace the relationship his country had forged with him and the responsibilities and burdens that accompanied it.[11]

Hillary was, therefore, worthy of his high status in the public imagination.

King saw a person beyond the image, but it is Hillary's own extensive writing that still provides the best entry into his world, moving beyond what he did to what he thought and why he acted in the way he did. In these works he becomes far more human and self-questioning. Yet none of the literature, whether academic or popular, looks critically at his work in the Himalaya or the Himalayan Trust that he set up to be the vehicle through which he carried out his aid programme. For Hillary, Khunde Hospital was an integral part of this work, and so this history also provides a case study for considering his work more broadly.

Hillary's early life was unremarkable. Edmund Percival Hillary was born on 20 July 1919 in a hospital in Auckland, the largest city in New Zealand, and grew up in the small town of Tuakau, about sixty kilometres south of Auckland, where his father ran a local weekly newspaper. One of three children, he had an elder sister June and a younger brother Rex. His mother had trained as a teacher and believed in the importance of a good education. After finishing at the local primary school he went to Auckland Grammar School, which was thought to be one of the best academic schools in the country.

10 Michael King, *The Penguin History of New Zealand* (Auckland: Penguin Books, 2003), 510.

11 King, *Penguin History of New Zealand*, 511.

In his two autobiographies, Hillary described his strict upbringing, clashes with his father's rigid views, his loneliness, lack of friends and a sense of physical inferiority. He thought he must have been a "difficult child".[12] Significantly, in view of Hillary's future relationship with Sherpas, he wrote of how his father had a "close" relationship with the Maori community and so the young Edmund grew up accepting "our Maori neighbours as an ordinary and normal part" of his life.[13]

When he was fifteen, the family moved to Auckland and eventually bought a house in Remuera Road, one of the best suburbs. This was a big surprise to Hillary, because in his daily life there never appeared to be any money for the children. Hillary did reasonably well at school and his mother encouraged him to go to Auckland University at the young age of sixteen, but after two "rather miserable" years studying mathematics and science Hillary left and went into the family beekeeping business.[14] "It was a good life—a life of open air and sun and hard physical work."[15] The family also had a period of involvement with a religious group, Radiant Living, becoming foundation members when it set up a branch in Auckland. He left after a few years, but during this time he "learned to speak confidently from the platform; to think more freely on important topics; to mix more readily with a wide variety of people."[16] These were all skills that Hillary needed after 1953.

Hillary did not begin climbing until during the Second World War, but by the late 1940s it was a very important part of his life.[17]

12 Hillary, *View from the Summit,* 40.

13 Hillary, *Nothing Venture, Nothing Win,* 19. He also noted that he could not remember any Maori being invited to his home, unlike his own relations with Sherpas.

14 Hillary, *View from the Summit,* 43–44.

15 Hillary, *Nothing Venture, Nothing Win,* 25–26.

16 Ibid., 27.

17 People climb mountains for many reasons. For a general account see Robert Macfarlane, *Mountains of the Mind: A History of a Fascination* (London: Granta, 2003). For a discussion of mountains in the New Zealand context see Eric Pawson, "The Meanings of Mountains", in *Environmental Histories of New*

As a young boy, Hillary—like Tenzing—had been a dreamer. [18] He read avidly about adventure. New Zealand's mountains became his personal adventure and he quickly rose to become one of the country's leading climbers. In 1946 he met Harry Ayres, New Zealand's "outstanding" mountain guide, and Hillary saw this as the turning point in his climbing career. [19] The two often climbed together and Hillary learned a lot from Ayres about the technical aspects of climbing. Ayres was highly skilled on ice. Hillary also "absorbed a great deal of his [Ayres] philosophy of safe but forceful mountaineering". [20] After the 1953 success, Colonel John Hunt, leader of the expedition, described Hillary as "quite exceptionally strong and abounding in a restless energy, possessed of a thrusting mind which swept aside all unproved obstacles". [21]

The Southern Alps were a good training ground for the rigours and ice of the distant Himalaya. Although the Everest story was mainly a British affair, New Zealand had connections that went back as far as the famous 1924 expedition. [22] Noel Odell, who was the last person to see George Mallory and Andrew Irvine alive near the summit of Everest, settled in New Zealand after the Second World War and became Professor of Geology at the University of

---

Zealand, ed. Eric Pawson and Tom Brooking (Auckland: Oxford University Press, 2002), 136–50.

18 See opening paragraph in chapter two of this book.

19 Hillary, *View from the Summit,* 59.

20 Hillary, *Nothing Venture, Nothing Win,* 78.

21 John Hunt, *The Ascent of Everest* (London: Hodder and Stoughton, 1953), 28. Hillary frequently used "restless" in his own writings and used physical activity to battle boredom.

22 Peter Hansen, nevertheless, refers to a distinctive New Zealand climbing tradition and that by the 1930s New Zealand climbing had become independent of British models. Peter H. Hansen, "Debate: Tenzing's Two Wrist-Watches: The Conquest of Everest and Late Imperial Culture in Britain 1921–1953", *Past and Present* 157, 1997, 159–77. Also see Philip Temple, *The World at Their Feet: The Story of New Zealand Mountaineers in the Great Ranges of the World* (Christchurch: Whitcombe & Tombs, 1969) and Norman Hardie, *On My Own Two Feet: The Life of a Mountaineer* (Christchurch: Canterbury University Press, 2006).

Otago.[23] His talks helped stimulate local New Zealand interest in the Himalaya. In 1951 British climber Eric Shipton's positive memories of New Zealander Dan Bryant on the 1935 Everest Reconnaissance led to Shipton agreeing to a request from the New Zealand Alpine Club and inviting two New Zealanders, from a group already in Nepal, to join him on the reconnaissance of Everest from the south.[24] One of these was Hillary. In 1952 he was part of Shipton's expedition to Cho Oyu.[25] Although Hunt replaced Shipton as leader of the planned attempt on Everest for 1953 and had not met Hillary, he invited both him and Lowe to join the team.

Hillary's success on Everest made him well known, but also acted as a catalyst. Philip Temple, in his account of New Zealand mountaineers on overseas expeditions, contrasted the Hillary of 1952 with that of 1954:

> He was no longer simply the strong, hearty companion, mildly ambitious for himself, with plenty of go; no longer the man who was often glad to follow a lead, taking an unsophisticated view of his surroundings. Everest proved that he could tackle and overcome the biggest problems and there was something to be said for his way of going about things. He was more certain, more confident, more experienced in organisation and leadership and more ambitious for himself and others.[26]

In the 1950s Hillary's world became a mixture of lecture tours, family life, writing, a little beekeeping and a lot of adventure. In 1954 he led a New Zealand Alpine Club expedition east of Everest to the Barun Valley, and between 1955 and 1958 was involved with the Commonwealth Trans-Antarctic Expedition, controversially leading the New Zealand team to the South Pole by tractor.

At this point in Hillary's life, there was no indication of the watershed that would occur during his next Himalayan expedition. In 1960–61 he returned to Nepal with a multi-purpose expedition

[23] Bryant, *New Zealanders and Everest,* 15–16.

[24] Hillary also wrote to Shipton. Hillary, *View from the Summit,* 76.

[25] To the dismay of the British, who saw Everest as their mountain, the Nepalese government gave permission for the Swiss to attempt to climb Everest in 1952.

[26] Temple, *The World at Their Feet,* 95.

which aimed to look for the yeti—the famous "abominable snowman" of the Himalaya, to conduct physiological research into high-altitude acclimatisation and to make an attempt without oxygen to climb Makalu, the world's fifth highest mountain. It was on this expedition that Hillary decided to do something to help the Sherpa who he believed had given so much to mountaineering. The change of direction would help channel some of Hillary's restless energy, would draw on his developing organisational skills and would require the determination that helped him get to the top of Everest. It would also alter fundamentally the focus of Hillary's life.

While Hillary had a lot of fun with his expeditions, he also describes his feeling a sense of "duty" to help the Sherpa.[27] Anthropologist Sherry Ortner discusses the "sahibs" of Himalayan mountaineering—as she calls the international mountaineers—and refers to the values of male, Western paternalism of responsibility towards the subordinate and weak.[28] Hillary's own use of the word "duty" implies a very strong sense of responsibility, but he never saw Sherpas as weak or subordinate. Sherpas were his friends. He did not feel sorry for them, but believed they lacked money and the educational opportunities to help themselves. As he was in a position to provide these, he believed he should. His father had been "passionate" about social justice, but helping one's friends is also, as Hillary's biographer Alexa Johnston writes, "fondly thought of as the Kiwi way".[29]

Hillary traced the beginning of his aid programme to the Sherpa to a conversation he had during the expedition. One evening in October 1960, in the extreme cold of the expedition's high-altitude campsite, Hillary asked the senior of his Sherpas how he could most

[27] Interview with Sir Edmund Hillary, Auckland, May 2002.

[28] Ortner, *Life and Death on Mt. Everest,* 46. *Sahib* (boss or master) is a Hindi term which Sherpas used to address or refer to the overseas members of the expedition.

[29] Alexa Johnston, *Sir Edmund Hillary: An Extraordinary Life* (Auckland: Penguin Viking, 2005), 25 and 222. New Zealanders are popularly known as "Kiwis". Johnston gained unprecedented access to Hillary's personal archives for her authorised and illustrated biography.

help them.[30] His *sirdar* (foreman) Urkien's choice was education, rather than medical care or agricultural improvement which Hillary thought were the Sherpa's "primary needs".[31] Views differ about this story, about who should be credited with the request for education and about when Hillary began to seriously think of helping the Sherpa, but this was, and remained, the story that he told.[32] Some schooling existed in the monasteries, but the only government school was at Namche Bazar and its fortunes varied.

Hillary had some reservations about providing education. Peter Mulgrew, a sub-lieutenant in the New Zealand Navy who had been with Hillary in Antarctica and was again with him in 1960–61, wrote of Hillary's reaction to Urkein's request for education for their children: "This greatly interested Hillary who had felt that it would be far better to leave the Sherpas alone".[33] Hillary was concerned about too much education, because this "could make the children misfits" in their own community.[34] Romantics did not want to see any alterations to the Sherpa way of life, but change was already occurring with the opening up of Nepal and visitors going to the Everest area. Hillary and his friends talked much about what they thought they could or should do. Michael (Mike) Gill, a climber and in 1961 still a medical student, best expressed their turmoil:

> It is so easy to be sentimental about the Sherpas . . . We sit back in our city homes with our books and television, water on tap, electricity . . . and we think mistily of those happy, healthy Sherpas living simply . . . The Sherpa has a more realistic view of his life: he knows that if blight strikes the potato crop he will have a hungry winter . . .
>
> Change and education of a sort have come to the Sherpas whether we think they need them or not. They look at these people who have so

30 Hillary, *Schoolhouse in the Clouds,* 2.

31 Peter Mulgrew, *No Place for Men* (Auckland: Fontana Silver Fern, 1975 [1964]), 153–54. Urkien had a few years earlier approached another New Zealand climber, Norman Hardie, about education for his sons. Norman Hardie, *In Highest Nepal: Our Life Among the Sherpas* (London: George Allen & Unwin, 1957), 69.

32 Ortner, *Life and Death on Mt. Everest,* 341 note 50; Fisher, *Sherpas,* 68–71.

33 Mulgrew, *No Place for Men,* 153–54.

34 Hillary, *Schoolhouse in the Clouds,* 23.

much more than they have . . . so much money that they can afford to do useless things like climbing mountains. They look and find that these foreigners are not obviously more able or intelligent than they are.[35]

Sherpas articulated the difference to be the opportunities afforded by education. In June 1961 Hillary built them a school in Khumjung, the largest village in Khumbu. Funding came from his expedition's American sponsors, World Book Encyclopedia of Chicago. Secular education was a powerful symbol and tool of modernity, but education, so Hillary, Gill and Mulgrew believed, would also help Sherpas cope and harness the changes.[36]

In 1961 Hillary did not envisage the wide-ranging and long-term involvement that would eventually develop between him and the Sherpas. "When I left Khumjung on June 13th", he wrote in the mid-1970s, "I little realised I was leaving behind what was to become a new way of life for me".[37] The new way of life would continue. Hillary had seen the school as a "one-off" project.[38] By 1966, however, he had constructed further schools, bridges, an airstrip, improved water supplies and provided short-term medical care. Furthermore, building schools was just the start of an ongoing support, since teachers had to be found and paid and school supplies provided. Despite Hillary's initial thoughts, his visit to the main monastery of the area at Tengboche that took place shortly before Khumjung School's construction, illustrated both the way he worked and also suggested that the school might not be a "one-off" involvement with helping the people and the area. Hillary had visited the monastery before, but he described how, with considerable ceremony, he was shown around by its head, the *rinpoche* ("precious" one).[39] Mountaineering expeditions visited Tengboche on

35 Michael Gill, *Mountain Midsummer: Climbing in Four Continents* (London: Hodder and Stoughton, 1969), 168–69.

36 Fisher also believed that the schools were the "crucial link between tradition and modernity". Fisher, *Sherpas,* 172.

37 Hillary, *Nothing Venture, Nothing Win*, 251.

38 Interview with Sir Edmund Hillary, Kathmandu, April 1997.

39 Edmund Hillary and Desmond Doig, *High in the Thin Cold Air* (London: Hodder and Stoughton, 1963 [1962]), 269–70.

their way to climbing Everest, or one of the other mountains, and their donations had enabled the monastery to provide a new roof. Hillary saw that the new roof had some rust in a few places and promised to try and get some paint; something he was able to do on his return to Kathmandu.

The paint and the school demonstrated that when Hillary said he was going to do something, he did so. Over the years many people have visited the area and said they wanted to help. Some people have provided considerable assistance, but in most cases and for various reasons nothing usually happened. Hillary carried out his pledges and his help was very practical. On his expeditions he gathered like-minded people around him to carry out his plans, and who could adapt to working in the difficult conditions of Khumbu. Walter (Wally) Romanes, a builder from Hastings in New Zealand, was on the 1960–61 expedition. Hillary had designed the Green Hut used in the expedition, but the "ingenious" Romanes built it "far better than I had ever expected".[40] At the end of the expedition, Romanes helped Hillary build Khumjung school.

While Hillary may have felt an obligation to help the Sherpa, this sense of duty did not form the basis of his relationship with Sherpas; the evident warmth of his affection, the respect he gave them and the way he worked with them as equals did not arise out of obligation. Hillary's relationship with Sherpas underpinned the whole Hillary/Trust programme in Nepal and continued to do so. He described them in the familiar language of the Western narrative of the Sherpa, but without idealising them or believing himself superior. He recognised that they were: "good and bad, strong and weak, honest and dishonest like the rest of us. But few of those who visit them can remain indifferent to their loyalty, affection and charm, or unimpressed with their remarkable toughness and courage."[41]

Hillary and his senior Sherpas sat around the fire together and he listened to what they were telling him. Despite having other

[40] Ibid., 168. The Green Hut was the lower of two huts used by the expedition. The other was the more famous Silver Hut that was the site for the high-altitude physiological research.

[41] Hillary, preface to *Schoolhouse in the Clouds*.

projects in mind and some doubts about the choice of assistance, Hillary agreed to their request.

Listening to Sherpas, undertaking practical projects and carrying out what he said he would do, were the hallmarks of Hillary's work in the area, but he also had another motive for wanting to help them. He was extremely conscious of the intensified Chinese presence just over the border in Tibet; this awareness pervaded books about the area written in the 1950s and early 1960s.[42] Hillary's response to the situation in Khumbu was again typical, although he also thought about larger issues. The Red Cross wanted to fly in emergency supplies to the refugees who were coming across the border.[43] Hillary's expedition built an airstrip at Mingbo (4,600 metres) and in return the Red Cross flew in the building materials for the school at Khumjung. The Red Cross had wanted the refugees to do the work "but I knew this would cause considerable resentment among the Sherpas, who were seeking work, too, and whose economy had been impaired by the flood of refugees and the cessation of trade with Tibet."[44] Hillary also knew of the "increased penetration of Chinese Communist propaganda and money across the border".[45] Widespread international concern at this time about the spread of communism was an important reason why Nepal was receiving increasing amounts of foreign aid, but little assistance had reached the areas near Nepal's long border with Tibet.

The aid to Sherpas provided through the school at Khumjung and the paint for the monastery at Tengboche had not been part of Hillary's 1960–61 Himalayan Scientific and Mountaineering Ex-

[42] Ibid., 7. Hillary does not discuss this in later accounts. Hillary's concerns at the time are clearly evident in documents, especially from the New Zealand High Commission in New Delhi. See Himalayan Climbing Expeditions & Schoolhouse Project, ABHS 6949 W4628 NDI 64/14/2 Part 2 [Archives New Zealand/Te Rua Mahara o te Kawanatanga, Head Office, Wellington, hereafter ANZ].

[43] Toni Hagen, a Swiss geologist who became involved with the Tibetan refugee programme of the International Committee of the Red Cross, does not mention Hillary's role. Toni Hagen, *Nepal: The Kingdom in the Himalayas* (New Delhi: Oxford and IBH, 1980 [1961]), 172.

[44] Hillary and Doig, *High in the Thin Cold Air,* 188.

[45] Hillary, *Schoolhouse in the Clouds,* 7.

pedition's objectives. His focus was that of the outsider who came to Nepal primarily for climbing, science and adventure.[46] The scientific endeavours of 1960 and 1961, whether the search for the yeti or the high-altitude physiological experiments, were also not for the benefit of either the local population or the area. Hillary became sick towards the end of the expedition, and afterwards he commented that if the effects of high altitude restricted his activities "he will devite [*sic*] himself to scientific work".[47]

Hillary's next expedition to Nepal, however, reflected humanitarian rather than scientific aims, although he would still continue to plan and enjoy adventures both in Nepal and elsewhere:

> The Himalayan Schoolhouse Expedition 1963 was an expedition with a difference. We planned to assault two great unclimbed peaks, members of the party were mountaineers of wide repute, yet our major program involved much more than this. We intended to repay in some measure the debt we owed to the Sherpas who live in the shadow of Mount Everest: we would build schools for them, pipe fresh water, and treat their diseases.[48]

46 In the late 1940s a few climbing expeditions gained Nepalese government permission to enter the country because they also had scientific objectives. See, for example, H. W. Tilman, *Nepal Himalaya* (Cambridge: Cambridge University Press, 1952), 4–5. Similarly, missionary Robert Fleming gained permission to enter Nepal to study the country's birdlife not evangelise. Jonathan Lindell, *Nepal and the Gospel of God* (Kathmandu: United Mission to Nepal, 1979), 134–35.

47 *Otago Daily Times* (Dunedin), 14 June 1961. From a collection of newspaper cuttings at "Sir Edmund Hillary: Everest and Beyond" exhibition, Otago Museum (Dunedin), 16 October 2004–20 March 2005.

48 Hillary, preface to *Schoolhouse in the Clouds*. A limited and sometimes inaccurate knowledge of the history of Hillary's work unfortunately mars Vincanne Adams' discussion of Hillary and the Himalayan Trust. For example, Louise and Belinda Hillary were killed on their way to Phaphlu Hospital not Khunde. Adams, *Tigers of the Snow and Other Virtual Sherpas,* 89–94. Adams (p. 90) rightly comments on the dual nature of his expeditions and believed the climbing ensured economic support from Western volunteers. Although initially Hillary had hoped to include a peak, the expedition that built Khunde Hospital had no climbing because of a ban by the Nepalese government at that time on mountaineering in the area. In practice Hillary chose people for his expeditions for the various skills they would contribute.

Hillary had suffered what appeared to be a "transient stroke" on Makalu in 1961 and would not go really high again, but it is unlikely that a need for a new challenge was the main reason for this different type of Hillary expedition.[49] After building the school at Khumjung Hillary began to get petitions from other villages asking for assistance.[50] Such requests for help, combined with Hillary's personal feelings that he should assist if he could, led him to continue. Adventures, practical projects, the companionship of friends and family, laughter and convivial Sherpa hospitality ensured that he also had a lot of fun on the way![51]

Translating a desire to help into effective action also required three further considerations: permission from the Nepalese government, finance and organisation. From the beginning of his work in Nepal, Hillary had to deal with people, organisations and supply issues in countries that were a long way from New Zealand and where communication could be difficult and limited. While Hillary procured the paint for Tengboche monastery from Kathmandu, building Khumjung school involved bringing in construction materials from India. In both cases he then had to organise transportation to Khumbu.

By the end of 1961, preliminary discussions had begun with the Nepalese government for both the climbing and aid objectives of the 1963 expedition. Hillary operated in a private capacity, but the Nepalese government required official endorsement of an expedition. The New Zealand government, through the Department of External Affairs in Wellington but particularly the New Zealand

---

Often climbing combined with the desired project skills but sometimes not. Hillary's brother Rex, who was a major contributor over many years to the Trust's building and maintenance programme, was not a climber.

49 Mulgrew, *No Place for Men,* Appendix—Medical Aspects, 192. Hillary was also sick in 1954.

50 For example, a petition from Thame village dated 27 October 1962 with the much quoted sentence "Though our children have eyes but still they are blind!" Hillary, *Schoolhouse in the Clouds,* 3.

51 Interview, Hillary, June 2002.

High Commission in New Delhi, was drawn into the process.[52] Hillary learned from these early encounters with officialdom, but a slow and often difficult process for obtaining approval came to be expected and would also occur in the case of the hospital at Khunde.[53]

While education was the main thrust of Hillary's early involvement with Sherpas, he did not abandon his belief that Western medicine would also help them. The medical experiences of overseas visitors to Nepal and the wider Himalayan region, their travel into often remote areas with no roads and the lack of Western medical services along their route, provide both the general background and the more immediate context that led Hillary to build Khunde Hospital in 1966.[54] As the epigraph to this chapter shows, Hillary distinguished the romantic image of Himalayan people from the harsh realities of their life and was aware of the considerable sickness he encountered as he travelled in the mountains. He knew that people had their own beliefs and practices and that they attributed a supernatural reason to most ill health.[55] To Hillary's way of thinking, this was understandable because the Sherpa lacked "medical knowledge". Like other overseas visitors, medical knowledge to Hillary was the system he was familiar with—Western medicine. On his own expeditions he saw how local people sought medical

[52] Secretary of External Affairs to the High Commissioner, 16 January 1962, Himalayan Climbing Expeditions & Schoolhouse Project, ABHS 6949 W4628 NDI 64/14/2 Part 2 [ANZ].

[53] Obtaining official approval was an area where the worlds of Hillary and foreign aid intersected, and is discussed in chapter four. Hillary remained an independent operator, raising the required finance from various sources, including government, and organising what became a substantial and ongoing commitment to Nepal. Hillary at times caused headaches in official circles, but the government could also bask in the reflected glory of Sir Edmund Hillary being a New Zealander.

[54] Given the lack of biomedical services in these areas and the consequent lack of archival sources, visitors' accounts provide an important avenue for information.

[55] Hillary, *Schoolhouse in the Clouds,* 111. A more common assumption by Western visitors was that nothing existed if there was no Western medicine.

care from foreigners and benefited from their medicines and from the expertise of doctors.

While local people usually carried little when they travelled, visitors from other countries were more heavily laden. In many areas there was nowhere to stay and no food to buy. Visitors would employ local people as porters to help with transportation. Part of the traveller's supplies was a medical kit that included medicines, dressings and equipment to deal with sickness and accidents that occurred along the journey, although this varied with the size of the group and the medical skills, if any, of its members. The kit was used to treat not only one's own problems, but also those of the group's employees; a large expedition could have hundreds of porters. Travel was slow in Nepal: most of it was on foot through a land with few roads and often very rugged terrain, with narrow tracks, rickety bridges or rivers to cross, and temperatures ranging from the heat and humidity of the lowlands to the freezing cold and limited oxygen of the highest mountains. As the group progressed through an area, and particularly when it stopped to camp, some of the local inhabitants would approach the visitors for treatment of various illnesses.[56]

Until the early 1950s the Nepalese government allowed few people from Western nations into their country and an even smaller number were able to venture beyond Kathmandu. The number of visitors increased during the 1950s and 1960s, but travel to areas such as Khumbu still required specific (additional) permission. In 1964 only twenty outsiders were reported to have visited visited Khumbu, one of which was a Hillary expedition.[57] Toni Hagen, a Swiss geologist who first went to Nepal in 1950 as part of a Swiss technical mission, was one of the few foreigners able to travel extensively throughout the country while compiling a geological survey of Nepal. He wrote that every foreigner was looked on as a "doctor Sahib".[58] In 1953 another British newspaper, the *Daily Mail,* sent reporter Ralph Izzard to cover the Everest Expedition in competition

[56] This continued and at times has been an issue in the provision of health services in Khumbu. See chapter three.

[57] Brower, *Sherpa of Khumbu*, 67.

[58] Hagen, *Nepal,* 127.

with *The Times* which had copyright to the expedition's dispatches. Izzard had to organise his own expedition in search of news:

> Medical supplies I purchased in abundance, not so much for myself (I was only to use Paludrine), but to patch up the coolies when necessary and because all Europeans travelling through the wilderness are expected to administer a pill or a plaster to all who may be met by the way and happen to need them.[59]

Expeditions that included doctors could provide more extensive medical services for the local population. Hunt described the scene in 1953 at their first base camp at Tengboche: "The arrival of an expedition invariably attracts the halt and the maimed, and Mike Ward has many 'cases' to examine. There are teeth to be pulled, sore eyes, ulcers, fevers and obscure stomach pains to be cured."[60] The rising number of climbing expeditions and other travellers to Nepal increased people's access to this type of medical practice. Hillary's expeditions in 1954 and 1960–61 contained doctors and followed this tradition of treating the local inhabitants in the areas they passed through.

Expedition medical practice, however, was a response to the lack of biomedical facilities in rural Nepal and to people asking for medical treatment. Inherently, it could only be a short-term measure. Usually, the expedition would see a patient, treat him/her and move on, not knowing whether or not the person got better. Accounts of these early expeditions only occasionally mentioned meeting a patient they had assisted earlier. At Junbesi in Solu, doctors on the 1963 American Mount Everest Expedition were confronted with a woman with severe burns whom they arranged to evacuate to Kathmandu where she was given skin grafts. She recovered and met the expedition on its return journey.[61] (The woman had tried

59 Izzard, *An Innocent on Everest,* 57. Malaria is a problem in the lowlands and Paludrine is an antimalarial drug. The more neutral term "porter" has replaced "coolie".

60 Hunt, *The Ascent of Everest*, 78.

61 Gilbert Roberts, "Health and Medicine", in *Americans on Everest,* by James Ramsey Ullman (Philadelphia and New York: J.B. Lippincott, 1964), 343–50.

to retrieve her sole yak from a burning shed.) While burn injuries were not uncommon among the local population who commonly used open fires, an expensive helicopter evacuation for treatment in Kathmandu was![62]

One of Hillary's aims for the 1963 Himalayan Schoolhouse Expedition was to go beyond this kind of temporary response to medical problems among local populations and set up a medical clinic in Khumjung. He wanted "not only to give immediate medical treatment to the Sherpas, but also to carry out a wider investigation with a view to establishing more long-range medical aid in the future."[63] By the time the expedition arrived in the village they had begun to implement one strand of this broader, long-term strategy—vaccination.

The approach that Hillary took in 1963 contrasts with the approach the American Everest expedition took in vaccinating the local population during an epidemic of smallpox, and illustrates the different direction Hillary was beginning to take. As an expedition passed through different districts, the threat of epidemic disease both for the group and the local communities was real. Movement from place to place and contact with people could both introduce and help spread an infectious illness. Smallpox was endemic within Nepal, but periodically became epidemic.[64] Hillary knew that smallpox might be a problem during his expedition, as the Americans had reported a case. In the Pharak village of Phakding, they had discovered a young porter with smallpox and isolated him.[65] Expedition members and the climbing Sherpas were already vaccinated but not other Sherpas or the lowland porters. The expedition's radio did not work, but through the radio at the military checkpost in Namche the expedition arranged for vaccine to be flown in from Kathmandu.[66] Meanwhile, the expedition saw no further cases of

[62] Ullman, *Americans on Everest,* 70.

[63] Hillary, *Schoolhouse in the Clouds,* 101.

[64] An endemic disease currently denotes a disease that is commonly found among the inhabitants of a particular place. The last recorded case of smallpox in Nepal was in 1975.

[65] The porter died. Roberts, "Health and Medicine", 348.

[66] Ullman, *Americans on Everest,* 82.

smallpox, and so continued its journey towards the Everest area. Above Namche it vaccinated five hundred people, although by the time the vaccine arrived the unvaccinated lowland porters had already left the expedition.[67]

Before Hillary left Kathmandu, he took the precaution of obtaining from the World Health Organization (WHO) representative in Kathmandu a smallpox vaccination set sufficient for at least two hundred people.[68] Hillary's expedition met its first case of smallpox in the small village of Surkye (about a half-day's walk south of Phakding), but when the expedition doctor Philip Houghton opened the vaccine package he found the set had already been used. With no easy means of communication with the outside world, nothing could be done quickly. As the expedition moved up the Dudh Kosi valley there were other cases and deaths, and fear of the disease was growing among the local population who began asking for help. Although some vaccination had occurred previously in the area, most people were unprotected.[69] Hillary resolved that a vaccination programme had to become a major part of the expedition and at Namche discussed the situation with the checkpost captain.[70] Hillary sent a radio message to Kathmandu and two days later, "with unprecedented alacrity", the Swiss Red Cross plane dropped the vaccine into Khumjung where the expedition was based.[71] The disease was spreading rapidly. Members of the expedition immediately began vaccinating the villagers of Khumjung and the nearby vil-

67 Ibid. Hillary mentions requests for vaccine from further afield as the epidemic spread. Hillary, *Schoolhouse in the Clouds,* 47–49. Nowadays lowland porters continue higher. This has health implications, because porters who normally reside at lower altitudes are susceptible to altitude sickness. Some die in the higher altitude of Khumbu. See chapter three.

68 Hillary, *Schoolhouse in the Clouds,* 40.

69 M. B. Gill, "The Sherpas: A Survey of an Isolated Mountain Community" (Department of Preventive and Social Medicine diss., University of Otago, 1961), 16. Sherpas with Hillary's expedition were not vaccinated at this stage. Hillary, *Schoolhouse in the Clouds,* 40.

70 Although Namche Bazar was the administrative centre of the area, government presence was limited in the early 1960s. Hillary mentions that the checkpost had a medical orderly. Hillary, *Schoolhouse in the Clouds,* 48.

71 Ibid., 42. Hillary later received a bill for 800 rupees (US$105).

lage of Khunde, vaccinating around three hundred people—over one-third of the population—during the first day. They then turned their attention to the other villages in the area. In total, expedition members gave over seven thousand vaccinations throughout the district. Hillary later wrote that of all the expedition's activities "the one most widely appreciated was undoubtedly the vaccination, and this hadn't been part of my original plans".[72] In his proposal to the Nepalese government for permission to build the hospital he said that not only would the hospital treat illness but would also introduce public health programmes.[73]

At the same time as undertaking vaccination, the expedition was also setting up a medical clinic in Khumjung. Hillary's account provided a vivid description of the way he worked. It showed his characteristic practical approach and how expedition members and villagers consulted and worked together. Above all, it reiterated how he listened to and was prepared to act on advice from Sherpas. The clinic began in a tent that measured just over three square metres, but it was soon evident that more space was needed for storage and to carry out procedures. Mingma Tsering, Hillary's sirdar, suggested that they take over one of the guest rooms opening off the walled courtyard in front of Khumjung *gompa* (temple). The room needed to be made suitable for use for the six months that the clinic would operate.

> After consultation with the village headmen we agreed to share the costs of renovation. The village put in a solid wooden floor and a raised sleeping bench. Then they plastered the walls with fresh clay and repaired the wood-shake roof.
>
> We, in our turn, lined the walls with bamboo matting and built a series of long shelves for the drugs and a couple of solid tables for operating

72 Ibid., 49. Hillary's vaccination activities during the epidemic created a favourable impression with the Nepalese in Kathmandu. Ian McIntosh to Hillary, 21 September 1963, Himalayan Climbing Expeditions & Schoolhouse Project, ABHS 6949 W4628 NDI 64/14/2 Part 2 [ANZ].

73 Sir Edmund Hillary, "New Zealand Hospital for the Sherpas", 22 October 1965, Himalayan Climbing Expeditions & Schoolhouse Projects, ABHS 6949 W4628 NDI 64/14/2 Part 3 [ANZ]. "Public health" here refers to preventive health.

> purposes. We screened the sleeping bench off from the main room so the doctors could have some privacy. A wood-burning stove was installed for comfort. We enlarged the window considerably to take full advantage of the view.[74]

The situation of the clinic was also significant. The suggestion to use a room at the gompa came from Mingma Tsering. No problem seemed to exist for the local community in having a clinic practising Western medicine within the complex of its Buddhist temple.[75]

The two, recently qualified, young New Zealand doctors who ran the clinic, Houghton and Gill, were faced with a variety of medical work that was both familiar and unfamiliar to those coming in from Western medical practice.[76] Each morning patients attended the clinic, although Houghton and Gill also made weekly visits to Namche to treat people. Many patients required teeth to be pulled, a lot had gastric problems, while most small children had runny ears and noses. A number of adults had hangovers from the large amounts of alcohol consumed at parties.[77] As might be expected in an area where the level of hygiene was poor, diarrhoea was common. The two doctors also saw cases of pneumonia, heart failure, chronic bronchitis, venereal disease and cancer. One person had a broken leg and one patient was diagnosed with leprosy. Antibiotics provided lifesaving cures for pneumonia, but for an elderly woman with breast cancer—a condition they were surprised to see—little

[74] Hillary, *Schoolhouse in the Clouds,* 104. The use of wood, whether for firewood or building, was not yet considered an environmental concern for the area. This was still the situation when the hospital was built. R. Willan, "Report on a Visit to the Khumbu by the Chief Conservator of Forests for Nepal", May 1966, Forestry [KH].

[75] For a discussion of spatial ideas in the Himalayan region, see Niels Gutschow, Axels Michaels, Charles Ramble and Ernst Steinkellner, eds, *Sacred Landscape of the Himalaya: Proceedings of an International Conference at Heidelberg 25–27 May 1998* (Vienna: Austrian Academy of Sciences Press, 2003).

[76] Hillary, *Schoolhouse in the Clouds,* 106–7, and Gill, *Mountain Midsummer,* 185–86. After the main expedition left, Houghton and Gill remained for a further three months during the monsoon.

[77] Parties and hospitality are an important aspect of Sherpa society. See Sherry B. Ortner, *Sherpas Through Their Rituals* (Cambridge: Cambridge University Press, 1978).

could be done except cleaning and dressing, since the clinic had insufficient medicines to try to effectively control the pain.

Tuberculosis was the most important fatal disease. While tuberculosis was a major concern in countries such as Nepal, this situation was similar to Western countries in the nineteenth century and in the second half of the twentieth century the diagnosis and treatment of tuberculosis was not a major part of Gill and Houghton's medical training.[78] The expedition saw the condition in its many and varied forms affecting lungs, joints, spine, eyes and skin.[79] A monk coughed up blood almost continuously, three young children had collapsed spines, and a young Tibetan refugee and his sister died within two months of feeling unwell.

Such distressing medical conditions reinforced Hillary's thoughts of the need for longer-term measures. He initially approached the Nepalese government in late 1963 for permission to open a small hospital in Khumjung, but as he was uncertain about funding he decided not to proceed with it in his application for an expedition in 1964.[80] This new expedition continued the smallpox vaccination programme started the previous year and began work among some of the Khumjung schoolchildren on a prophylactic programme to combat iodine deficiency diseases, as well as offering the more usual expedition general medical care to the local population.[81] Such activities both promoted biomedicine and continued its association in the Khumbu context with Western travellers. Hillary's team also built an airstrip at Lukla, which would greatly facilitate the transport

78 At this time urban South India served as a global "laboratory" for the study of tuberculosis and its treatment. Sunil Amrith, "In Search of a 'Magic Bullet' for Tuberculosis: South India and Beyond, 1955–1965", *Social History of Medicine* 17, no. 1, 2004, 113–30.

79 Unsurprisingly, Sherpas did not recognise the many manifestations of tuberculosis as a single disease. Tuberculosis within a biomedical framework is, in any case, often a difficult disease to diagnose.

80 Hillary to Ian McIntosh, 21 January 1964 and McIntosh to Bishwa Pradhan, Royal Nepalese Embassy, New Delhi, 31 January 1964, Himalayan Climbing Expeditions & Schoolhouse Project, ABHS 6949 W4628 NDI 64/14/2 Part 2 [ANZ].

81 Max Pearl, "Kiwi in the Khumbu", *New Zealand Medical Journal* 64, 1965, 584–88. Pearl was the expedition doctor.

of building materials and supplies, shortening the journey from a seventeen-day walk through rugged terrain with a large number of porters to an approximately one-hour flight and only a two-day "carry".

The hospital at Khunde had become Hillary's biggest project. In October 1965 Hillary wrote to Ian McIntosh at the Department of External Affairs in Wellington and enclosed his application to the Nepalese government for approval to build a small hospital at Khunde, which he planned to construct between September and December 1966.[82] Also included were three petitions from the local village councils to support his proposal.[83] New Zealand did not have diplomatic representation in Nepal, and so Wellington forwarded the application to the New Zealand High Commission in New Delhi to approach the Nepalese government through the Royal Nepalese Embassy in New Delhi.[84]

One of the questions that visitors frequently ask when they go to the hospital is "Why is the hospital at Khunde?"[85] Hillary's first approach to the Nepalese government in 1963 indicated that at that time he envisaged building a small hospital at Khumjung where he had built the first school. Khumjung was the largest village in Khumbu with 93 houses, when anthropologist Christoph von Fürer-Haimendorf carried out his research in 1957, compared with only 45 in Khunde.[86] Land was available, however, on the sunny slopes at the edge of Khunde village near a permanent water supply, whereas Khumjung's water supply dried up in spring.[87] Khunde

82 Hillary to McIntosh, 15 October 1965, Himalayan Climbing Expeditions & Schoolhouse Projects, ABHS 6949 W4628 NDI 64/14/2 Part 3 [ANZ].

83 These are referred to in the files, but the originals were forwarded with the proposal and have not been viewed by the author. Petitions from local people became a recognised part of the local ritual of asking for assistance.

84 Secretary of External Affairs to the High Commissioner, 22 October 1965, Himalayan Climbing Expeditions & Schoolhouse Projects, ABHS 6949 W4628 NDI 64/14/2 Part 3 [ANZ]. New Zealand's High Commissioner to India was also accredited as its Ambassador to Nepal.

85 Personal participation.

86 Von Fürer-Haimendorf, *The Sherpas of Nepal*, 5.

87 Hillary improved water supplies to both villages in 1963.

was the home of Mingma Tsering, and while he was the main driver for the hospital being situated there he also had the support of the village and the headman.[88] Khunde was only a 20-minute walk from Khumjung and the two villages shared the gompa. Khunde and Khumjung are the central villages of the area and between them contain one-third of the population. In his background document for the hospital project, Hillary described Khunde as "the central village".[89]

Visitors today wonder why Hillary did not choose Namche Bazar, the administrative and tourist centre of the area. Ghazali Musa, in his survey of travel health experiences in this area, not surprisingly found it "strange that sick people have to go further and climb higher in order to obtain treatment".[90] In 1957 Namche was smaller than Khumjung with 73 houses. Situated in an amphitheatre on the route to Tibet, it was a trading village with little land for agriculture—or for a hospital. In the 1950s and early 1960s government presence was limited and tourism was minimal. A file note on Hillary, who visited the New Zealand High Commission in New Delhi in September 1964, mentioned his plan for a "hospital-cum-first-aid post at Namche Bazar", but it is unlikely that Hillary seriously considered this location.[91] The government had just es-

[88] Personal communication, Diane McKinnon, November 2005. Diane and her husband Dr John McKinnon were the first volunteers at Khunde Hospital (1966–68).

[89] Hillary, "New Zealand Hospital for the Sherpas", 22 October 1965, Himalayan Climbing Expeditions & Schoolhouse Projects, ABHS 6949 W4628 NDI 64/14/2 Part 3 [ANZ].

[90] Ghazali Musa, "An Investigation of Travel Health Experiences in High Altitude Destinations: Case Studies of Sagarmatha National Park (Nepal) and Tibet (China)", (Ph.D. thesis, University of Otago, 2001), 295. Unfortunately neither he nor the current doctor at Khunde Hospital at the time of his visit, whom he approached about the issue, understood the historical context for the situation of the hospital. Musa's supposition (p. 296) that the government sited their medical clinic in Namche because of the hospital at Khunde ignores the fact that the government clinic was built first.

[91] Note for File: Sir Edmund Hillary, 9 September 1964, Himalayan Climbing Expeditions & Schoolhouse Project, ABHS 6949 W4628 NDI 64/14/2 Part 2 [ANZ].

tablished a medical clinic in the village, most Sherpas involved with Hillary's expeditions came from other villages and in 1964 Hillary's expedition had faced problems there when building a school.[92]

Hillary submitted his project proposal, but he still had substantial sums of money to raise. He estimated the hospital and first year's running costs would be £15,000.[93] Originally he had tried to persuade the New Zealand government to support the project under the Colombo Plan, through which some New Zealand aid was already going to Nepal, but was unsuccessful.[94] Hillary, therefore, had to look for alternative sources. His wife, Louise, wrote of how trying to find the necessary finance dominated the lives of the Hillary family and that it was "a worrying time".[95] Hillary set up the Sherpa Hospital Appeal Committee under his chairmanship to raise funds through a public appeal in New Zealand. Money began to trickle in. He and Louise also organised a business-house appeal with Louise making the appointments and Hillary visiting each business: this raised £4,500. The turning point came when the Lions Clubs (a service organisation) of the Auckland Provincial District decided to back the project and raised over £8,000 by organising lectures and selling tickets. Substantial contributions were also donated by New Zealand businesses in the form of building materials, food, medi-

92 It is not clear when Hillary learned of the government clinic's existence. Even though he did not think much of the government clinic, he was unlikely to have set up his project in competition with the government. His way of working did not include criticism or competition. The steep 400-metre walk between the two villages also located the hospital in a different area. Relations at this time with the Nepalese authorities were sometimes difficult. Mingma Tsering was also keen to avoid unreasonable demands being made of the hospital's limited resources. Personal communication, Diane McKinnon, November 2005.

93 Hillary, "New Zealand Hospital for the Sherpas", 22 October 1965, Himalayan Climbing Expeditions & Schoolhouse Projects, ABHS 6949 W4628 NDI 64/14/2 Part 3 [ANZ].

94 Hillary to McIntosh, 13 September 1963, Himalayan Climbing Expeditions & Schoolhouse Projects ABHS 6949 W4628 NDI 64/14/2 Part 2 [ANZ]. The Colombo Plan came into operation in 1951 and aimed to stimulate development in the Asian region through capital aid and technical assistance. See chapter four.

95 Louise Hillary, *A Yak for Christmas* (New York: Doubleday, 1969), 50–51.

cines and equipment. Finally, assistance also came from his American sponsors in Chicago, Field Enterprises Educational Corporation and Sears Roebuck, and the sale of expedition press rights.

In March 1966 Hillary received approval from the Nepalese government to build the hospital, although he was unhappy about their proposed customs duties.[96] The expedition, however, proceeded as planned and built the hospital in six weeks during the northern hemisphere autumn of 1966.[97] The construction team of New Zealanders and Sherpas married Sherpa building practices and skills in building rock walls and using pit-saws with those of New Zealand which employed timber frames and trusses, corrugated aluminium, glass and Western plumbing.[98] The hospital was officially opened on 18 December 1966. Ten days later Hillary left the area and the hospital in the hands of New Zealand's Volunteer Service Abroad (VSA) volunteers, Dr John McKinnon and his wife, Diane.

Hillary and Khunde Hospital: An Important Relationship

After Hillary's group left, the hospital's connection to Hillary and New Zealand became increasingly stretched. If one considers the hospital as occupying a space within Hillary's world, the concept of worlds allows the different geographical spaces to be linked; it then becomes important to examine the mechanisms by which this position was maintained. Even while Hillary remained in Nepal, communication was difficult and slow. Khunde Hospital was geographically isolated. Hillary's first challenge had been to build the hospital, but the second and more difficult task was the ongoing issue of keeping the hospital running so that staff could provide

[96] Shardul S. Rana, Joint Secretary, Ministry of Foreign Affairs, to Hillary, 22 March 1966, Himalayan Climbing Expeditions & Schoolhouse Projects, ABHS 6949 W4628 NDI 64/14/2 Part 3 [ANZ].

[97] Brian Ahern, "A Hospital for Kunde", *New Zealand Alpine Journal* 22, no. 1, 1967, 13–19; interview with Neville Wooderson, Khunde, April 1998. I would like to thank Neville Wooderson for a copy of the plans of the hospital.

[98] The construction team consisted of Hillary, Brian Ahern, Stuart King, Neville Wooderson, Phu Dorje, Tenzing Niendra and Pemba Tharkay.

the expected medical services. That they continued to do so was a significant achievement. It owed much to the work of the staff who managed the hospital at a local level, but also to Hillary who continued to remain responsible for ensuring that the staff had the means to carry out their medical work. The hospital became part of a wide range of projects and activities that he and other members of the Trust administered and serviced. Later, when the Canadian organisations became involved, ultimate responsibility for the hospital remained with Hillary and the Trust.

Such long-term involvement was not Hillary's intention in 1966—although it would be equally true to say that at the time he had not determined the extent of his ongoing commitment. Hillary was aware that the Nepalese government "now insists that any new project should be guaranteed for a minimum of five years".[99] This was a lot of money for Hillary to raise and his background document to the Nepalese government outlined that the hospital was "to be fully equipped and stocked with drugs" and that he would raise funds for the "salary and expenses of the hospital staff and the operating costs of the hospital for the first full year of operation" which he estimated would be £3,000.[100] At the end of the year, however, there was no indication that he was not going to continue. In 1967, Hillary was planning such issues as staffing, supplies and maintenance.

These activities required approval from the Nepalese government. Hillary's dealings with them show that from the beginning, and throughout, he treated Khunde Hospital as an integral part of his broader programme.[101] In 1968, his expedition restocked the

[99] Hillary, "Himalayan Schoolhouse Expedition" outline to Minister of External Affairs, Wellington, 5 August 1963, EA W2824 Economic and Technical Assistance to individual countries—Nepal: Sir Edmund Hillary's Himalayan Projects, 118/13/13/14 Part 1 [ANZ].

[100] Hillary, "New Zealand Hospital for the Sherpas", 22 October 1965, Himalayan Climbing Expeditions & Schoolhouse Projects, ABHS 6949 W4628 NDI 64/14/2 Part 3 [ANZ].

[101] See, for an example in this early period, Hillary's proposal to the Nepalese Foreign Minister, 28 July 1969, Himalayan Climbing Expeditions & Schoolhouse Projects, ABHS 6949 W4628 NDI 64/14/2 Part 3 [ANZ].

hospital and installed new overseas volunteers, built an additional classroom at Khumjung School and a team carried out further research on iodine deficiency among Sherpas.[102] In addition, Hillary had an interest in Nepal beyond the Sherpa. In 1968 he tested the navigability of Nepalese rivers by jet boat with a view to assessing the potential of river transport as a way to solve Nepal's transport problems.[103]

Hillary was actively involved with implementing his programme and visited Nepal regularly to undertake projects and monitor the work. The letters of the hospital's second volunteer couple, Dr Richard and Lesley Evans, described the considerable organisation required to get them, other members of the group and all the supplies to their destination during their two-week walk into Khumbu with Hillary.[104] They also witnessed villagers petitioning him to assist, the ritual surrounding such occasions and Hillary's awareness of what was expected from such gatherings.[105] At other times he would review his existing projects.

Hillary's ideas and philosophy infused the programme.[106] He had outlined a few years earlier in *Schoolhouse in the Clouds* his views about the way overseas staff would work at the hospital he wanted to build for Sherpas. He described how he had observed aid programmes for a number of years in different countries, but while large amounts of money were being spent he saw that there was also resentment among recipients. He believed that:

102 See chapter three for an analysis of the problem of iodine deficiency in Khumbu and its ongoing treatment and prevention.

103 Hillary, *Nothing Venture Nothing Win,* 295–301; Joyce Hamilton, "Woman's Eye-View of Trekking with Hillary in Nepal", *New Zealand Woman's Weekly,* 10 February 1969, 6–9. Joyce Hamilton was the wife of Jon Hamilton whose father, Bill Hamilton, had invented the jet boat.

104 Dr Richard and Lesley Evans to their family [Evans papers].

105 The notion of a lay protector or patron existed within Sherpa society. See chapter two.

106 In practice this could be quite ad hoc and "seat of the pants". Personal communication, Jim Wilson, January 2006. Chapter four discusses the wider international aid context.

> We should not expect people to be continuously grateful for what is being done for them—the giver-receiver relationship is always a tricky and dangerous one, and most aid is strongly flavored with self-interest. Whereas gratitude has something of inequality about it, goodwill is an active and growing idea that a proud man need not feel ashamed to entertain.[107]

Yet he believed goodwill was something that was "frequently overlooked or ignored". "The basic fact is that *people* create goodwill—money cannot do it on its own." The emphasis was Hillary's. He wrote that he was impressed by the American Peace Corps volunteers, who were also working in Nepal:

> With worth-while motivation, the volunteers live simply in town and village, learn the local language, work with their hands and minds alongside the local people, and at the same time build up a fund of goodwill that does much to counteract the side effects of more grandiose projects.[108]

By the 1960s an international volunteer movement had become widely established in Western countries.[109] In 1963, Hillary became the first President of the recently formed New Zealand Council for Volunteer Service Abroad, which aimed to send young New Zealanders to work abroad as volunteers in development projects in the Third World. Hillary's scheme for overseas staff at Khunde was initially operated through Volunteer Service Abroad (VSA), as the organisation quickly became known. The volunteers went through the VSA selection procedure and VSA was their employer. Hillary saw a considerable advantage for the volunteers in this arrangement, because it gave them the same recognition with the Nepalese and other governments that volunteers with similar organisations from

107 Hillary, *Schoolhouse in the Clouds*, 5–6.

108 Ibid. Dr John Cunningham's account of the first years of the British Nepal Medical Trust's work expressed similar approval. John S. Cunningham, *Kingdom in the Sky* (London: Souvenir Press, 1975).

109 For the New Zealand context and a survey of New Zealand volunteers, see Keren Clark, *The Two-Way Street: A Survey of Volunteer Service Abroad* (Wellington: New Zealand Council for Educational Research, 1978).

other countries received.[110] Financially, VSA provided transport to and from Nepal and insurance for the volunteers' belongings. Hillary's organisation was the sponsor and paid other volunteer costs such as food, accommodation and transport while in Nepal.

In practice VSA had little to do with Khunde Hospital volunteers' activities, and unlike other countries where VSA volunteers were placed, Nepal had no agreement with VSA.[111] Furthermore, before the prospective volunteers went through the VSA process, candidates had usually had preliminary contact with Hillary and/or Dr Max Pearl who ran the medical side of Hillary's programme. Dr John McKinnon was a climber and had been part of Hillary's 1964 expedition. Dr Richard (Dick) Evans, who was in the same year of medical school as McKinnon, was contacted by Pearl when McKinnon's intended replacement decided not to go.[112] In the late 1970s, a disagreement between the Trust and VSA about the suitability of one couple led to the Trust assuming all responsibility for volunteer selection and maintenance.[113] Dr James (Jim) and Hilary Jerram were the last of the VSA volunteers at Khunde Hospital. In practice, the "Dear Successor" letters suggest that little changed for the volunteers.[114] Members of the Trust also continued an ongoing amicable relationship with VSA.[115]

The overseas volunteers went to Khunde Hospital for approximately two years. This length of stay enabled the volunteers to settle in, learn something about the people and the area and carry out

110 Hospital Handbook, 1976, chapter eight, no page numbers [KH].

111 Neville Peat, *The VSA Way: 25 Years of Volunteering Overseas* (Wellington: Compatriot Press for Volunteer Service Abroad, 1987), 27. The volunteers periodically wrote to VSA and submitted material for VSA publications.

112 Interview with Dr Richard and Lesley Evans, Christchurch, September 2004.

113 Interview, Hillary, June 2002.

114 Dear Successor file [KH]. These letters were an opportunity for the incumbent volunteers to tell their successors directly about things they needed to know for coming to Khunde.

115 Personal communication, Dr John and Diane McKinnon, November 2005. Although Hillary resigned as President in 1976, he was elected a Life Member. Diane McKinnon and Pearl were on the VSA Council and in 1984 Diane became chairperson of VSA.

useful activity. Reasons for wanting to go to Khunde varied, but a search for outdoor adventure was often high on the list. The early volunteers were in their twenties and the doctors were in the early stages of their careers. Doctors Selwyn and Ann Lang were both second-year house surgeons in Auckland in 1969 and were planning to be ship doctors, but could not get placement on the same ship. Then the opportunity came to go to Khunde. They were contacted by Pearl, and with the help of a supportive family left for Nepal five weeks after their interview.[116] After they returned to New Zealand, they began their specialist training. Many of the volunteers were climbers or enjoyed the outdoor environment. Some expressed ideas of being keen to work in developing countries or of wanting to help others.[117] People had not only to want to go and work at Khunde, but to be prepared to accept the lack of pay and basic living conditions associated with being volunteers. This varied pattern of reasons for wanting to go to Khunde continued, both before and after the Trust took over the appointments and similarly when the SEHF in Canada became involved. Doctors David Murdoch and Lynley Cook had already been to Nepal and had also worked in the Khumbu area visiting Khunde Hospital, but Cook recalls sitting on the verandah, looking out at the peaks and thinking that two years at Khunde was one job she would not do because it was so demanding.[118] In 1991, however, she and Murdoch became Khunde Hospital volunteers. During the 1990s some of the volunteers sent to Khunde were older, such as ourselves, and the doctors had more medical experience with some having public health training.

The Trust had an important role in supporting the volunteers, both in terms of everyday physical needs and their overall well-being. In contrast to most other VSA volunteers, those who were at Khunde Hospital went as couples. A Trust document stated:

[116] Interview with Drs Selwyn and Ann Lang, Auckland, May 2002. Despite the short time before their departure the Langs still went through the full VSA selection procedure. Ann's sister was also a VSA volunteer.

[117] Being a volunteer was also a particular form of aid and will be discussed in chapter four.

[118] Interview with Dr Lynley Cook, Brighton (New Zealand), December 2002.

> Two years is a long time to be away from one's own family, friends and culture and there are times when a couple will feel lonely and homesick.
>
> It is this isolation and length of stay that makes us require the doctor always to be one of a couple and that the couple be mature, independent and stable.[119]

Marriage was not a pre-requisite for consideration, but in only one case was the couple unmarried during their stay at Khunde.[120] Only one of the volunteers had to be a doctor, although from the early 1980s it was more common for both to be medically qualified. Oral sources and correspondence, as well as Dr Elizabeth Harding's book, reveal the stresses and strains experienced by the volunteers.[121] Causes varied, as did individual circumstances and temperaments, but amidst the enormous enjoyment and satisfaction experienced at Khunde a common theme occurred of repeated and often prolonged stress whether due to the place, food, illness, the people, the work, the Trust or the SEHF or just the general unfamiliarity and challenges to be faced.

Two years, however, was not long in terms of sustaining policies or programmes. The volunteer doctor was responsible for providing medical care and running the hospital at the local level, but the fact that most of the volunteers were young also meant that their medical experience was not extensive.[122] An overview of the way Khunde Hospital has functioned since it opened nevertheless reveals considerable continuity and stability. This stemmed in part from the ongoing health needs and wants of the local population, the environmental challenges and Hillary's aim that the hospital would "enable the sick of the Khumbu area to receive basic medical

119 "The Kunde Couple", no date and anonymous, Dear Successor [KH].

120 Keren Clark comments that, during the period she surveyed (1963–72), Nepal was one of the few countries where VSA volunteers did not marry someone from the host population. Clark, *The Two-Way Street,* 138. At the time, however, the only volunteers were at Khunde Hospital and were already married.

121 Elizabeth Harding, *You Are A Brave Man: A Kiwi Odyssey in the Himalayas* (Auckland: Random House, 1996).

122 All the doctors at times were challenged medically.

treatment and also make possible the initiation of public health programs".[123] The major policy initiatives such as the prevention and treatment of iodine deficiency, immunisation, family planning, going out into the community and health education were all begun in the hospital's early days.[124] Variation occurred when the individual volunteers interpreted the respective roles of treatment and prevention in different ways and with the particular mix of issues confronting each set of volunteers at any given time. Continuity and stability too depended significantly on the relationships between the incumbents at Khunde (whether appointed from New Zealand or Canada), with previous volunteers and with the Trust's Medical Sub-committee, which played an important role through selection, induction and continuing communication.

Another feature of these relationships that were often ongoing was the long-term involvement of people: not only of Hillary himself but also of many of the other Trust members or those connected with Trust activities. This influenced all aspects of the organisation. Thirty years later, of the original 11 people on the application for the incorporation of the Sherpa Trust Board on 14 September 1966, Hillary, Gill, June Mulgrew, Jim Wilson and Murray Ellis were still actively involved with the work, four had died, one was socially associated and one had resigned.[125] Many of the Khunde volunteers also continued their involvement with the Trust's work.

One of the results of these long associations was an ageing of the Trust. Hillary was forty-seven years old when he built Khunde Hospital and actively involved with the physical work of his building projects. In the late 1990s, when he was almost eighty, he con-

[123] Hillary, "New Zealand Hospital for the Sherpas", 22 October 1965, Himalayan Climbing Expeditions & Schoolhouse Projects ABHS, 6949 W4628 NDI 64/14/2 Part 3 [ANZ].

[124] Chapter three discusses the significant influence of the first doctor, John McKinnon.

[125] Application for Incorporation of the Sherpa Trust Board as a Board, 14 September 1966. I would like to thank Dr Mike Gill for giving me a copy of this document. The Sherpa Trust Board became the Himalayan Trust Board on 9 April 1971. Murray Ellis remained involved until his death in February 2005 as did Hillary until January 2008.

tinued to run the Trust and visit Nepal, but he was unable to tolerate Khumbu's high altitude for more than a few hours. Khunde Hospital volunteers who in the mid-1960s were in their mid-twenties were correspondingly older. The party that was held after a Trust annual general meeting was still fun but was a more sedate affair than in earlier years. Hillary's and other Trust members' Sherpa friends also went back a long way. In some cases, for both, these were inter-generational.

Hillary's expeditions were predominantly male. In New Zealand, both men and women were active in climbing and in 1953 Mt Cook, New Zealand's highest mountain, had its first all-female ascent. In contrast, until the 1970s Himalayan mountaineering was an "overwhelmingly" male sport.[126] Writing in 1979, after his journey up the Ganges River in India, Hillary reflected on the male composition of the expeditions he organised:

> One thing I have slowly come to realise is that wives of the 1960s and 70s are not the same creatures as those of the 1940s and 50s when I began going off on expeditions. In those days one expected a wife to stay pluckily at home caring for small children and generally keeping the home fires burning. Times have changed, and I find increasingly that when wives are around I need to treat them with some circumspection if I happen to be proposing a new trip.[127]

He noted the solicitousness of other expedition members towards their wives as departure neared. Wives and children joined up with his expeditions at times, but came as associates rather than members.

[126] Ortner, *Life and Death on Mt. Everest,* 217. Ortner earlier (pp. 149–50) discusses how the 1950s and 60s saw a number of contradictory trends in mountaineering, with on the one hand some climbers "seeking a kind of mystical communion with the mountains and with the Sherpas", but on the other hand the strengthening of the military approach to mountaineering with the organisation of large expeditions and the "hypermasculine sahib". Also see Hansen, "Confetti of Empire".

[127] Edmund Hillary, *From the Ocean to the Sky* (New York: Viking Press, 1979), 37. Also see Ortner, *Life and Death on Mt. Everest,* chapters six to eight, for discussion of these changes.

This masculine environment was carried over into the Trust, although in practice the type of people Hillary needed for his projects, such as climbers and tradespeople, tended to be male.[128] Wilson noted in a 1988 Trust newsletter which he edited that "Jim's wife, Ann, used to attend Trust meetings as an associate but now declines in protest at the male dominance and chauvinist bias of the Trust—note above how many men are members and how many wives merely associates!"[129] Despite their active part in Hillary's work while in Nepal, the female volunteers at Khunde Hospital were in a similar position on their return to New Zealand. Jim Wilson's lighthearted, though pointed, remark would have surprised none of those present at the meeting he was describing. It would also make no difference. Wilson wrote of the Trust's annual general meeting, held as usual at Hillary's home in Auckland:

> The Himalayan Trust is a diverse band of firm and sometimes fiery friends bonded together by experience of and fascination by Nepal, and by strong affection for and loyalty to Ed. This latter bond—loyalty to Ed—does not preclude criticism of Ed at times, or of others of our number, but always it is criticism within strong links of love and shared goals so meetings, while never dull, are never acrimonious.[130]

The medical aspect of Hillary's work came within the sphere of a medical sub-committee. Hillary, while responsible for the hospital, had little to do with its running. The committee, like the organisation as a whole, was an informal group. It was largely composed of former medical volunteers and was particularly concerned with the practical work involved with supporting Khunde Hospital, such as arranging supplies and dealing with issues raised by the volunteers who ran the hospital. Dr Max Pearl was chairman until his sudden

[128] Personal communication, Gill, November 2005. The great majority of Gill's class at medical school were also male.

[129] Jim Wilson, Himalayan Trust Newsletter, 1988, 14 [Wilson papers]. The newsletter was circulated to benefactors, those who had worked for the Trust or, for a limited period, people who were subscribing Friends of the Trust.

[130] Wilson, Himalayan Trust Newsletter, 1988, 13. In practice, as befitting a bunch of strong-minded individuals, they sometimes were.

death in 1980; he was succeeded by McKinnon, who after leaving Khunde had specialised in ophthalmology and practised in Nelson in the South Island of New Zealand.

Pearl's influence on the medical and general work of the Trust was considerable. Hillary relied on him for all kinds of advice and believes that if he was dependent on anyone in the Trust it was Pearl.[131] Hillary saw him as "sensible and enthusiastic" about Sherpas. Pearl was 13 years old when he came out to New Zealand in 1936 with his family—as refugees from Germany. In 1947 he graduated in medicine from the University of Otago and set up a general practice in Auckland.[132] Keen to meet Hillary, he was introduced through mutual acquaintances several years later and became doctor for Hillary's 1964 expedition.[133] Pearl subsequently became a close friend of Hillary and this good relationship, helped by both living in Auckland, undoubtedly assisted in the running of Trust affairs.

The Trust's medical work increased in prominence in the 1970s. In 1975 (under the New Education System Plan that brought most schools and colleges into an integrated national structure under government control) the Nepalese government assumed responsibility for financing and administering the schools that the Trust was running. This reduced Trust involvement in education. Support continued, but Hillary wrote in his annual report for a meeting of the Himalayan Trust Board in June 1975 that "As a consequence of the changes in our school responsibility the Trust will find its main emphasis turning to medical work which will vastly increase with the opening of the Solu Hospital."[134] Unlike Khunde Hospital, the

[131] Interview, Hillary, June 2002. Unfortunately Pearl's papers were destroyed after his death; only those kept by others remain. A few letters are at Khunde Hospital.

[132] Obituary, *New Zealand Medical Journal,* 12 November 1980, 364–65.

[133] Interview with Betty Joplin, Auckland, October 2002. Joplin was a friend of Louise Hillary, and did Hillary's secretarial work since first typing the manuscript in 1958 for *No Latitude for Error* (London: Hodder and Stoughton, 1961), Hillary's book about the 1955–58 expedition to Antarctica.

[134] Sir Edmund Hillary, Annual Report 1 July 1974 to 30 June 1975 [Hillary papers]. Documents relating to the Himalayan Trust in New Zealand were held at the home of Sir Edmund Hillary.

Solu (Phaphlu) Hospital, which was situated in the more populous lower part of the district some four days walk from Khunde, was built with financial support from the New Zealand government. Hillary also wrote that he did "not feel qualified to handle many of the medical problems that are arising".[135] On looking to the future, he saw much for the Trust still to do in Nepal. Funds were coming in to do this, but that he would need more assistance from other Trust members.[136] The minutes of the next meeting of the Trust in April 1976, reported that "After considerable discussion on the increasing hospital responsibility, on staff problems, and on co-ordination of hospital activities" it was resolved to reform the "hospital Sub-Committee".[137] The volunteers in Nepal were directed to channel official Trust medical business through this sub-committee which had its structure strengthened. While Pearl continued as chairman, McKinnon became deputy chairman and Dr Ann Lang its secretary. They also had the power to add to the membership and Hillary would be an ex-officio member.

Not surprisingly Hillary added to his 1975 annual report that his heart was "heavy". The building of the Solu Hospital had brought enormous personal tragedy for Hillary. On 31 March 1975 his wife, Louise, and their younger daughter, Belinda, were killed in a plane crash just after take-off from Kathmandu on their way to Phaphlu. Hillary's happiness, that was so evident in the autobiography that he had just completed, was shattered. Work continued in Nepal, but it was an unhappy time for all.

While the provision and continuing support of the overseas staff was one important area that kept Khunde Hospital closely tied to the world of Hillary and the Trust, finance, supplies and maintenance and construction were additional essential components in Hillary's long-term achievement of the hospital providing an ongoing medical service. While some of the projects, such as a bridge over the Dudh Kosi in 1964, were conceived in terms of a single input of

[135] Hillary, Annual Report, 1 July 1974 to 30 June 1975.

[136] The Sir Edmund Hillary Foundation was set up in Canada at this time. See chapter four.

[137] Minutes of a meeting of the Himalayan Trust Board, 22 April 1976 [Hillary papers].

finance, materials or labour, the schools and the hospital from the start required further involvement. In July 1969 Hillary signalled his further commitment to Khunde Hospital when he applied to the Nepalese foreign minister for approval to carry out assistance projects in 1970. In this proposal he guaranteed to continue providing both the teachers' salaries at the eight schools he had helped build and also the operating costs for Khunde Hospital for a further five years until the end of 1974. [138]

The organisation and support of Hillary's early projects were centred on expeditions from New Zealand to Nepal. The focal point for activities was Hillary's home in Auckland and he worked with the key people involved on any particular scheme or problem. This personal and informal style was maintained, although the structure of the New Zealand organisation became more formal in 1966 with the incorporation, under the provisions of the 1957 Charitable Trusts Act, of the Sherpa Trust Board. In 1971 it became the Himalayan Trust Board, by which name it continues to operate, although it is usually called the Himalayan Trust or the Trust. In January 1972 Hillary signed an agreement on behalf of the Himalayan Trust Board, referred to in the agreement as the "Trust", with the government of Nepal which established the formal basis for the next three years of Hillary's work in Nepal. [139] Appendix A of the Agreement covered both the school and hospital programmes and specifically referred to Khunde Hospital. For the duration of the Agreement, the hospital's "maintenance, provision of medical supplies, equipment and the provision of medical staff" was to be the responsibility of the Trust. [140] With subsequent renewals, it continued to be the basis on which the hospital existed in Nepal—notwithstanding the involvement of other donors. These dealings with the Nepalese government were undertaken mainly by Hillary, or individual Trust members such as Pearl, and did not involve Khunde Hospital staff.

[138] Hillary to the Foreign Minister, H.M. Government of Nepal, 28 July 1969, Himalayan Climbing Expeditions & Schoolhouse Projects, ABHS, 6949 W4628 NDI 64/14/2 Part 3 [ANZ].

[139] The wider aid context and circumstances surrounding the signing of this agreement will be discussed in chapter four.

[140] Trust Agreements [Himalayan Trust office, Kathmandu, hereafter HTK].

In 1966 and for the first few years thereafter, most things the hospital required came from overseas. When Hillary approached Neville Wooderson to see if it was possible to install some plumbing at the proposed hospital, he warned him that at Khunde "he couldn't just pop down the road" if he needed something.[141] Attention to detail was important and required considerable planning and organisation— something that Hillary was very good at. Hillary eventually sent twelve tons of materials for the hospital by sea from Auckland to Calcutta. There they were loaded on to trucks for the road journey to Kathmandu where the expedition experienced considerable delays and incurred heavy costs before they could clear customs.[142] The supplies were then flown to Lukla and carried by porters up to Khunde.

By this time Hillary visited Nepal at least annually to carry out new projects and support existing ones. The 1970 expedition illustrated clearly the way in which Hillary was approaching and running the Nepal programme and the detailed forward planning that was required. His application in July 1969 to the Foreign Minister of Nepal divided the proposed work into two parts.[143] The existing schools throughout the district required some maintenance and the hospital at Khunde required medical and food supplies to be restocked. He also wrote that the local *panchayat* (village councils) had "requested our assistance" for a number of new projects and sought approval to build or improve three schools in Solu, set up a technical training section at Khumjung school, pipe fresh water to Tengboche, Phortse and Khumjung and help to rebuild the terrace at the front of the gompa at Thame. At Khunde Hospital, Hillary wanted to add an extra room at one end of the building to enlarge the doctor's flat and another at the other that could be used for inpatients. Hillary had raised the necessary funds through giving a lecture tour in the USA and Canada in 1969, with further finance coming from the employees of World Book Encyclopedia. Most of the building

141 Interview, Wooderson, 1998.

142 Ahern, "A Hospital for Kunde", 13–19; interview, Wooderson, 1998.

143 Hillary to the Foreign Minister, H.M. Government of Nepal, 28 July 1969, Himalayan Climbing Expeditions & Schoolhouse Projects, ABHS 6949 W4628 NDI 64/14/2 Part 3 [ANZ].

materials, medical equipment, medicines and food supplies were donated by individuals, groups and companies in New Zealand. The appendix to Hillary's application outlined the work at the hospital and detailed the materials to be brought into Nepal and those that would be bought in Kathmandu.[144] Ordinary nails, plywood, paint and glass were available within Nepal, while plumbing supplies, fibreglass insulation, plastic skylights, aluminium ridging and nails and a cast iron wood burning stove and chimney were to be brought in. An official permit was requested for the timber needed for construction.

At this point Hillary's key person in Nepal for the implementation of his projects was Mingma Tsering of Khunde. He was also an important link with the local community for the overseas volunteers at the hospital.[145] Mingma Tsering had worked as a climbing Sherpa on Hillary's 1960–61 expedition and had been on the unsuccessful attempt to climb Makalu. Hillary described that he was "very impressed" with Mingma's "loyalty and common sense" and appointed him sirdar for the 1963 expedition.[146] Mingma could neither read nor write, but had a "fantastic memory". Above all he was responsible for talking with the headmen and committees in the various villages. Hillary and Mingma Tsering worked together closely. Mingma would advise Hillary on the suitability of projects and Hillary saw him as a "good judge", doing little that Mingma had not agreed with. Once a project had been decided upon and materials worked out, Mingma then organised the local labour and supplies. Hillary recalled that Mingma could be "bossy" with him—but that he "needed" to be.[147] The friendship between these two people was the key relationship in understanding Hillary's work in

[144] Appendix D, Hillary to the Foreign Minister, H.M. Government of Nepal, 28 July 1969, Himalayan Climbing Expeditions & Schoolhouse Projects, ABHS 6949 W4628 NDI 64/14/2 Part 3 [ANZ].

[145] This mediating role of key Sherpas, both in the sense of providing a link with the community and at times resolving difficulties, is discussed in chapters two and three.

[146] Interview, Hillary, June 2002.

[147] Ibid.

Nepal.[148] Its warmth was underscored by Ann Wilson's painting of Mingma hanging in Hillary's home draped with a respectful *khata* (scarf). Hillary's world met that of Sherpas through Mingma.

Initially Hillary was relatively free to work on his own in cooperation with the local people, but changes were occurring both in Khumbu and nationally. The Nepalese government sought to modernise and develop the country, but also ensure Nepalese authority in a process that entailed the involvement of multiple international aid donors in a multiplicity of projects.[149] Although Hillary was just a small player in the donor field, he was nevertheless part of the much wider aid scene developing in Nepal. His need for contact with organisations and people in Kathmandu grew. The most significant factor in the way Khunde Hospital was supported from the mid-1960s to the late 1990s was the hospital's decreasing isolation within Nepal and the increasing role of a small Trust organisation in Kathmandu.

Hillary received considerable help from the British Embassy in Kathmandu as he began his work in Nepal.[150] The earliest address for Khunde Hospital was through the Embassy. Trust people, including the volunteers, often stayed there. In a letter to Brian Lendrum, the New Zealand High Commissioner in New Delhi, Hillary referred to Brigadier Gordon Richardson acting as "our agent in Kathmandu".[151] In October 1969 Richardson wrote to Indian Oxygen Ltd in Calcutta about oxygen cylinders that had been sent for refilling but had not as yet been returned, and that the isolated

148 Mingma Tsering died in 1993. The length of their friendship again demonstrated the importance of long-term relationships, not only among the overseas members of the Trust but also with Sherpas.

149 See chapter four.

150 The involvement was voluntary and any files held by the Embassy during this period were not kept at the 30 years review. Letter from Miss M.T. Ryan, Records and Historical Department, Foreign and Commonwealth Office to author, 11 August 2003. Information about the support from the British Embassy comes from oral sources, files from the New Zealand High Commission in New Delhi and the writings of Hillary and other Trust members.

151 Hillary to Brian Lendrum, 8 June 1968, Himalayan Climbing Expeditions & Schoolhouse Projects, ABHS 6949 W4628 NDI 64/14/2 Part 3 [ANZ].

and high-altitude Khunde Hospital had sent more cylinders and was now "completely without oxygen". [152] This letter illustrated the kind of assistance being given, the problems faced by the hospital and why ongoing support was crucial to Khunde Hospital's ability to provide medical services. With Hillary's expanding programme, this support role could only increase. At the end of October 1969 New Zealand's Deputy High Commissioner, Denis Dunlop, following his visit to Nepal, wrote to Arthur Kellas, the British Ambassador, that "I went around with Ed Hillary a bit and I certainly realise the burden he imposes on the poor Brigadier", but he added a little later "I am sure Ed realises the situation and will recognise his obligations as best he can". [153]

Hillary did indeed understand the situation. Dunlop also mentioned in the letter Hillary's discussion with Richardson about renting a room elsewhere to relieve pressure on storage facilities and "possibly of depending a little more on the services of Elizabeth". [154] Elizabeth Hawley was American, and had arrived in Kathmandu in September 1960 as correspondent for Reuters News Agency and *Time* and *Life* magazines. [155] The reply from Kellas to Dunlop in November confirmed that Hillary had "as you expected, engaged the services of Elizabeth Hawley, who is very capable". [156] Her work for Hillary began with paying scholarship money to Sherpa students who had come to Kathmandu for further schooling, handling the

152 Brigadier G. S. N. Richardson to Indian Oxygen Ltd., 9 October 1969, Himalayan Climbing Expeditions & Schoolhouse Projects, ABHS 6949 W4628 NDI 64/14/2 Part 4 [ANZ]. Such letters demonstrate the importance of the New Zealand High Commission files.

153 D. F. Dunlop to A. R. H. Kellas, 31 October 1969, Himalayan Climbing Expeditions & Schoolhouse Projects, ABHS 6949 W4628 NDI 64/14/2 Part 4 [ANZ]. On 24 December, the New Zealand Prime Minister Keith Holyoake wrote to Kellas thanking him for their support of Hillary's work.

154 Ibid.

155 Interview with Elizabeth Hawley, Honorary New Zealand Consul, Kathmandu, June 2003. For a recent biography, see Bernadette McDonald, *I'll Call You in Kathmandu: The Elizabeth Hawley Story* (Seattle: The Mountaineers Books, 2005).

156 Kellas to Dunlop, 19 November 1969, Himalayan Climbing Expeditions & Schoolhouse Projects, ABHS 6949 W4628 NDI 64/14/2 Part 4 [ANZ].

post and organising the mail bags for the hospital. These she would take out to the airport for the flight to Lukla.[157] The Trust and Khunde Hospital used her personal box number as its address—as it continues to do today.

What Hillary had done, as he explained in a letter to Rex Cunninghame, the New Zealand High Commissioner, was "to separate our dealings at the diplomatic level from the ordinary routine of running the operation".[158] Elizabeth Hawley became the "Executive Officer" in Nepal for the Trust, while Hillary appointed John Claydon as his "Representative" to handle negotiations with government departments and countersign customs exemptions and other forms. Claydon was a pilot who was with Hillary's 1955–58 expedition to Antarctica. When Claydon's civil aviation work in Nepal with the Asian Development Bank finished and he returned to New Zealand, Hillary needed a new "Representative". With no permanent official New Zealand presence in Kathmandu, he had to turn elsewhere. "The duties of the 'Representative' are not particularly arduous but it is desirable that he should be readily available in Kathmandu", wrote Hillary to Cunninghame in 1972. He continued:

> We have had a long and happy association with the British Embassy and Mr. Terence O'Brien has kindly agreed to take on the responsibilities of being our 'Representative'. Mr. O'Brien in fact suggests that we nominate the 'British Ambassador' rather than any particular Ambassador by name. I am sure you will agree that this is a very happy solution to our problem.[159]

In Hillary's absence from Nepal, the British Ambassador signed the renewals of Khunde Hospital's agreement with the Nepalese government in 1980, 1983 and 1986.

157 Records have not been kept in Kathmandu for this early period of operations. Overall there are few written archives of the Trust in the office in Kathmandu.

158 Hillary to R. Cunninghame, 3 July 1972, Himalayan Climbing Expeditions & Schoolhouse Projects, ABHS 6949 W4628 NDI 64/14/2 Part 4 [ANZ].

159 Ibid.

Staff at the hospital, however, increasingly dealt with Elizabeth Hawley. Dr Paul and Glen Silvester's "Dear Successor" letter in June 1975 described the difficulty of getting things done in Kathmandu, but "What Liz can't do in Kathmandu for you just isn't possible!" [160] Much of the work was done by Kumar, who was her "outside man". [161] He obtained the food and medical supplies for the hospital and went to the post office or the bank. Elizabeth Hawley also dealt with the volunteers' personal affairs. The relationship was not necessarily easy. Canadian volunteer doctors, Penny Dawson and Jamie Uhrig, referred to her as "Miss Hawley" when they wrote to the incoming volunteers in 1982, and stressed the need to always be "precise" in their dealings with her. [162] Although she held the title of Executive Officer, she did not function as such. Policy decisions about the hospital and the Trust were made by the New Zealand organisation. In a 1988 letter to the Nepalese Ministry of Forests regarding a proposed forestry project, Hillary wrote that "we regard the Himalayan Trust in Kathmandu as a liaison office and not an Executive office being used largely for the exchange of information and advice between New Zealand and Nepal and vice versa." [163]

The development of an executive role for the Trust's Kathmandu office arose with Hillary's increasing reliance on Ang Rita Sherpa. [164] When Hillary offered him employment in the Trust office, Ang Rita, like Mingma Tsering in Khumbu, already had a long association with Hillary and the Trust. Youngest son of the famous artist Kapa Kalden, he had been in the first class at Khumjung School in 1961. He was an outstanding student and his School Leaving Certificate result in 1969 was the highest in Nepal. Ang Rita planned to study medicine with a view to working in one of the Trust hospitals.

160 21 June 1975, Dear Successor [KH].

161 Interview, Elizabeth Hawley, 2003.

162 10 December 1982, Dear Successor [KH].

163 14 July 1988, letter from Hillary to B. N. Khunjeli, Secretary, Ministry of Forests, HMG Nepal, Trust Agreements [HTK].

164 Fisher, *Sherpas*, 98–105. Also see Himalayan Climbing Expeditions & Schoolhouse Projects: Khumjung Hospital, ABHS 6949 W4628 NDI 64/14/2 Part 5 [ANZ] regarding his applications for medical training.

He received a Burmese government scholarship, but unfortunately student unrest in Rangoon in 1975 twice led to the government closing the universities. Ang Rita's career changed direction, but he was dissatisfied with positions in the trekking industry or hotel management. In 1986 Hillary brought him to work for the Trust and he rose to become in the 1990s the key executive person in Nepal for Hillary's work. Ang Rita's description of his job, written for anthropologist James Fisher, described a broad range of duties in which supporting the hospitals was an integral part of the wider Hillary programme. He saw his main responsibilities as:

> looking after many scholarship students enrolled in the various college campuses, managing supplies and their transport to hospitals and schools in Solu-Khumbu, coordinating arrangments with HMG officials, organizing construction materials for new projects, etc. In the fall of 1988 I spent a month in England in a fund-raising program with British Venture Scouts.[165]

By the mid-1990s, Khunde Hospital staff dealt mostly with Ang Rita. Although his title was "Chief Administrative Officer" his role developed the executive capacity that Elizabeth Hawley's role did not.[166] She retained her position, but like Hillary was in her seventies. Her active role decreased. She became, however, New Zealand's honorary consul in Nepal and has a considerable knowledge of Nepalese affairs.[167] Hillary believed that while Mingma Tsering was the right man for his work in Khumbu, Ang Rita had the multiple linguistic skills and education for dealing with bureaucracy and the changing situation in Nepal.[168]

The Trust office in Kathmandu was concerned with the whole Hillary programme, closely liaising with him, whether he was in

165 Fisher, *Sherpas*, 103–4.

166 Interestingly, for someone who has been closely involved with Hillary's work, she has hardly visited Khumbu since she went to Nepal in 1960. Mountaineering historians are grateful for the comprehensive data she continues to collect from expeditions.

167 Previously the New Zealand government had made use of her services as an Aid Liaison Officer.

168 Interview, Hillary, June 2002.

New Zealand or elsewhere such as the period between 1985 and 1989 when as New Zealand's High Commissioner to India he was living in New Delhi. [169] Hillary continued to direct activities and retained financial control. A considerable part of each year was spent fund-raising and involved extensive travel, particularly to Canada and the USA, that became harder as he got older. [170] Money was sent to Kathmandu where Elizabeth Hawley operated the Trust's accounts and would oversee the disbursement of funds.

From the Khunde Hospital staff's point of view, Hillary and the organisation, whether the Trust or the SEHF, provided the money through the Kathmandu office that they needed to run the hospital. They did not have to raise the funds. At Khunde, the staff managed the everyday accounting and control of expenditure at the hospital. Hillary did not set a budget, but monthly and quarterly accounts were sent to him and when he was unhappy he communicated this to the volunteers. The finances of the hospital were presented to Trust members in his financial report at the annual general meeting. The hospital was costed as an individual project, but presented within the Trust's overall expenditure, even when, from the late 1970s, an increasing amount of the funds for the hospital came from the SEHF in Canada and its successful project applications to the Canadian International Development Agency (CIDA). [171]

New Zealand and Canada, however, were a long way from Nepal, and Khunde was isolated within Nepal. From the beginning this made communication difficult. The 1963 smallpox epidemic had already highlighted the problem. As noted earlier, Hillary had to wait to call for vaccine until he reached the military checkpost at Namche and asked if he could use their radio. [172] This delay of one day was short in comparison to what might be expected in many

[169] Hillary was New Zealand Prime Minister David Lange's inspired choice to reopen the High Commission that had been closed in 1982. It was also Hillary's first "9-to-5" employment.

[170] The effort was sometimes taken for granted within the Trust. Conversation, Hillary, Auckland, May 2002.

[171] Chapter four discusses the setting up of the SEHF and CIDA involvement. Hospital staff also sent regular financial statements to the SEHF.

[172] Hillary, *Schoolhouse in the Clouds*, 42.

remote areas. Radios required government permission and in this border area the Nepalese government was reluctant to grant approval. In the 1960s relations in the wider region between India and China were uneasy, and when the hospital was built the Nepalese government had banned climbing by overseas expeditions along the border.

Letters were the main form of communication between the hospital and Hillary and usually took weeks to reach their destination in either direction. The regular correspondence from December 1969 to December 1971 between the Langs and their families show that both parties became used to the long turn-around of letters and managed to transact a considerable amount of business.[173] Their families were also in contact with Hillary and Pearl. From the hospital's inception a mail runner was employed, although in the early years this was not a permanent position. At times other intermediaries, such as a person on a flight to or from Kathmandu, would be used. Mani Ram, a Rai (the largest ethnic group in Solukhumbu) from the village of Deusa, began working for the Trust in 1984 and became its visible face along the route. He carried letters, other messages, money and assorted small items. The round trip between the Trust office and the hospital took between ten and fourteen days, with one or two nights in either Kathmandu or Khunde. The mail runner remained the most reliable system for the Trust. It also operated all year, unlike flights that became very scarce during the monsoon season.

Hillary tried to obtain radio communication for the hospital. In his application for the expedition in 1970, Hillary sought permission to install radio transceivers which could link into a Nepalese radio facility in Kathmandu.[174] The hospital has had radio communication at times, but with varying effectiveness and limited usefulness.

173 Lang papers. I am very grateful for being allowed to look through the original correspondence from both Selwyn and Ann and both families, as well as assorted other documents. Together they provide a rich "snapshot" of their two years at Khunde. Ann died in March 2006.

174 Hillary to the Foreign Minister, H. M. Government of Nepal, 28 July 1969, Himalayan Climbing Expeditions & Schoolhouse Projects, ABHS 6949 W4628 NDI 64/14/2 Part 3 [ANZ].

The situation did not change until early 1995 when Khunde Hospital was given the single telephone line for Khunde village. Although expensive, the arrival of a telephone enabled quicker communication to be made locally, with Kathmandu and if necessary overseas. In April 1997 the hospital acquired email. The combination of telephone and email transformed the communication situation for the hospital.[175] Despite changing technology the arrival of the mail runner at Khunde remained an exciting event for the overseas staff, but the transportation of larger items from Kathmandu continued to be often slow and fraught with difficulties along the route.

Communication problems occurred when something happened which required a rapid response or advice. However well-prepared the volunteers were before they went to Nepal, and however much assistance they were given by senior local staff, all volunteers ran into problems at times.[176] Misunderstandings and frustrations resulted. Other Trust members realised, and the volunteers discovered, that Hillary was not the best communicator.[177] In 1976 the Trust's medical sub-committee had designated Ann Lang to write once a month from New Zealand to both hospitals and the volunteers were also to write once a month to the New Zealand organisation to try and forestall problems.[178] A further dimension to communication issues was the arrival of the first Canadian volunteers at Khunde in 1981. Selected and appointed by the Sir Edmund Hillary Foundation of Canada, the volunteers nevertheless entered an institution that was largely run through New Zealand. The compilation of a Hospital Handbook in 1976 had brought together in one document a large amount of information about a wide range of subjects that were helpful to the volunteers. Nevertheless, the revised edition of the Handbook in 1985 by Khunde doctors Keith Buswell and

175 The rise of Maoist activities in other parts of Nepal after 1996 had not yet affected the hospital's communication system in the late 1990s.

176 Trust medical personnel also visited. See chapter four.

177 Dealing with the increasing number of doctors within the organisation was also not easy for Hillary.

178 "Report on the Main Points covered by Medical Committee on 4th and 5th September", assorted papers [KH]; personal communication, Gill, November 2005.

Elly Kroef could unequivocally state that "without doubt there have been more problems and misunderstandings in the area of communications than in any other part of the Trust's operations over the past fifteen years. There are various reasons for this." [179]

Another key aspect of organisational support for the hospital was the provision of medical, food and other supplies. As a result of its location, transport costs have always been a significant item for the hospital—as it was for other organisations and businesses that were gradually established in the area. Both airfreight and carriage by porters were expensive. Although from the beginning some drugs were bought in Kathmandu, most medical supplies in the early period were brought from New Zealand with Trust members gathering donations from drug companies and the free samples given out to general practitioners. [180] By 1975 the focus had shifted to obtaining the hospital's medical supplies largely from within Nepal, using a basic range of items manufactured by the Royal Nepal Drug House and UNICEF supplies for tuberculosis, vaccination and family planning that were channelled through various government departments. [181] The pharmacy at the United Mission to Nepal's (UMN) Shanta Bhawan Hospital was also helpful, but in 1976 their pharmacist had to inform the Trust that they could no longer purchase drugs for the hospital because their own import licence was not large enough for their own needs. [182] Supplies could also be bought at retail outlets, but tended to be expensive.

This framework has largely continued, but with the particular configuration varying at any one time. The medical committee in New Zealand would help when the hospital was unable to obtain an item from more local sources. Sometimes the availability of supplies from Royal Drugs was very limited, while in 1987 complicated regulations, imposed by the Nepalese government after the

179 Kunde Hospital Handbook, revised 1985, 1: chapter seven, no page numbers.

180 Kunde Hospital Annual Report, 1 November 1969 to 21 October 1970; personal communication, Diane McKinnon, November 2005.

181 21 June 1975, Dear Successor [KH].

182 Paul Williams, pharmacist, Shanta Bhawan Hospital, Kathmandu to McKinnon, Himalayan Trust, assorted papers [KH].

1986 Chernobyl nuclear explosion in Russia, made it difficult to order from overseas drug companies. [183] Hospital staff did an annual stock-take, or half-yearly from the early 1990s, and sent their order down to the Kathmandu office which would then liaise, purchase and despatch to Khunde. [184] It was a function that, because of their isolated situation, hospital staff could not handle on their own from Khunde.

Initial reliance on overseas sources was also significant for food and other supplies for the hospital. From his climbing and expedition experiences, Hillary believed that good food supplied more than the physical means to live. [185] Food was important to the volunteers; it was psychologically important to a feeling of well-being in difficult circumstances. At the hospital, the use of a greenhouse boosted the supply of vegetables and extended the growing season. As more types of food became available in Nepal these were used to supplement Khumbu sources. They were ordered and bought in Kathmandu and then sent to Khunde along with medical and other supplies. While increasingly less food came from New Zealand, gradually the leftover "treats" from expeditions also dropped: expeditions had begun to sell food to local people who would then use it to stock their shops and sell on to the rising number of trekkers in the region. Prices have risen throughout the period and are high in relation to non-tourist areas. [186] In practice, the weekly market in Namche Bazar was more important for the hospital than the shops with fresh and non-perishable food items being brought up by porters from the lowlands along with other supplies.

A further area where Trust personnel in Kathmandu played an important support role, both for the hospital and for individuals, was

[183] Kunde Hospital Annual Report, August 1987 to August 1988.

[184] Kunde Hospital Annual Report, 1 June 1991 to 31 May 1992. The change was made by the volunteers to try and prevent over-ordering.

[185] Food is often unappealing at high altitude. Hillary had carried some of his favourites on the higher stages of Everest, including a heavy tin of apricots in syrup, "although cold reason told me that most of this food wasn't really essential". Hillary, *High Adventure,* 203–04.

[186] For inflation in Khumbu see, for example, Brower, *Sherpa of Khumbu,* 88–89.

in the area of patients referred for treatment in Kathmandu. In the early 1990s the Handbook's advice for volunteers was: "Needless to say, any referrals to Kathmandu hospitals and specialists should only be made when necessary. Teaching [Hospital] and Bir [Hospital] are the current preference, largely because they offer a reasonable standard with lower costs." [187] By then, many Khumbu people were used to visiting or living for extended periods in Kathmandu, but for others and especially those from more remote areas, going to Kathmandu was a daunting experience. Patients, both in Khunde Hospital and in Kathmandu, also needed someone to provide food and help look after them. The Handbook's advice continued that "Whenever someone is referred to Kathmandu they need to have at least one friend/relative to accompany them. Ang Rita handles most arrangements and, if possible, the patient would first report to him at Dilli Bazaar." [188]

The remaining support function for the hospital for which Hillary and the Trust in New Zealand were responsible was construction and maintenance. This practical work was the reason for Hillary's initial involvement in helping the Sherpa and remained an important focus for Hillary and the Trust. The sending of a "work party" from New Zealand to different parts of the Solukhumbu district enabled many of the Trust members to keep in regular contact with Nepal and different Sherpas. Hillary acknowledged that he got the credit for a lot of the work done by others. [189] Hillary's brother, Rex, first visited in 1970 and then went 21 times in 26 years, often spending months during the monsoon on a variety of projects

[187] Handbook revision by Drs David Murdoch and Lynley Cook, undated and no page numbers, Handbook [KH]. It continued:

> A letter should be sent with the patient for Ang Rita detailing where they are to go and what expenses the Trust should meet. In general, how much of the expenses the patient meets is judged individually and always in consultation with Kami and/or Mingma. There are many wealthy people who can afford to meet all costs, but many more can only afford a fraction if anything. Most people at least pay their transport costs to and from Kathmandu.

[188] Ibid. The Trust office was, and remains, in Dilli Bazar.

[189] Hillary, *View from the Summit,* 289.

throughout the region.[190] Again the pattern was of initial reliance on overseas expertise and supplies, followed by an increasing local contribution. Unlike construction, maintenance was an ongoing part of running a project but it was a task that saw even longer practical involvement from overseas Trust personnel.[191] At Khunde Hospital, Mingma Temba increasingly took on this role.

In 1998, as in 1966, Hillary was still important to the functioning of Khunde Hospital. His personal and practical involvement decreased as he got older, as Khunde's isolation lessened within Nepal and as more was dealt with in Nepal through the increasing expertise of local staff and the developing role of the Kathmandu office of the Trust. Nevertheless, even if the money increasingly came from Canada, in Nepal it remained the Trust's responsibility to ensure that Khunde Hospital had the means to carry out its medical work.

Why Was Khunde Hospital Important to Hillary?

While Hillary and the Trust have played a vital role in enabling the hospital to carry out its work, Khunde Hospital and its staff in return have been important for Hillary and the Trust programme. As Alnoor Ebrahim has discussed in his recent study of NGOs and organisational change, the relationship between those who fund and those who run the projects is one of interdependence.[192] Also, good publicity about the hospital promoted both the hospital and Hillary's programme as a whole. (Similarly, in Canada it publicised the activities of the SEHF and CIDA.)

From the beginning, providing medical services was never the staff's only responsibility, although at times their other roles created tensions within the Trust. Only one of the overseas volunteer couples had to be a doctor which meant that, although the second volunteer would support the doctor's medical work in many ways,

190 Interview with Rex Hillary, Auckland, October 2002. Rex Hillary died in September 2004.

191 The apparent lack of initiative shown by local Sherpas regarding maintenance continued to puzzle Hillary. Interview, Hillary, June 2002.

192 Alnoor Ebrahim, *NGOs and Organizational Change: Discourse, Reporting, and Learning* (Cambridge: Cambridge University Press, 2003).

the other volunteer could also take on other roles such as teaching. When both volunteers were doctors the various duties were to be divided. Initially, Hillary had influence in the running and the curriculum of the schools that he had built throughout the district. These taught the standard Nepalese curriculum but with "extras". Hillary recruited teachers from Darjeeling, but also expected the volunteers at Khunde to teach English at the nearby Khumjung School. [193] Diane McKinnon was a teacher and her time was divided between helping at the hospital and the school. [194] She also taught English in the evenings at the hospital. [195] Her successor, Lesley Evans, was a trained speech therapist and had spent a year working with Tibetan refugees in India teaching English to orphaned children. [196]

Until 1981, the only female doctor at the hospital was Ann Lang. Both she and husband Selwyn were doctors; Ann took on the teaching role as well. The medical workload was low and she enjoyed the work at the school. Selwyn wrote that, as well as teaching conversational English to the senior students:

> [Ann] helps in the handicraft centre, where weaving, carpet-making, sewing, carpentry, painting, and the chipping of mani (prayer) stones is taught by visiting 'experts', and visits the other Hillary-assisted schools, as often as possible, to help the school committees and staff sort out their problems. Night classes, for adults and children not attending school, are also popular and frequently eventful. [197]

Although Ann did her share of the medical work, Hillary's and the local people's perception was that Ann provided a supporting role at the hospital. When the Hospital Advisory Committee was

[193] Being able to speak English was an important attribute when seeking employment in the growing tourist industry in the area.

[194] Louise Hillary, *A Yak for Christmas,* 45.

[195] Personal communication, Diane McKinnon, November 2005.

[196] "They'll be Living on Top of World—in Nepal", newspaper cutting written by staff writer Dorothy Braxton, source and date not given but p. 15 [Lang papers].

[197] Selwyn Lang, "From Our Man on the Spot", unpublished and undated [Lang papers].

established in 1970, Selwyn was the chairman and she the secretary.

When the Nepalese government took over the schools in 1975, Hillary's and the Trust's role decreased, but the volunteers continued teaching. Dr Rob and Leigh Riley wrote in their "Dear Successor" letter in 1977 that with the New Educational Plan the school's schedule was "tight" and that "your presence in the school is as much a favour to you as to the kids".[198] Nevertheless, two years later the Jerrams considered that the teaching remained important and that the role might expand as the school had gained permission to become a high school.[199] Teaching also gave the doctor's wife a place in the local community apart from being known as the Khunde doctor's wife.[200] Nevertheless, for someone who was not trained as a teacher, as the Jerrams wrote, this role could be "challenging".[201] In 1981, the first Canadian volunteers, Drs Penny Dawson and Jamie Uhrig, reversed this division. Both were doctors, but Uhrig took on the teaching responsibilities.[202] In 1981 the teaching role was three and a half hours daily, but by the end of the decade the teaching input to the school was four hours per week and only for health education.[203] By the mid-1990s teaching inputs from the hospital ceased altogether.

A number of aspects were involved in this decline of the teaching role. Both volunteers in this period were often doctors, the amount of medical work increased and the attitudes of the volunteers varied. Also, their overseas teaching methods did not fit in with the more structured Nepalese teaching style and examination requirements. The hospital's annual report for 1985–86 referred to the advantages in terms of the medical work of having two doctors, but for teach-

198 19 June 1977, Dear Successor [KH].

199 28 June 1979, ibid.

200 Ibid.

201 Ibid.

202 10 December 1982, ibid.

203 16 February 1981, ibid.; Kunde Hospital Annual Report June 1989 to May 1990.

ing it was "not optimal".[204] With both the previous couples the enthusiasm for teaching "seems to wane rather early". Equally the school appeared less than enthusiastic. The volunteers took the opportunity of their association with the schools to run health education classes, but the 1994–95 annual report indicated that the health education classes by the volunteers had only occurred after "badgering".[205] This could have been because of the volunteers or because of internal pressures within the school or school system. Either way, the volunteers were unlikely to be told directly the reason behind an apparent reluctance to use their services, but they became aware that things did not seem to be going according to plan.[206]

The volunteers were also important for Hillary because they could provide local representation for the Trust programme. During the early 1970s the volunteers oversaw, in the absence of Hillary or other members of the Trust, the construction of new projects. Subsequently, they were involved in their ongoing administration. Many of these projects were increasingly distant from Khunde. In 1972 Dr Lindsay Strang, who was also a climber, crossed over the high Tesi Lapsa pass (5,755 metres) into the Rolwaling Valley to the village of Beding. He described school-building as not really his "forte" and that he was "redundant" because of the skills of Mingma Tsering and his team of Sherpas.[207] The preliminary work had already been done by Trust members McKinnon and Murray Jones. Strang did, however, take the opportunity to vaccinate 75 per cent of the local population against smallpox and tuberculosis. The following year Strang noted in his annual report the increasing amount of work from the administration of 14 schools. He "strongly recommended that this burden of the administration be soon taken over by some other Himalayan Trust representative because the actual medical responsibilities are ever increasing."[208] Visits to what was

[204] Khunde Hospital Annual Report, 1 August 1985–31 July 1986.

[205] Khunde Hospital Annual Report, February 1994–January 1995.

[206] Participant observation. In our case we hoped our children could join some of the sports activities, but somehow it never happened.

[207] Draft of a proposed article for the New Zealand Alpine Club, Articles and Letters from Ex Kunde Doctors (Early) [KH].

[208] Kunde Hospital Annual Report for the Year Ending 31 October 1973.

generally referred to by Khunde doctors as "downvalley"—the area beyond Lukla that was outside the hospital's normal patient catchment area—and school inspections could take him away from the hospital for ten days. His wife, Genevieve, had post-graduate nursing experience and he believed could cope with much of the medical work, but this was not always the case. He believed that it was an "unwelcome responsibility" for a volunteer without any medical training to be left in solo charge for more than one to two days. Even with capable and experienced local staff, as happened in the 1980s and 1990s, some medical problems were beyond their skills. Some were also beyond those of the doctor.

The situation for the volunteers changed in the mid-1970s when first the Nepalese government took over responsibility for the schools and then a second Trust hospital at Phaphlu in Solu opened in early 1976. These developments meant that the Khunde Hospital volunteers did not have to travel to the lower part of the district. Nevertheless they remained involved in the Trust's overall programme. Dr John and Sue Reekie wrote to Strang in New Zealand in 1981 how "we have had to police the present system ourselves as Shyam states that he is unable to do this without official school supervisor status."[209] They found trying to encourage better teaching standards and attendance a "considerable hassle" with "very limited" success. The Khunde volunteers also represented both the hospital and the wider Trust programme in other developments in the area, such as the Sagarmatha National Park that was established in 1976 as a bilateral aid programme between the New Zealand and Nepalese governments.[210]

Hospital staff were also important administratively for Hillary as they complemented the practical role of Mingma Tsering. All paperwork, payments and accounting for both the hospital and other

[209] 23 August 1981, Trust Letters, 1981–82 [KH]. Shyam Pradhan Krishna was the long-serving headmaster of Khumjung School which over the years increased in size and became first a middle school and then a high school. At times the hospital volunteers did not appreciate the political difficulties of his position as to what he could and could not do.

[210] Hillary played a major—and at times contested—role in the establishment of the Everest area as a national park.

Trust work in Khumbu took place through the hospital. Canadian volunteers, Ian Schokking and Catherine Hagen who were both doctors, estimated in 1990 that they were spending between them five to ten hours per week on administration and accounting.[211] The Hospital Handbook detailed the separate accounts the volunteers needed to keep for the hospital, schools, building projects, banking, and the recent addition of forestry. Receipts and expenditure were to be summarised monthly and sent every three months to the Trust. The end of the financial year was 30 June and "it is important to get these accounts out as quickly as possible".[212]

Whichever way it was viewed, the non-medical role of the volunteers was also an area of potential conflict, particularly when the ideas and views of the volunteers differed from those of Hillary or other Trust members. On the one hand, the volunteers spent two years living in Nepal at a "grassroots" level and were bound to have their own ideas. They would not have been appointed in the first place to Khunde Hospital, given the demands of the post, if they had not been able to function independently. On the other hand, the volunteers lacked the long-term knowledge and understanding of the way Hillary worked and his involvement in Nepal with its difficulties and constraints. The New Zealand volunteers also had little knowledge or understanding of the Canadian relationship. Not surprisingly, tensions developed and periodically surfaced.[213]

Often the different views were tolerated within the Trust organisation and remained an internal issue, but sometimes they became more serious. The communication difficulties exacerbated the problems that rarely related to the medical work being done. In early 1990, for example, the volunteers were critical of a proposed Himalayan Trust forestry project in the area and expressed their concern. They wrote that they believed that "when our monitoring process leads us to disagree with Trust policy, we feel we should

[211] Kunde Hospital Annual General Report, June 1989 to May 1990.

[212] Kunde Hospital Handbook, 1985, 1: chapter nine [KH].

[213] Examples occur throughout the correspondence and files.

have a voice with the Trust Forestry Sub-Committee".[214] Their criticism was not received well, either in New Zealand or Canada. Both Hillary and Zeke O'Connor, President of the SEHF which was the principal funder for the forestry scheme, wrote how the finance and administration of the proposed project were not the volunteers' responsibility.[215] McKinnon, the chairman of the Medical Sub-committee, wrote in a more conciliatory tone and described some of the background difficulties to the project that had occurred before their arrival and that it was "in the light of these difficulties that the current project has developed".[216] A few months later he again wrote:

> I hope that some of the flak created by purely written style communication has settled down with the arrival of Zeke and Ed in person. Nobody doubts your good intentions. As I have said many times it is difficult to have real dialogue by correspondence so having Trust members and yourselves on the ground to nut things out will I am sure clear the air and generally make for a constructive future.[217]

Another area in which Khunde Hospital gave considerable support to Hillary's work was in terms of positive publicity. The hospital was seen as being successful and doing a good job. The Everest area was small but had a high international profile. As a result Khunde Hospital has had frequent mentions in a variety of media. While some academic research, especially that of Adams and Draper, criticised the hospital or aspects of it, popular accounts, whether references in books or articles in widely read magazines such as the *National Geographic*, were favourable. The hospital also featured in films about the area. A BBC documentary, *The Sherpas of Everest*, showed the renowned British climber Eric Shipton meeting Hillary along the trail, described Hillary's aid projects in the area and

[214] 20 February 1990, letter (confidential) to Zeke O'Connor, John McKinnon and Mike Gill, Correspondence 89–91 [KH].

[215] 22 January 1990 and 28 February 1990, June 89 – (incoming correspondence . . .) [KH].

[216] 5 January 1990, Correspondence 89–91 [KH].

[217] 16 April 1990, June 89 – (incoming correspondence . . .) [KH].

visited Khunde.[218] The documentary, filmed at the end of 1969, said the hospital was the only one for "hundreds of miles", was built with funds raised in New Zealand and sustained by donations from around the world. It referred to some of the health problems of the area and filmed the volunteers during the handover period between the Evans and the Langs. It showed footage both of their medical work and of Lesley Evans and Ann Lang teaching a class of children at Khumjung. Khunde Hospital was clearly portrayed both in its own right and as part of the wider Hillary and Trust programme and showed both the volunteers' medical and wider role.

This publicity was important in attracting support for the Trust's ongoing work, because Hillary, unlike most aid donors, downplayed his personal role.[219] While Hillary was the first to provide such ongoing help to Sherpas in Khumbu, aid projects have multiplied in recent years. Hillary's name on plaques and information boards over which he had influence was conspicuous in its low profile or absence. He preferred to draw attention to the work rather than to himself.[220] This was illustrated in his attitude towards the name of the hospital. In his project proposal to the Nepalese government, Hillary referred to a "New Zealand Hospital for Sherpas".[221] McKinnon in 1967 called it "Kunde Hospital".[222] Evans, however, in his reports to the Department of Health called it first

218 *The Sherpas of Everest,* produced and directed by Ned Kelly, 50 min., BBC Bristol, *The World About Us* series, 1971. The programme first screened in New Zealand at the end of May 1971 and was accompanied by an article in the *NZ Listener* by Selwyn Lang who had accompanied Hillary on an inspection visit. Selwyn Lang, "The Highest Schools in the World", *NZ Listener,* 24 May 1971, 10–11.

219 An important factor in considering aid is the promotion such work gave to the donors and is discussed in chapter four.

220 In terms of fundraising, however, he was prepared to use his name.

221 Hillary, "New Zealand Hospital for the Sherpas", 22 October 1965, Himalayan Climbing Expeditions & Schoolhouse Projects, ABHS 6949 W4628 NDI 64/14/2 Part 3 [ANZ].

222 J. R. McKinnon, "Health Problems of Khumbu: A Review of the First Nine Months Work at Kunde Hospital". This report was sent with letters dated 10 October 1967 to Dr Joshi, Director of Health, and to the Editor, *Journal of Nepal*. In a letter to McKinnon dated 24 March 1968, Hillary used

the "Hillary Sherpa Hospital" and then the "Hillary Hospital".[223] By the hospital's annual report for 1969–70, the name had officially become "Kunde Hospital" and was shown as such in the Trust's agreement with the Nepalese government signed in early 1972.[224] During Hillary's visit in 1970 he removed the "Hillary Hospital" sign which was replaced with an English-Nepali version for "Kunde Hospital".[225] Hillary was also very aware of the sensitivities of the Nepalese authorities. In a letter to Brian Lendrum, the New Zealand High Commissioner to India, he wrote "I am aware that the Nepalese are a bit jealous of the Sherpa aid—its [*sic*] not that we are really doing all that much in a financial sense but we get rather overmuch publicity for it."[226] In many respects, Hillary did not need to further advertise his role as he remained newsworthy throughout the whole period.[227]

Publicity for Hillary's ongoing work attracted visitors to the hospital. The hospital was listed in guidebooks, both as a resource if ill and as a place to visit. Jamie McGuinness described Khunde, in his *Trekking in the Everest Region,* as "well-known for its excellent hospital" which offered "exceptional services for a 'bush' hospital",

---

"Khunde Sherpa Hospital" in the address. Illustration in Johnston, Sir Edmund Hillary, 174–75.

223 Hillary Sherpa Hospital Report, 23 August 1968 to 27 February 1969 and Hillary Hospital Report, August [1969] to 12 December 1969.

224 The Hillary connection was still employed at times. The proceeds of a fundraising event by the Lions Clubs of Auckland and Remuera at the Embassy Theatre in Auckland on 8 August 1971, attended by both Hillary and Tenzing Norgay, were "for the maintenance and operation of Hillary Hospital, Kunde, Nepal". I would like to thank Alexa Johnston, curator of the "Sir Edmund Hillary Everest and Beyond" exhibition at Auckland Museum, 25 October 2002 to 28 February 2003, for a photocopy of the function booklet.

225 23 April 1970, notes [Lang papers].

226 Hillary to Lendrum, 15 January 1970, Himalayan Climbing Expeditions & Schoolhouse Projects, ABHS 6949 W4628 NDI 64/14/2 Part 4 [ANZ].

227 Alexa Johnston noted Hillary's surprise in October 2002 on first seeing nine cases of awards and medals on display at the Auckland Museum exhibition "Sir Edmund Hillary: Everest and Beyond". Johnston, *Sir Edmund Hillary,* 216.

acknowledged that this was a Himalayan Trust project which was staffed by overseas volunteer doctors and wrote that people were "most welcome to have a look around" depending on "how busy everyone is".[228] From the Trust's perspective, the hospital was established to provide medical services to the local population. Visitors to the area both made demands on the hospital and the staff as well as assisting financially and medically. The wider Trust programme derived benefit from these tourists who saw or experienced the Trust's work, but the pressures created by rising numbers of visitors and patients also led to an ambivalent response from the volunteers and the Trust about how to deal with this issue.[229] The situation was difficult, but in the peak of the trekking season the small number of staff and limited facilities of the hospital struggled to cope with incessant visitor demands and an increasing local patient workload.

Conclusion

More than thirty years after being established, Khunde Hospital remained as it had begun—an integral part of iconic New Zealander Sir Edmund Hillary's private aid programme for the people of the Everest area of Nepal. Hillary became an international celebrity after his success on Everest in 1953, but a few years later used the ongoing fame to assist the mainly Sherpa population through education, health services and a broad range of other projects which were implemented through a small NGO that he established in New Zealand, the Himalayan Trust. What began as a short-term and limited involvement became long-term and changed the direction of his and his family's life.

This chapter has highlighted the individual nature of Hillary's aid programme; the important role that Hillary has played in the case of Khunde Hospital nevertheless illustrates many of the ways in which donors influence aid projects whatever their size. Without

[228] Jamie McGuinness, *Trekking in the Everest Region,* 3rd ed. (Hindhead: Trailblazer Publications, 1998), 162.

[229] The medical problems of tourists are discussed in chapter three, while chapter four considers tourists as aid donors.

Hillary the hospital would not have been built. To do so he had to overcome considerable challenges from the physical environment, the area's remoteness and Nepalese politics and bureaucracy. Yet in many ways it is easier to raise money for a tangible, emotional and "one-off" project such as building a hospital to provide health services in an area that does not have them, than to find ongoing funds for running costs such as maintenance and supplies, or to ensure the hospital has the necessary staff. Yet without these—and the continuing commitment to ensure their provision—no project can function as intended. Those working at Khunde Hospital knew that they could rely on Hillary and the Trust or the Sir Edmund Hillary Foundation to meet these physical needs for running medical services. The involvement of the SEHF from the later 1970s reduced the financial pressure on Hillary and the Trust in New Zealand, but did not alter Hillary's own sense of responsibility for the hospital. This commitment, however, did not translate into intrusion into the medical sphere which was left to the staff at Khunde supported by the Trust's medical sub-committee.

While Khunde Hospital was a central part of Hillary's assistance to the people living in the Everest area, good publicity about the hospital enhanced Hillary's overall programme and reputation. Nevertheless, while the relationship was two-way the dominant influence was Hillary's and his ideas and his way of working suffused the whole programme. While this suggests the top-down model and is probably illustrative of how international aid works, especially when the hospital was built in the 1960s, Hillary promoted a different way of doing things based on his personal views about giving and receiving aid. Trust and respect, words that are often spoken but less readily put into practice, were at the heart of Hillary's long relationship with the Sherpa. For Hillary, how he worked was no less important than what he accomplished, and these standards applied not only to himself but also to those around him. That he was prepared to listen to his Sherpa friends and respond to their requests rather than assume he knew best and tell them what he thought they needed, was evident from the beginning when he agreed to build them a school.

Hillary's programme in Nepal was carried out through the Himalayan Trust, beginning as, and remaining, an informal group with many people being involved to varying extent throughout. This was the way he liked it. The long-term associations provided considerable continuity, but each relationship was also different, reflecting different personalities, interests and their involvement with Hillary. The Trust's annual general meeting in September 1998 and the arrival of further guests for a party in the evening encapsulates this world of Sir Edmund Hillary and the Himalayan Trust and Khunde Hospital's place within it.[230] Despite increasing emphasis on the work of NGOs in the 1990s by international aid funders, the development of complex relationships and more stringent and pervasive administrative arrangements (which will be discussed in chapter four), Hillary and the Trust had remained remarkably independent both in Nepal and overseas to continue with their ways of implementing aid and working with the recipients of their assistance in a partnership begun in the early 1960s.

The meeting was held as usual at Hillary's home in Auckland on a Saturday afternoon. The gathering of Trust members and associates included: family, such as son Peter; those, such as Murray Ellis whose links with Hillary went back to the 1950s and before the beginning of Hillary's work in Nepal; and others, such as former Khunde Hospital volunteers Dr Lindsay and Genevieve Strang, who had become involved along the way.[231] The hospital featured in Hillary's two-page chairman's report, which mentioned that major maintenance work had been carried out at the hospital through the activities of a volunteer Trust work-party and reported on the progress of Kami Temba's medical training in Fiji. The medical sub-committee reported on their earlier meeting held to discuss the ongoing work and support of Khunde and Phaphlu hospitals. Unlike early Trust meetings, this one in 1998 included Ang Rita, a Sherpa who had benefited from the Trust's work in his home community and was now the organisation's key person in Nepal. He

[230] Minutes of the Annual General Meeting of the Himalayan Trust, 19 September 1998 and Chairman's report [Hillary papers].

[231] The Strangs were at Khunde from 1971 to 1973.

had come to New Zealand from Kathmandu and represented the increasing importance to the Trust and to the hospital of the office in Kathmandu, whose development also reflected the many changes occurring within Nepal.

Despite Hillary's advancing age in 1998 (he was now 79 years old and had been ill during the year preventing his usual northern spring visit to Nepal) Hillary announced in his report that "I have drawn up still another five year plan and I am confident that the Himalayan Trust and its friends will be able to carry this out to fruition." Hillary's personal and practical involvement may have decreased, but his presence within the organisation had not and his personal workstyle (of listening to, working with and respecting the wishes of his Sherpa friends) that had defined his work from the beginning continued to influence the whole programme, including the provision of health services from Khunde Hospital.

2

Khunde Hospital and the Sherpa of Khumbu

Life was hard and death "always close" in the Khumbu of Tenzing Norgay's childhood.[1] His family was poor. He knew that he was "not made to be a farmer or a herder" and he had already tried being a monk.[2] In late 1932, eighteen years old and having already run away from home once before, he and a group of eleven other "boys and girls" set off across the mountains of East Nepal for Darjeeling in British India where they hoped to earn money and "see the world".[3] Khumbu was remote; but people travelled between Darjeeling and Khumbu and Tenzing had heard about the mountaineering expeditions. He wanted to join them. Twenty years later Tenzing stood on the summit of Everest and, like Hillary, became internationally famous. So too did the Sherpas and their home near the highest mountain in the world.

Until 1950, the Nepalese government had allowed no Westerner to visit Sherpas in their mountain home of Khumbu, but in the course of the next fifty years the area became one of Nepal's leading destinations for overseas visitors. The expansion of tourism fuelled Khumbu's economic development. As James Fisher and Stanley

1 Tenzing Norgay (as told to) James Ramsey Ullman, *Man of Everest: The Autobiography of Tenzing* (London: The Reprint Society, 1956 [1955]), 34. The book was also published as *Tiger of the Snows: The Autobiography of Tenzing of Everest* (New York: G. P. Putnam's Sons, 1955). See also Ed Douglas, *Tenzing: Hero of Everest, A Biography of Tenzing Norgay* (Washington DC: National Geographic, 2003), and Judy and Tashi Tenzing, *Tenzing and the Sherpas of Everest* (Sydney: HarperCollins, 2001).

2 Tenzing Norgay, *Man of Everest*, 35 and 43.

3 Ibid., 44.

Stevens argue, Sherpa society had never been static.[4] During the first half of the twentieth century, for example, major changes occurred in Khumbu, such as the introduction of celibate monasticism and the establishment of the potato as the staple food. At the heart of Sherpa dealings with the West from the 1950s onwards was their encounter with modernity. While education laid the foundation, health services provided from Khunde Hospital were part of this changing world of Khumbu.[5] Sherpas saw both positive and negative impacts in what happened in their homeland, but remain positive about what they viewed as necessary "modernisation". While many of the early visitors later became saddened by the changes and loss of the old subsistence way of life, the transformation of Khumbu has been accompanied by continuity in traditional beliefs and practices and in some cases an intensification of Sherpa culture.[6]

Sherpa fame and Western fascination not only brought visitors to the area to see and experience the physical and cultural environment of the Sherpa, but has also produced its own genre of Sherpa studies.[7] Investigators from around the world have examined at different times, from many standpoints and disciplines, a wide variety of issues concerning the people and the place, although concern with questions of continuity or change dominate most discussions about Sherpas. Many studies refer to Khunde Hospital and many scholars list the hospital and the volunteers in their acknowledgements. As with the association of Hillary and the Trust with Sherpas, many

4 Fisher, *Sherpas*; Stevens, *Claiming the High Ground.*

5 For biomedicine as an expression of modernity in healing practices, see Linda H. Connor, "Healing Powers in Contemporary Asia", in *Healing Powers and Modernity: Traditional Medicine, Shamanism, and Science in Asian Societies,* ed. Linda H. Connor and Geoffrey Samuel (Westport: Bergin & Garvey, 2001), 3–21.

6 For this view of sadness at these changes see particularly, but not exclusively, Christoph von Fürer-Haimendorf, *Himalayan Traders: Life in Highland Nepal* (London: John Murray, 1975) and *The Sherpas Transformed: Social Change in a Buddhist Society of Nepal* (New Delhi: Sterling Publishers, 1984). On change and intensification of Sherpa life, see Fisher, *Sherpas,* 66.

7 Vincanne Adams comments that "In some ways, a history of anthropology of the Sherpas follows a discursive genealogy of anthropology itself". Adams, *Tigers of the Snow and Other Virtual Sherpas,* 28.

of the researchers too have shown long-term involvement.[8] With an interest often lasting decades, considerations of time infuse the ethnographies and an investigator's own involvement becomes part of the research.

In this chapter I consider Sherpa encounters with Khunde Hospital during a period of just over thirty years and argue that Sherpa beliefs and practices about sickness informed, and continue to inform, a person's responses to the hospital, and that, as elsewhere in the Himalayan region, people used the hospital as part of a plural strategy for dealing with ill health. I further argue that while Khunde Hospital was an integral part of Hillary's aid programme and Hillary's world, it was also an integral part of the wider development of the Khumbu region, both by being part of the change (by bringing in a different medical system with outside personnel and offering employment) and also being affected by the transformation that was occurring around it. The rising level of education, the development of tourism, increasing affluence and the area's decreasing isolation all had an impact on the hospital.[9] Khunde Hospital was not a "site" where a new medical system was introduced and displaced the old. Sherpa beliefs and practices and those of Western medicine continually engaged with each other as individual people confronted each episode of illness and decided whether or not using Khunde Hospital was the right option.

My discussion of "Sherpa beliefs and practices" is not intended to homogenise the considerable internal and regional variation that existed, and continues to exist, within and between different groups of Sherpas in Khumbu, Solu or Rolwaling, or further afield in Kathmandu or Darjeeling.[10] Nor am I writing an ethnography

[8] Sherry Ortner notes that "after thirty years of varied ethnographic research among the Sherpas, one can no longer give a simple account of their style or ethos". Sherry B. Ortner, *High Religion: A Cultural and Political History of Sherpa Buddhism* (Delhi: Motilal Banarsidass, 1999 [1989]), 6.

[9] The following chapter on Khunde Hospital as a Western medicine project will consider how those offering the new medical services reacted to the local community's responses to the hospital.

[10] A range of literature exists for other groups of Sherpas, but for a comparative ethnography of different groups of Sherpas see Ramesh Raj Kunwar, *Fire of*

of Sherpas. I am, however, using existing ethnography and oral information in conjunction with other primary sources to support my historical analysis of Khunde Hospital.

The first section of this chapter examines "traditional" views of Khumbu Sherpas about the causes and treatment of sickness.[11] It provides the foundation from which to consider Sherpa responses to the hospital. Ideas about illness and its cause form a key part of the belief system of any society and are often linked to views about a much wider range of misfortune.[12] This section, which is more descriptive, also draws heavily upon my experience of living and working at Khunde Hospital. Much of the discussion is written using the present tense rather than the historical past, because the traditional ideas referred to remain current and dynamic and highly relevant to the provision of health services from the hospital, whether patients come from the villages of Khumbu, live in Kathmandu or travel overseas. Sherpa ideas of disease causation are fundamentally different from those of Western medicine. Sherpas inhabit a world that is full of various types of beings that can be dangerous if offended or ignored, but can also be appeased through appropriate measures. Sickness is not seen in isolation; hence Sherpas respond to the origin of problems in their business or personal affairs, sickness to humans or animals, or poor crops in much the same way. Dealing with such forces remains an integral part of Sherpa life. Sherpa responses to Tibetan and Western medicine prior to the opening of Khunde Hospital in 1966 are also discussed.

The second part of the chapter analyses Sherpa encounters with Khunde Hospital. While knowledge of the existence of Western or modern medicine had spread throughout the wider region, Khumbu remained in the 1960s relatively isolated within Nepal and from the

---

Himal: An Anthropological Study of the Sherpas of the Nepal Himalayan Region (New Delhi: Nirala, 1989).

11 My use of the term "traditional" does not imply a system that is unchanging or unchanged. Craig Janes also suggests there is no satisfactory term to refer to non-Western indigenous medical systems. Janes, "The Health Transition, 1803–20.

12 Cecil Helman, *Culture, Health and Illness: An Introduction for Health Professionals,* 3rd ed. (Oxford: Butterworth Heineman, 1994), 7.

outside, particularly from the Western world. Despite such awareness, and the recent opening of a small government health post in Namche Bazar, in many respects the opening of Khunde Hospital still presented a "first contact" situation. How people reacted to Khunde Hospital was about the way people used a particular institution and its services and also their response to the introduction of modern medicine. This type of medicine was used pragmatically and selectively (it still is). Despite people's increasing attendance at the hospital, it was, for the most part, on Sherpa terms. Sherpas have incorporated Western medicine and the hospital into Khumbu life in a way that has not displaced other avenues for dealing with sickness and other activities. Khunde Hospital also always had a wider role in the community because of its connection with Hillary's work in the area. It was not just a place to go to when sick.

The last section of the chapter draws on the limited written Sherpa sources and considers Sherpa views about their changing world and the integral place that modern medicine and Khunde Hospital have come to occupy in Khumbu.

Sherpa Beliefs and Practices About Sickness

Both written and oral evidence is available to consider the subject of Sherpa beliefs and practices about sickness, but while most oral sources are Sherpa most written ones are not. Anthropologists have researched and written about Sherpa beliefs since the 1950s. That they remain interested is testament to the continuing relevance of the various traditional Sherpa explanations and actions, but neither Vincanne Adams nor John Draper, who have carried out the most extensive research, had Sherpa ill health as their first concern.[13] I wish to draw on their research, but privilege the oral and limited written testimony of Sherpas, and the ideas and experiences of the overseas volunteers at Khunde Hospital, about how Sherpas thought

[13] See Introduction. In her doctoral research Adams focused on the interdependence of healing and economic participation of Sherpas in the rise of tourism, while Draper examined power and the control of knowledge as it related to sickness. Adams, "Healing Buddhas and Mountain Guides"; Draper, "Beyond Medicine".

about and dealt with ill health.[14] These were the groups who were directly involved in the sickness encounter between Sherpa beliefs and practices and Western medicine as practised from Khunde Hospital from the end of 1966.[15]

Central to Sherpa interpretations of events of misfortune is their understanding of Tibetan Buddhism. The Nyingmapa tradition is the oldest in Tibetan Buddhism and has the closest links with the animist traditions of pre-Buddhist Tibet. Draper contended that because the religious elite of the monasteries possessed the greatest religious knowledge, ordinary people could not exercise real choice about what to believe or do, for example, when sick.[16] While many households as well as the monasteries held religious texts, which

[14] For a similar interpretation of Sherpa beliefs and practices about sickness, see a short article by Canadian volunteer doctors at Khunde Hospital Penny Dawson and Jamie Uhrig, "Sherpas and Sickness", *Alpine Journal* 89, no. 333, 1984, 80–83.

[15] I found it very difficult to decide how to relate the wealth of ethnographic information to the construction of Sherpa beliefs and practices that we worked with at Khunde Hospital. In 1999 I wrote a short piece summarising my ideas. Kami Temba Sherpa, now Dr Kami Temba Sherpa, read it through and made corrections. He also identified the one point where I had used additional information from a book to supplement what I had been told. Draper relates a similar experience. In his discussions with people about sickness, he found that cause rather than symptom was particularly important. He attempted to explain this through the idea that everything in the universe is interconnected, an idea often found in Western discourses on Buddhism. When he went through his notes towards the end of his fieldwork he wrote that:

> I was struck by how often I had imposed esoteric notions such as the notion of interconnectedness on to my informants; had blithely assumed that Western interpretations of Buddhist theories of si[c]kness would be familiar to the Sherpas, (and would be understood and accepted by all Sherpas equally). More detailed examination of my notes, however, revealed that no Sherpa—lay or otherwise—had ever explained things exactly this way to me, and, no matter how hard I subsequently tried, no Sherpa ever did. Draper, "Beyond Medicine", 167–68.

[16] John Draper, "Lama Knows: Religion and Power in Sherpa Society", in *Tantra and Popular Religion in Tibet,* ed. Geoffrey Samuel, Hamish Gregor and Elisabeth Stutchbury (New Delhi: International Academy of Indian Culture and Aditya Prakashan, 1994), 79–134.

were written in Tibetan, lay Sherpas hired monks from the monasteries to read these texts for a variety of ceremonies. Draper believed the laity did have knowledge of spiritual matters, but distinguished between "factual" and "interpretive" religious knowledge.[17] The religious elite controlled access to the latter. They could interpret the supernatural realm of sickness. While people appeared to have agency, their choices were actually constrained because they did not control this knowledge.[18] In practice, Sherpas were not particularly bothered, because they gained the religious benefit by having the reading done or by attending a religious festival. The emphasis on monastic practice, as Ortner has examined, was recent and part of the rise in importance in Khumbu of celibate monasticism.[19] In 1960 von Fürer-Haimendorf had described a society where most village rites were still carried out by village lama and laymen. He estimated that over 30 per cent of adult males in the community were literate and that the laity understood the Tibetan of these texts.[20] Again in practice, having a detailed knowledge probably did not make much difference to what people did when they were sick, because their course of action when choices were limited (as they were in Sherpa society prior to the arrival of Khunde Hospital) was likely to have been the same.

Three aspects of Sherpa Buddhism have particular relevance when dealing with ill health: the belief in rebirth, the idea of fate and the concept of merit. People did not require a detailed knowledge of the religious texts to understand the basic principles. Every activity of the body or the mind or speech, whether conscious or unconscious, had its inevitable consequence in a person's present or future life.[21] For a Sherpa, his or her fate in the life to come de-

[17] Draper, "Lama Knows", 100.

[18] Ibid., 108.

[19] See Ortner, *High Religion* and Ortner, *Life and Death on Mt. Everest,* chapter three, for the period after the founding of Tengboche monastery in 1916.

[20] Christoph von Fürer-Haimendorf, "The Role of the Monastery in Sherpa Society", *Ethnologica* 2, 1960, 12–28.

[21] Terry Clifford, *Tibetan Buddhist Medicine & Psychiatry: The Diamond Healing* (Delhi: Motilal Banarsidass, 2001 [1984]), 8.

pended on the balance between merit and sin.[22] A person acquired merit through good deeds, but morally negative actions were sinful. Life was like a ledger. At the end of one's life, a person hoped the balance was tipped in favour of the virtuous and he or she would be reborn in a better life. Good deeds also helped a person prevent sickness and other misfortune in their present life.

Everyone has his or her own personal *lha* (god). The lha is a person's protector, but if someone forgets to respect it properly, does not put up prayer flags or does not perform sufficient *puja* (worship) then it becomes angry and as a consequence is feared. Severe backache is always blamed on one's lha, but an unhappy lha can also cause a sudden death or disaster to befall a family, as the following event illustrates.[23] One evening in the late 1990s a woman was returning with some of her family members from a neighbouring village to her home in Khunde when she fell off the narrow track and was severely injured. Many villagers helped rescue her and she was carried to Khunde Hospital. The family believed the woman's lha was upset and had caused *hrindi* (ghosts) to push her off the trail.

Various agents can cause problems for the individual and explanations vary considerably between villages and individuals. Identifying the responsible outside agent takes precedence over dealing with the illness as it manifests in the human body. This underlying cause also tends to be the basis for the classification of disease.[24] Illnesses will be linked by Sherpa perceptions of cause. As these differed from those of modern medicine, then their views about the

[22] Von Fürer-Haimendorf, *The Sherpas of Nepal,* 271–72. Lay Sherpas use "sin" as their English translation for such ideas.

[23] Personal participation.

[24] Draper believed the classification inadequate for people to understand the importance and severity of their condition, and thereby control the treatment. Draper, "Beyond Medicine", 170. N. J. Allen, however, in his study of the Thulung Rai of east Nepal cautions against looking for clarity and consistency where they may not exist. For example (p. 528), he found no importance appeared to be attached to the precise description of symptoms. N. J. Allen, "Approaches to Illness in the Nepalese Hills", in *Social Anthropology and Medicine,* ed. J. B. Loudon (London: Academic Press, 1976), 500–52.

seriousness of particular illnesses could also vary.[25] The ones that people most worry about are those that can cause something nasty to happen suddenly, such as death.[26]

Sometimes an agent acts alone, but often, as in the story above, there is more than one to cause problems. The most feared type of ghost is the *nerpa* (malignant spirit of a dead person). People believe that the spirit of a dead person will usually go straight to its next life, but if left wandering can cause periodic havoc. Someone who has met with a violent death, or who has not received the correct funeral rites, is thought to be more at risk of becoming nerpa.[27] Nerpa can be either male or female, and Sherpas consider them the cause of much major sickness, or the fatal blow to someone already weakened from another cause. The classic sign that someone's illness is due to nerpa is that the symptoms are similar to those experienced by the dead person. The implications of such worries for seriously ill people and their families in their dealing with Khunde Hospital are discussed in the next section.

Other agents of illness and misfortune can bring about a wide range of problems. A *pem* (a type of "witch" spirit) is seen in contrast to nerpa, as it is something that works through a number of living rather than dead women, although occasionally it can be a man.[28] A pem is usually held responsible for prolonged diarrhoea and vomiting illnesses that are common in places such as Khumbu.[29] The type of situation that leads to someone getting a disease due to pem is one where the person is having food or drink which the

[25] Chapter three discusses disease in Khumbu from a Western medical perspective.

[26] Interviews with Kami Temba Sherpa, Suva (Fiji), May–June 1999.

[27] The appropriate religious ceremonies help the spirit avoid the obstacles along the way.

[28] Draper was unhappy about pem being "glossed as witchcraft" as he believed there are significant differences. He defined pem as "the unconscious projection of negativity", such as greed or envy, on to one's neighbours and kin. Draper, "Beyond Medicine", 189.

[29] From a Western medical perspective, such places would be considered as having limited hygiene that leads to contaminated food and drink, resulting in diarrhoea and vomiting.

pem wants but is not offered.[30] Pem can also present problems for women in labour, who try to avoid being seen by another woman. Pem can prolong the event, make it worse and even turn a male foetus into a female one. People will try and avoid contact with women suspected of being pem, but if this is unavoidable they will be nice to the person, not wanting to upset the spirit that has taken hold of the woman. As Sherpas believe the spirit is to blame rather than the person, these people do not receive the harsh treatment that they might suffer in many other cultures.[31]

Spirits can also be associated with places. A *lu* (serpent spirit) is one that lives "underneath" the earth in contrast to the lha which lives "above"; its home may be found near water, special trees and beside or downstairs in houses.[32] The third lake in the Gokyo valley is home to a powerful lu which local people visit in the hope of receiving help to become rich or, if they have fertility problems, to conceive. A lu differs from nerpa or pem in that it is potentially benevolent if treated properly, but if neglected or offended turns harmful. People consider an offended lu the likely cause for skin infections such as the very common impetigo or sores, arthritis and joint pains. The lu may have been upset because the person spat or urinated on or near its home. An angry lu is also an explanation for iodine deficiency disorders (IDD), such as goitre and cretinism.[33] Draper describes how people believe that when they drink the water from the streams this makes their blood flow thicker and causes bulges in the neck.[34] This belief is extended to explaining the high level of cretinism in the village of Phortse. Phortse is situated behind the sacred mountain of Khumbu Yul Lha (usually called Khumbila). As people go behind rocks, houses or mountains to urinate, the streams in Phortse are very well urinated which makes the lu even angrier and so the results are more serious.

[30] Hospitality involving food and drink is an important feature of Sherpa life. See Ortner, *Sherpas Through Their Rituals,* 68–74.

[31] Von Fürer-Haimendorf, *The Sherpas of Nepal,* 264.

[32] Personal communication, Kami Temba, 1999.

[33] See chapter three.

[34] Draper, "Beyond Medicine", 164. The region's soil, not water, is low in iodine.

These spirits and gods are deemed "unseen" causes of problems. In contrast to this is poisoning, which is regarded as "seen".[35] Draper estimated that "perhaps 1 in 4 Sherpas in the Thame valley have been considered poisoned at some time in their lives" and that his informants thought that the percentage could be even higher in the villages of Pangboche and Phortse or in Pharak.[36] Poisoning usually causes a gastric problem. If a person has abdominal pain accompanied by jaundice for a long period, he or she believes they are going to die from being poisoned.[37] Unfortunately, in the case of liver disease, which presents with such symptoms, they may well do so. If a person considers they have been poisoned, they or their family know that someone had intentionally harmed them.[38] The poison is thought to be a white powder, which is slipped under the poisoner's fingernail into a victim's drink of tea or *chang* (local beer). In the rituals of hospitality, this would not be noticed.[39] Animals can also die from being poisoned.

As well as specific agents causing illness and other misfortunes, a number of other beliefs are also important to the provision of health care by Khunde Hospital. The notion of *lhungtar* (luck) affects all aspects of a person's life.[40] The day of one's birth, month and year are important astrological data that influence a person's luck. Sherpas also believe that there are ages when a person is more likely to suffer bad luck, and also days and months of the year, or even whole years. It is unwise to travel on an unlucky day, or to have a wedding or build a house in an unlucky year. Local people's perception of many deaths in Khumbu in 1997–98 did not occasion surprise and reinforced their belief in their idea of "black" years.[41]

35 Interview with Ang Rita Sherpa, Kathmandu, June 2003.

36 Draper, "Beyond Medicine", 193.

37 Interviews, Kami Temba, May–June 1999.

38 Interview, Ang Rita, 2003.

39 Ibid.

40 "Luck" is the English word Sherpas use, but its English usage implies a degree of chance that is absent from a Sherpa understanding of the concept.

41 Personal observation. The exact number was not known because registration of deaths is not compulsory.

The activities or places that can result in a spiritual pollution known as *thip* also affect health.[42] The worst are being near a place where a baby is being born or near a dead body. Low caste people are polluting, as are unwashed plates. Thip can lead to various problems for an affected individual, including sickness. It causes conjunctivitis ("sticky eyes"), nose-bleeds and cold sores in the mouth.[43] Thip provides another explanation for iodine deficiency disorders as it is also blamed where people are seen as mentally "slow". People considered the woman to be at fault when a baby was born a cretin.

Lastly, some idea of the infectious nature of an illness and immunity exist in Sherpa society.[44] People believe, for example, that the very common *chamba* (the common cold/mild headache/cough) spreads from person to person as does chickenpox and measles.[45] Smallpox was also viewed in such a manner. Those who had smallpox were isolated and bodies were not cremated in the usual Sherpa custom. When two girls died in the Thame area during the 1963 epidemic their bodies were buried away from habitation and no funeral arrangements were held.[46] Measles has a high mortality in countries such as Nepal, but people understood that if a person survived measles he/she would not be affected by the disease again.

In response to these various causes and ideas about sickness, Sherpas use a number of strategies. They can try and prevent illness or other problems occurring by increasing their store of luck,

42 Also see Sherry B. Ortner, "Sherpa Purity", *American Anthropologist* 75, 1973, 49–63.

43 The descriptive labelling of a condition along the lines of its symptoms is common amongst Sherpas using the hospital.

44 I am using "infectious" to describe an illness that is seen to spread among people. See Margaret Pelling, "The Meaning of Contagion: Reproduction, Medicine and Metaphor", in *Contagion: Historical and Cultural Studies,* ed. Alison Bashford and Claire Hooker (London: Routledge, 2001), 15–38.

For a discussion (based on research in Africa) that argues that serious disease can usually be understood within a non-supernatural framework, referred to as "indigenous contagion theory", see Edward C. Green, *Indigenous Theories of Contagious Disease* (Walnut Creek, London: AltaMira Press, 1999).

45 Draper translates as "flu", but chamba is closer to the common cold rather than influenza. Influenza is a serious illness. Draper, "Beyond Medicine", 321.

46 Personal communication, Dr Kami Temba, June 2005.

so that he or she is in a better position to combat the various forces working against them. Good health and long life are part of this overall view of living. The prayer flags on houses are changed at least twice a year. The new ones will bring good luck, but keeping the old ones will not.[47] Religious ceremonies are held throughout the year, some for the benefit of the whole village while others are for the individual person or the family. For example, on the fifteenth day of *Mani Rimdu* local people visit the monastery to receive the lama's blessing and the *rilbu* (long-life pills).[48]

Other measures are used to ward off attacks by malevolent beings or to evade illness. Houses have low doorways to prevent the entry of a ghost which cannot bend its back.[49] The nerpa often follows its living family members along the trail when they go visiting, and so people try and stop it by placing on the track a piece of thorn bush with a pile of stones on top. Thread-crosses which function as ghost traps are another device.[50] Children are particularly vulnerable and parents must be careful. A charcoal spot placed on a child's nose prevents him or her being seen by ghosts at night.

If a person becomes ill, then a number of options are available. In some cases people do nothing or self-treat. People are very familiar with the symptoms of chamba and no further action is required unless a person does not get better. *Pang* in Western medical terms is seen as a type of depression that mainly affects women. It particularly occurs after childbirth, but melted butter is rubbed through the woman's hair immediately after the birth to try and prevent the problem occurring. Pang tends to run in families and can affect a woman's chances in marriage. The woman becomes lethargic, shuns light, stays inside and eats. It is seen as a sickness and may take two to three years to clear, but people believe it will clear of its own accord without the sufferer or family having to take any

[47] Personal communication, Ang Rita, September 2005.

[48] Ngawang Tenzin Zangbu (as told by), *Stories and Customs of the Sherpas,* ed. Frances Klatzel (Kathmandu: Mera Publications, 2000), 70.

[49] This is less evident in modern tourist lodges. Most tourists are taller than Sherpas.

[50] See Réne de Nebesky-Wojkowitz, *Oracles and Demons of Tibet* ('s-Gravenhage [The Hague]: Mouton & Co, 1956), 369–70.

action.[51] In the rugged terrain of Khumbu broken bones are common, but unlike many societies nobody specialised in dealing with the problem. Some experienced yak-herders gained a reputation for looking after animals and some people made splints, particularly for long bone fractures.[52] Many people, however, remained deformed. This led Hillary to believe the Sherpas had no traditional skills in bone-setting.[53] People attribute broken bones to being down on one's luck, although if a fall is unusual they may seek an explanation elsewhere. Both animals and humans may take a medicine made from a rock found in India.[54] Today this medicine can be bought in Kathmandu, but twenty years ago the inhabitants of Khumbu used to have to make the journey to the Indian border near Biratnagar.

For many conditions, or when someone does not get better, a person can consult a number of different types of healer. The person may think the cause of their problem is a spirit, but it is the *lhawa* (spirit medium) who can find out more specifically which spirit is to blame and what action should be taken to appease that spirit and enable the patient to recover.[55] While lhawa were active among Khumbu Sherpas, Ortner found no practising Sherpa lhawa

[51] Sherpas do not have the major distinction between physical and mental health that developed in biomedicine.

[52] Interview Kami Temba, May–June 1999.

[53] Hillary, *Schoolhouse in the Clouds,* 110.

[54] In Sherpa this is called *gymtsal,* but it is also widely known throughout Nepal.

[55] The literature on Himalayan shamanism is considerable. On Sherpa shamanism, see Adams, *Tigers of the Snow and Other Virtual Sherpas,* 184–94; Draper, "Beyond Medicine", 214–32; Sherry B. Ortner, "The Case of Disappearing Shamans, or No Individualism, No Relationalism", *Ethnos* 23, no. 3, 1995, 355–90; Robert A. Paul, "Some Observations on Sherpa Shamanism", in *Spirit Possession in the Nepal Himalayas,* ed. John T. Hitchcock and Rex L. Jones (Warminster, England: Aris and Phillips, 1976), as well as references throughout the Sherpa ethnographic literature. For a study of shamanism among the Yolmo of the Helambu region, based on the author's own participation, see Robert R. Desjarlais, *Body and Emotion: The Aesthetics of Illness and Healing in the Nepal Himalayas* (Philadelphia: University of Pennsylvania Press, 1992). The Yolmo (p. 7) now like to identify themselves to outsiders as "Sherpa".

in Solu in the mid-1960s.[56] The lhawa, who is usually male but may be female, will visit the patient's home, although he/she does not have to see the patient. The central feature of the lhawa's healing ceremony is the trance, but unlike other Himalayan shamans the Sherpa lhawa does not make the journey to the world of the spirit.[57] Instead, the offending spirit enters the body of the lhawa. Healing occurs by finding out what the offended spirit wants; the spirit is usually hungry or thirsty and would like its favourite food or drink. This is brought and then consumed by the lhawa. Afterwards the spirit is expected to go away. The lhawa returns to his normal self and asks the spirit to follow him out of the house, after which ceremonies are performed just outside the patient's property and the spirit is sent on its way.[58] If a patient fails to recover, the lhawa will suggest another attempt either to appease the spirit or to look for another spirit that is 'keeping' the patient sick.

A *mindung* ("junior" lhawa) can also identify a malevolent spirit but does not have the power to go into a trance. A mindung is more likely to be consulted when a full-fledged lhawa is unavailable, but is also much less expensive.[59] Draper frequently refers to mindung. He carried out most of his research in the Thame area, which is not on the main tourist trail and has been slower to derive economic benefits from the increasing tourism in the area, but he does not make clear whether people's use of a mindung was related to cost factors or to a full lhawa being unavailable.[60]

People who are sick can also go and see a lama, but only some senior monks are able to perform this role and not all of these have

56 Ortner, "The Case of Disappearing Shamans", 355.

57 Von Fürer-Haimendorf, *The Sherpas of Nepal,* 256.

58 If a pem or nerpa is the suspect, the lhawa makes a dough from flour, shapes it into a person, adds food, sticks, thread and fire from live coals, places it on the trail in the direction of the house of the suspect and then burns it with butter.

59 Interview, Kami Temba, Suva, June 1999.

60 Draper, "Beyond Medicine"; Ivan G. Pawson, Dennyse D. Standford and Vincanne A. Adams, "Effects of Modernization on the Khumbu Region of Nepal: Changes in Population Structure, 1970–1982", *Mountain Research and Development* 4, no. 1, 1984, 73–81.

the full version of the required books.[61] The lama's methods differ from those of the lhawa. The lama throws dice, and then correlates the results of the dice, the onset of the illness and the patient's year of birth with his books.[62] He will ask about the patient's symptoms; like the lhawa he does not need to see the patient. An experienced lama will then interpret this information in relation to what is written in his texts. Treatment and management vary with the illness. The lama will suggest holding one of many different types of puja, that may last from a few minutes to several days and require varying numbers of monks; he may give the patient a necklace that has been blessed; or a patient may have to appease an offended god, do maintenance work on a trail, local *chorten* (Buddhist monument) or *mani* (prayer) wall, or make a good luck tree and plant it high on a mountainside or ridge. A lama has some specific treatments such as holy water to remove thip, some old, brightly dyed butter from the altar to rub on a painful area, or give a herbal pill made by a very notable lama to promote general good health. People consider his *ngaa* (a lama's breath with spit) very important, but only certain lama have this power. The ngaa works with animals as well as humans.

While the perceived cause or causes of the problem will determine which type of healer to approach, the perceived severity of the problem will influence whether or not a person will seek assistance.[63] A person who has severe chest pain will go straight to a lama to look for a cause.[64] On the other hand, if someone has mild sores that are thought to be caused by a lu the family will burn butter at home as an offering to the lu. If the sores get worse then the person or their family may consult a lhawa.[65] As a general rule, a lama will be consulted if a person's lha or thip is suspected to be the cause of some misfortune, but in the case of a spirit being thought to be the cause of the problem, then the person or family will call the lhawa.

61 A lama is a religious teacher. Sherpas refer to most monks as *tawa.*

62 This process is known as *soontaag.*

63 The use of "perceived" is both deliberate and significant. It is important not to assume that because a disease is considered severe by Western medicine it is considered in the same way by others.

64 Interview, Kami Temba, Suva, June 1999.

65 Ibid.

When the source of the misfortune is not clear, and especially if the patient is very sick, people tend to consult both.

The inhabitants of Khumbu also had another option when sick; they could consult an *amchi* (a practitioner of "Tibetan" medicine).[66] This medical system emphasises the relationship of the mind to the body, which is seen as a whole, and the body to the universe.[67] It blends spiritual, "magical" and rational healing practices. The body is composed of three humours; health arises when these are in a state of balance, disease when they are not. The humours are influenced by natural factors such as diet or seasonal changes, but also life activities, psychological conditions, astrological and "unseen forces", and spiritual or karmic conditions existing from a person's present or previous life.

The position of amchi medicine in Khumbu provides an example of changing dynamics within existing medical systems and shows that these could occur independently of the encounter with Western medicine.[68] Oral sources indicate that prior to 1950, when the Chinese intensified their presence in Tibet, Khumbu not only did not have Western medicine but also did not have its own amchi.[69] Trade does not appear to have been a means for the spread of Western medicine in Khumbu, because people going on trading trips to Tibet would buy Tibetan medicines for various symptoms and bring them back for later use. While medicinal and aromatic plants grew in Khumbu, local use was limited. Instead they were

66 In the wider Himalayan region, such as Bhutan, use of the word "Tibetan" to describe this type of medical system can be inappropriate. See Alex McKay with Dorje Wangchuk, "Traditional Medicine in Bhutan", *Asian Medicine Tradition and Modernity* 1, no. 1, 2005, 204–18. In Khumbu, "Tibetan" can be used as it denotes both medical system and place of origin, but amchi in Nepal face registration issues and emphasise an older and broader Himalayan heritage.

67 Clifford, *Tibetan Buddhist Medicine & Psychiatry,* 3–9.

68 Charles Leslie's work from the late 1970s was particularly influential in challenging the view of the static nature of other medical traditions. C. Leslie and A. Young, eds., *Paths to Asian Medical Knowledge* (Berkeley: University of California Press, 1992).

69 Interview, Kami Temba, 1999.

harvested and then sent to Tibet for processing.[70] When Tibetan demand declined, Khumbu people stopped collecting the plants.[71] Some amchi settled in Khumbu, but people consulted them less frequently than other practitioners. Some amchi were also lama, and people believed that amchi medicine was empowered through the lama's personal power.[72] Khumbu Sherpas recognised amchi medical practice as different from their own, but because of their shared Tibetan origin did not perceive of it as being alien or as different as Western medicine.[73]

Western medicine, nevertheless, was another option for people to employ when sick. Khumbu Sherpas would usually have come into contact with this type of medicine before the building of Khunde Hospital through foreign expedition work outside Nepal.[74] During the first half of the twentieth century climbing expeditions increasingly sought out Sherpas because of their ability to cope with high altitude. Prior to 1950, people had had to walk for ten days through the mountains to Darjeeling in northern India and then look for employment.[75] In the 1950s, as Nepal allowed more travel

[70] Interview, Dr Lhakpa Norbu Sherpa, Dunedin, January 2005. Dr Lhakpa Norbu was the first Sherpa to be awarded a Ph.D.

[71] Ibid. The demand for Tibetan medicine has increased, particularly in the West, but in Khumbu tourism provided an alternative income to plant collection.

[72] Interview, Ang Rita, 2003. People going on lengthy pilgrimages feared getting sick and would often carry amchi medicines as well as lama medicine in their *dablam* which was a shrine-shaped box for protective prints, relics and religious medicine that people wore on a cord and tucked in one's clothing. Ang Rita described people taking amchi medicines more on religious faith than for their chemical properties.

[73] Interviews, Dr Kami Temba and Ang Rita, 2003. Adams described similarities between the practice of biomedicine and amchi medicine but that Sherpas often saw them as the same. Adams, "Healing Buddhas and Mountain Guides", 139.

[74] See chapter three for the development of biomedicine in Nepal.

[75] While some expedition Sherpas lived permanently in Darjeeling, others retained Khumbu as their main place of residence. In December 1935 Ang Tharkay and Ang Tsering were recruited by Major Morris in Darjeeling, but were then asked to go to Solukhumbu to find "porteurs" (porters) for an expedition the following year to Everest. Ang Tharkay, *Memoires d'un Sherpa,*

by visitors from Western countries, the focus for expedition activity and recruitment shifted to Nepal. Expeditions also treated people as they passed through different areas.

Some expeditions also gave a few employees some basic training in health issues and some left a few medicines for later use, but sources about Sherpa involvement are scattered in expedition accounts and are relatively few. Tenzing related in his autobiography that on his first expedition in 1935, a reconnaissance trip to Everest led by Eric Shipton, the celebrated British Himalayan explorer and mountaineer, "I was assigned to the expedition doctor, and from him I learned many things about sickness, injuries, and first aid that were of much use to me in later years."[76] In an example of Khumbu Sherpa involvement, New Zealand climber Norman Hardie, who spent several months living in Khumjung in 1955, described how Urkien, his sirdar, was called out at three o'clock one morning to see a sick woman returning from an expedition.[77] Urkien came from Khumjung and, as well as climbing, had been a medical orderly on his first expedition the previous year, the 1954 New Zealand Alpine Club Expedition to the Barun valley led by Hillary.[78]

Hardie went to Khumjung because he wanted to learn about the Sherpas "who have contributed so much to the success of the greatest mountaineering expeditions".[79] His was not an academic undertaking; and his book *In Highest Nepal: Our Life Among the Sherpas,* was overshadowed by anthropologist Christoph von Fürer-Haimendorf's study *The Sherpas of Nepal: Buddhist Highlanders* which was published in 1964. Like many anthropologists of his era, von Fürer-Haimendorf saw Sherpas in terms of a society under threat in a modernising world, but Hardie's account remains of interest because, in contrast to von Fürer-Haimendorf whose focus was on the "Other" in their world, Hardie also observed Sherpa encoun-

recueillis par Basil P. Norton, translated into French by Henri Delgove (Paris: Amiot Dumont, 1954), 71.

76 Tenzing Norgay, *Man of Everest,* 62.

77 Hardie, *In Highest Nepal*, 119. Hardie had just climbed Mt Kangchenjunga as part of the successful first ascent of the world's third highest mountain.

78 In 1955 he was one of the Sherpas on the Kangchenjunga expedition.

79 Hardie, *In Highest Nepal,* 5.

ters with his own world.[80] On one occasion Hardie was puzzled by the actions of some of the expedition Sherpas in Khumjung. In an example that illustrates how beliefs about human sickness were part of a broader system, Hardie witnessed a ceremony by a lhawa who was called to find out both why Gyalgen's cow would not give milk and then to cure Annalu's sore knee and thigh.

> I wondered about the attitudes of Annalu, Gyalgen and Urkien, all of whom willingly accept the advice of doctors on expeditions; when I questioned them they said that on an expedition they are under the influence of the leader's and doctor's gods, but in their own village they have to revert to their old methods of approaching the earliest Tibetan lamas.[81]

Such an explanation nevertheless also illustrates that Sherpas operated in different worlds, in this case the world of the foreign-dominated mountaineering expedition and their own world in Khumbu. Once Sherpas had returned to their villages they would have had few, if any, of the resources of Western medicine to treat illness, but this explanation of following the expedition's "ways" when on an expedition was repeated, although in a different context, when Tenzing responded to criticism after the Everest climb in 1953: "As we Sherpas say, I was 'eating their salt.' They had run the expedition; why should they not handle this in their own way? So I sent no message, and I told the other Sherpas not to break the news until it was official."[82] Such acceptance of expedition ways was not always the case. Ortner shows how Sherpas negotiated to improve their position within expeditions.[83]

Although Sherpas did use expedition medicine, they also adopted a plural approach to treatment when sick. On Tenzing's second expedition in 1936, with Shipton to Garwhal in the central Himalaya, he became ill and had to be carried.

[80] Also see Robert Miller, "High Altitude Mountaineering, Cash Economy, and the Sherpa", *Human Organization* 24, no. 3, fall 1965, reprinted in *Himalayan Research Bulletin* 17, no. 2, 1997, 17–22.

[81] Hardie, *In Highest Nepal*, 122–24.

[82] Tenzing Norgay, *Man of Everest,* 274.

[83] Ortner, *Life and Death on Mt. Everest.*

> They told me that what I had was bilious fever, and some natives of the region said that if I ate a special sort of moss that grew on the stones it would help me. So I tried it. I boiled some moss in hot water and swallowed it, and then I vomited so much that I thought all my insides were coming out. But the fever went away. After that I was weak, but not sick any more, and able to go on.[84]

Ang Tharkay, who achieved fame as sirdar on the successful French expedition to Mt Annapurna in 1950, was born in Khunde in 1909.[85] On his first expedition to Everest in 1933 he suffered from frostbite.[86] The expedition doctor advised him to cut and gather wood and use his hands and legs as much as possible to restore circulation. Ang Tharkay explained in his autobiography that he and the other Sherpas did not understand the sense of this treatment. A friend then suggested "cauterisation", a treatment that was current among Sherpas.[87] Ang Tharkay was surprised to find that it brought some relief and he was able to continue.

Sherpas sometimes received medicines from expeditions for future use. Hardie wrote about a group of expedition Sherpas returning from the lower Indian altitudes who were not only given antimalarials but "one of their senior men had other supplies to cover a number of ills".[88] This group experienced only minor problems, but among another group of nine, who had begun walking home in the monsoon and had no medicines, five died. The wet conditions of the monsoon made it "the worst time for dysentery, malaria and many other complaints".[89] In the early 1960s, in an example showing the initiative of local people, the teachers from the school that Hillary built at Khumjung started going up to Everest Base Camp

[84] Tenzing Norgay, *Man of Everest*, 66–67.

[85] Judy and Tashi Tenzing, *Tenzing and the Sherpas of Everest,* 24.

[86] Ang Tharkay, *Memoires,* 63–64.

[87] This was probably moxibustion. Conversation with Dr Tenzin Namdul, Tibetan medicine practitioner, at the 10th Seminar of the International Association for Tibetan Studies, Oxford, September 2003.

[88] Hardie, *In Highest Nepal,* 120.

[89] Ibid., 119.

and approaching expeditions for medicines.[90] They then returned to the village, and from their living quarters provided treatment for the local people.

Contact with expeditions increased during the twentieth century, but some Sherpas were also exposed to Western medicine through other avenues. Ang Lhamu, Tenzing's second wife, accompanied him to England in 1953, but this was her second visit.[91] She was born in Darjeeling, although her family came from Khumbu, and had worked as an *ayah* (maidservant) looking after the two children of a British family. In 1938 the family returned to England, where for several months Ang Lhamu lived in the centre of London in a hotel near Hyde Park. During this time she became ill and was admitted to hospital. In 1953 she said that her most vivid memory of the earlier visit was lying in bed in hospital while learning how to use a gas mask. Unfortunately by the time she recovered, her employer had left England. Ang Lhamu was now unemployed, and she had to make the long journey back to India alone.[92] The example of Ang Lhamu was unusual, but would have been talked about among Sherpas in Darjeeling. In a community where communication was principally by word of mouth, this was the acknowledged means for spreading information. From Darjeeling such information could spread back to Khumbu as people travelled between the two areas.[93]

Another example was the young rinpoche at Tengboche monastery, the most important monastery in Khumbu. The rinpoche was born in Namche Bazar in 1935, but at the age of five years he was chosen and taken to Tengboche to be raised as the reincar-

[90] Conversation with Shyam Pradhan Krishna, Khunde, 1996. He went to Khumjung as a teacher in 1965. I do not know how extensive this practice was or for how long it continued as I was unable to follow this up with Shyam who died in 1998—a casualty of the "black" year. The McKinnons at Khunde Hospital were unaware that this was occurring.

[91] His first wife, Dawa Phuti, had died in 1944.

[92] Tenzing Norgay, *Man of Everest,* 48 and 96.

[93] In Khumbu, word of mouth remains the principal means of communication.

nate lama and head of the monastery.[94] He recalled that when he was about six years old he had to go to Kathmandu for a smallpox vaccination. Although this appears to be an isolated example, Alex McKay emphasises how the endorsement of such practices by the lay and religious elite was important in the spread of biomedicine in an area.[95]

Migration may also have brought some contact with Western medicine, whether through hearsay or actual use. Sherpas in Darjeeling had a variety of occupations. When Ang Tharkay arrived around 1930 he was employed for three months carrying stone during the building of the Victoria Hospital.[96] A few Sherpas joined the Gurkha battalions of the British Indian Army.[97] Toni Hagen, who travelled extensively in Nepal, wrote that returning Gurkha soldiers brought home goods and talked about conditions in other countries where smallpox was not necessarily fatal and that "modern medicine" had effective "remedies".[98] The first teacher at Hillary's school in Khumjung was Tem Dorje Sherpa, who came from Darjeeling. Previously he had been in the British Army where he had learned a little about Western medicine. He then applied this knowledge when he went to Khumjung.[99]

94 Ngawang Tenzin Zangbu, *Stories and Customs of the Sherpas,* 57–58. The age of a child can be confusing which has implications for biomedical health programmes, such as the current international polio eradication campaign. The "under five years" category needs in practice to include those children who are six years old in Sherpa terms.

95 Alex McKay, "'The Birth of a Clinic'? The IMS Dispensary in Gyantse (Tibet), 1904-1910", *Medical History* 49, 2005, 135–54. IMS refers to the Indian Medical Service.

96 Ang Tharkay, *Memoires,* 54. The exact date is not provided.

97 Ortner, *High Religion,* 160 and 217; Dash, *Darjeeling,* 72; conversation with Kami Temba, Suva, 1999. I was not aware of any Sherpa living on an army pension in Khumbu.

98 Hagen, *Nepal,* 126.

99 Conversation with Shyam Pradhan Krishna, Khunde, 1996. Tem Dorje had a considerable impact on personal hygiene practices among the children which reinforced the work of the hospital staff. Personal communication, Diane McKinnon, 12 February 2006.

The increasing presence of foreigners coming into Khumbu during the 1950s and early 1960s, although still small, accelerated the contact. In his preface to *The Sherpas of Nepal*, von Fürer-Haimendorf wrote of his wife that: "To many she endeared herself also by ministering to their medical needs, and their faith in her remedies enabled her to achieve several notable cures, not the least acclaimed of which was the successful mending of the broken leg of a yak." [100] Despite the fact that each medical system was based on a different perception of the cause, people using the treatments did not necessarily see conflict. The nature of the contact also began to change from being very temporary when an expedition passed through the area to something longer term. Hillary's expedition set up a clinic in Khumjung for six months in 1963. [101] It functioned throughout the monsoon when poor weather limited flying in the mountains and made Khumbu inaccessible except on foot.

At the same time as the local inhabitants were coming into increasing contact with visitors from outside the country, the Nepalese government and structures of the state were strengthening their presence in this border region and beginning to integrate it more fully within Nepal. Until the 1940s, when the central government set up an office in Namche Bazar, officials had only occasionally visited. [102] The village developed as the administrative centre of the area. Part of this expansion of state services included the setting up of a small health clinic in 1964, but it was not used much by the local population. Staffed by non-Sherpa paramedical health workers who did not know the area, who spoke a different language, who followed a different religion and who ate different food, this government clinic in the 1960s was no less foreign to Sherpas than the overseas expeditions.

Sherpa Encounters with Khunde Hospital

For most people, the provision of health services from Khunde Hospital would bring their first experience of Western medicine.

100 Von Fürer-Haimendorf, *The Sherpas of Nepal,* xv–xvi.

101 See chapter one of this book.

102 Stevens, *Claiming the High Ground,* 54–55.

By 1966, many people in the area, and particularly those that travelled, were aware of Western medicine and a few may have tried it, but until this time its availability in Khumbu was too limited to be in a position to challenge or replace existing Sherpa beliefs and practices. The hospital with its shiny roof was a symbol of the considerable change occurring in the lives of Khumbu Sherpas, but the prayer flags that continue to flutter from the pole at the front of the hospital or the Tibetan calendar that hangs in the hospital's office are evidence of the ongoing importance of the values of the local community in the work of the hospital.

The initial response to the hospital was curiosity. People were also "thankful".[103] Hillary was cast as a sponsor or protector *(jhindak)* who would receive merit for providing the hospital.[104] Although the relationship appears unequal and paternalistic, Sherpas embed it in, as Ortner discusses, "profoundly egalitarian assumptions".[105] Hillary will help them succeed and so they will become more equal. Tenzing described the relationship between Sherpas and "sahibs" as one of "good companions".[106] The Sherpas on an expedition were not servants. As noted in chapter one, this view fitted in with how Hillary saw the relationship. Many people helped with building the hospital, as they had done with other Hillary projects, and while the overseas members of the expedition brought in some new skills, such as plumbing, and equipment, Sherpas were the experts in using the abundant local rock.[107]

The official opening of the hospital provided the opportunity for a good social gathering and attracted people from throughout the area. Local women dressed in their finery and the current doctor, Kami Temba Sherpa, remembers coming as a child from Thame,

[103] Personal communication, Dr Kami Temba, 2005.

[104] See Ortner, *Life and Death on Mt. Everest,* 83–88, and Adams, *Tigers of the Snow and Other Virtual Sherpas,* 164–65.

[105] Ortner, *Life and Death on Mt. Everest,* 83.

[106] Tenzing Norgay, *Man of Everest,* 138.

[107] Hillary expected help with projects from the local community; such assistance and networks of assistance were and continue to be a feature of Sherpa society. Adams relates changes in these practices to economic factors. Adams, "Healing Buddhas and Mountain Guides".

three hours walk away.[108] Louise Hillary's book, *A Yak for Christmas,* provides a detailed and enthusiastic account of the occasion, describing people's excitement at the helicopters landing nearby with their official overseas guests from Kathmandu, Tibetan traders selling their wares and the rinpoche from Tengboche monastery taking photos with his camera which an expedition had given to him.[109] The senior government official came up from Namche and lent a loudspeaker system for the proceedings. His speech in Nepali demonstrated the government's limited hold in the region at this time as it had to be translated into Sherpa.

Many of the key features of this occasion, therefore, embodied the changes that were beginning to transform Khumbu and that would accelerate with the area's increasing economic development and decreasing isolation. Yet the visitor who appeared to create the most excitement was the elderly and revered lama from Thamo who was greeted at the hospital and then was settled at a place nearby by his staff. Louise Hillary wrote that:

> Before the day was out six or seven hundred people must have gone before him, made their obeisance, been blessed and given a little ribbon for their neck, a small ball of tsampa, and a sip of water or chung. The queue leading to the Thamo lama was sometimes a hundred feet in length, with whole families waiting patiently for their turn.[110]

With a sharp eye for business, the Tibetan traders set themselves up between the hospital and the Thamo lama. After the hospital's lay opening the lama's assistant "announced that the lama would like to bless the building".[111] This he proceeded to do. In 1963 this lama had rejected the offer of smallpox vaccination, and so his blessing in 1966 gave an important religious sanction to the new institution. The events of the day did not suggest any conflict.

The building as a physical structure met with a mixed response. People were very impressed with the plumbing that produced hot

108 Ahern, "A Hospital for Kunde", 18.

109 Louise Hillary, *A Yak for Christmas,* 88–99.

110 Ibid., 93. Tsampa is a flour made from ground barley.

111 Ibid.

water out of taps inside the building.[112] Sherpa houses did not have running water and the hot water would have been very welcome in the freezing cold of a Khumbu winter. People were less keen on the toilets, because a few years later volunteer doctor Ann Lang wrote home that "Mingma is fed up with our smelly toilets and yesterday he arrived with a large contingent of Sherpas to build two new ones."[113] Longdrop toilets in any case need replacing, but earlier the McKinnons had shown that they were happy to learn from local custom when they had leaves delivered to the hospital and adopted the local practice of throwing down some after each use of the toilet.[114] This is very effective in reducing smell. People also found that the bamboo matting of the long-stay ward, which creaked and cast shadows at night, gave plenty of scope for fears about the hospital's ghosts.[115] They also had different ideas about approaching the hospital "space", since the McKinnons decided to put a latch on the door of the clinic to prevent people from just walking in and the Evans wrote that they were considering doing the same with the door to their flat.[116]

With the opening of the hospital, Khumbu had two biomedical centres providing primary care services and so the local population now had a choice. As Pieter Streefland pointed out in his article about the spread of "modern Western medicine" in Nepal, people coming into contact with this system met "depending on time and place, totally different forms, aspects and message-bearers".[117] In other words, modern Western medicine had "many faces". Khumbu exemplified the diversity that Streefland referred to by bringing together in one small area many of these faces of medical practice. Khunde Hospital represented one of these, the government clinic

112 Interview, Wooderson, 1997.

113 29 January 1971 [Lang papers]; interview, Selwyn and Ann Lang, 2002.

114 Personal communication, Diane McKinnon, 12 February 2006. Sherpa toilets are emptied in the spring to provide fertiliser for the potato fields.

115 Conversation with Mingma Temba Sherpa, Khunde, January 1997.

116 Dr Richard and Lesley Evans to their family, 3 October 1968 [Evans papers].

117 Pieter Streefland, "The Frontier of Modern Western Medicine in Nepal", *Social Science & Medicine* 20, no. 11, 1985, 1156.

another. In deciding whether or not to use Khunde Hospital people would have to make choices both between systems and between different versions of the same medical system. Both the responses to Khunde Hospital as biomedicine, and to a particular version of its practice, are important in considering the place of the hospital in the world of Sherpas in Khumbu.

Patients

The basic question for people to decide was whether or not to use the hospital's services. Outpatient and inpatient records and annual reports provide evidence of whom and which diseases the hospital treated, and from where the patients came, but they are insufficient for an analysis of issues relating to class or status. (I discuss the medical aspect of these patient figures in the next chapter, but here I consider them from the point of view of the local community's response to the hospital.) Most people were treated as outpatients. Between January and June 1967, 1,066 people went to the hospital. [118] Of these, 376 (35.27 per cent) were adult males, 378 (35.46 per cent) were adult females, 147 (13.79 per cent) were males under the age of 16 years and 165 (15.48 per cent) were females under 16 years. All were Sherpa except for 53 classified as Nepalese, four coming from Tibet and three trekkers. [119] All but seven of these other Nepalese patients were male and 40 per cent came from outside Khumbu.

Thirty years later the statistics seem both similar to and different from the earlier pattern. During the first six months of 1997 outpatients totalled 3,381 of whom 1,358 (40.16 per cent) were adult males, 1,259 (37.24 per cent) were adult females, 457 (13.43 per cent) were males under the age of 16 years and 307 (9.1 per cent) were females under 16 years. [120] The number of outpatients had trebled; adults continued to dominate the figures. For both adults and children the proportion of female patients had decreased. Just

118 The outpatient register started from 1 January 1967, nearly two weeks after the official opening, and so the first patients are not recorded.

119 Sherpas living in Khumbu are, of course, Nepalese.

120 Kunde Hospital and Village Clinics Annual Report 1997.

over 68 per cent of the outpatients were Sherpa with the number of other Nepalese rising to 28 per cent. [121] Despite the vast increase in tourism there were only 112 tourist outpatients which represented just 3 per cent of the total number of consultations at the hospital. Khunde Hospital remained primarily a service for the local population, whether Sherpa or other Nepalese ethnic groups. The patient's current place of residence showed that 67.46 per cent of outpatients came from the three closest main villages of Khunde, Khumjung and Namche Bazar, 17.46 per cent came from the Thame and Everest valleys where the main settlements were between three and five hours walk from the hospital and 14.32 per cent came from the lower valleys. [122] While the hospital also provided inpatient facilities for serious cases or for people who lived a long distance from the hospital, most of the time the hospital only had a few inpatients at any given time. [123]

Two major issues arise from this statistical profile. Firstly, it reveals what had been happening at the hospital; it refers to the people who chose to use Western medicine by going to the hospital, although young children would have had the decision made for them. Secondly, although the figures suggest increasing use being made of Western medicine, a view of an inevitable and relentless one-way trend is problematic because many people did not use the hospital or used it for some health issues but not others. Also, when the non-Sherpa patients are removed from the overall total, the increase in use by the people permanently living in the area is smaller. To look at how Western medicine has been accepted in Khumbu it is necessary to look at why people chose to use this type of medi-

121 The changing demographic profile of patients reflected the development of the area. Most of these patients were temporary residents and the permanent residents remained predominantly Sherpa.

122 In this annual report, trekkers and Nepalese whose home was elsewhere in Nepal were included in the totals. We found it more useful to note residence as the place from which a patient's journey to the hospital originated. See chapter three of this book for the implications for monitoring and evaluating the hospital's activities of such inconsistency in the record-keeping.

123 I found no inpatient register for the period before October 1970, although the numbering of patient admissions indicates there were records.

cine or why they decided to look elsewhere for help when sick.[124] This requires looking beyond the hospital's statistics and considering other sources.

Information about non-use, medical pluralism and the use of multiple therapies can be gleaned from other hospital documents, correspondence from the overseas volunteers and oral sources. The local Sherpa hospital staff are particularly valuable resources for finding out both about the current situation and changes that have occurred. Another important avenue for information is the field research that has been carried out by a number of anthropologists among different groups of Sherpas. What people did when they were sick was often part of the researcher's gaze. Use of the hospital signified increasing modernisation among Sherpas, use of lama and lhawa supported the resilience of Sherpa beliefs and practices. In addition to the ethnographic information and analysis, the fact that several different studies were carried out over a long period of time also enables them to be used as written historical sources, which is particularly valuable when otherwise dealing largely with oral material.

From the beginning the local community adopted a mixed response to using the hospital's services. McKinnon in 1967 believed that those keenest on the hospital's services were the families who already had had contact with expedition medicine.[125] While some people used the hospital and others did not, people were selective about when and how they would use the hospital. Some women went to the hospital for antenatal care, but during his time no woman delivered at the hospital. He saw several acute surgical conditions but "all patients have refused hospitalisation when seriously ill".[126] Nima Yangen, his assistant nurse, remembers that people initially did not believe in the hospital.[127] She said that sometimes

124 In this book I focus on Sherpas. Other Nepalese groups have a different encounter with Khunde Hospital which also need to be examined, particularly as the proportion of these patients has increased significantly in recent years.

125 McKinnon, "Health Problems of Khumbu in Nepal," 141.

126 Ibid., 143.

127 Interview with Nima Yangen Sherpa, Kathmandu, July 2003.

"Dr John" got angry and sometimes he would go out and get a patient who had not come back, but when he and Diane left everyone in the village cried.[128] With only a few patients coming each day, Nima Yangen did not consider the hospital a busy place. She and McKinnon, however, visited the villages, and so the hospital would have been busier when they were there than a simple daily average of 5.89 patients during the first six months suggests.[129]

The most important factor in a person's decision to use the hospital was whether the hospital's treatment was considered effective.[130] Among Sherpas in Khumbu, it was a patient's perception of the efficacy of treatment from Khunde Hospital that was important.[131] People did not believe that going to the hospital was the best course of action for all illness. The pattern of use revolved around the issue of whether or not they saw a value in going to Khunde Hospital. This could be perceived in various ways and so "effective" meant different things to different people. The most obvious test of effectiveness was that if using Khunde Hospital resulted in a person getting better, then increasingly people were prepared to try the hospital.[132] Pills relieved a headache or an extraction removed the pain from a rotten tooth. People also wanted to become completely

[128] Hillary was there and was both surprised and impressed. Hillary, *Nothing Venture, Nothing Win,* 272.

[129] Nima Yangen's other experience of a medical institution was the much larger Shanta Bhawan Hospital in Kathmandu.

[130] Understandings of "efficacy" vary and this is reflected in the literature.

[131] For a similar view, see Helen Lambert, "Plural Traditions? Folk Therapeutics and 'English' Medicine in Rajasthan", in *Western Medicine as Contested Knowledge,* ed. Andrew Cunningham and Bridie Andrews (Manchester: Manchester University Press, 1997), 191–211; McKay, *Their Footprints Remain*. I am very grateful for being allowed to read McKay's draft manuscript and for comments. Also see Susan Heydon, "Change and Continuity: A History of Kunde Hospital, Solukhumbu, Nepal", *Himalayan Research Bulletin* 12, no. 2, 1997, 27–30 and "Sherpa Beliefs and Western Medicine: Providing Health Care at Khunde Hospital, Nepal", in *Soundings in Tibetan Medicine: Anthropological and Historical Perspectives. Proceedings of the Tenth Seminar of the International Association for Tibetan Studies, 2003,* ed. Mona Schrempf (Leiden: Brill, 2007), 65–87.

[132] Interview, Dr Kami Temba, 2003.

well rather than improved. A person with a bad cough expected no cough at night rather than a slight cough. As research among other groups has also indicated, the speed of the cure was also an important consideration. Western medicines were believed to act more quickly than other kinds.

Conversely, if someone believed the hospital was neither going to be able to cure the problem nor was it the right course of action, then he or she stayed away. Dr Richard Evans, who succeeded McKinnon in 1968, was very aware that while people who used the hospital were supportive, many people must have been against hospital treatment as they never came near. [133] When visiting villages he would ask if there were other sick people. Draper showed the cautiousness of the local response during his research in 1986 and 1987 when he collected information on four hundred episodes of illness among Thame valley people. Even if, as Draper acknowledged, the 5 per cent who said they used Western medicine was unrealistically low, only 7 per cent gave it as their preferred choice. [134] Twenty years after the hospital's opening, going there was not the main recourse when sick. These findings, I believe, question Adams's views about the degree of modernisation and altered beliefs among Sherpas. [135]

Obstacles faced people in their choice about whether or not to use the hospital. One difficulty was that sick people did not want to be seen walking through villages. Sickness was viewed as failure, and so they did not want to be seen to be sick and have people talking about them. [136] When a person walks along the trail other people always ask where the traveller is going or where have they come from. Sickness also weakened a person's resistance to attacks by pem or nerpa which could aggravate their problem. People were

133 Interview, Dr Richard and Lesley Evans, 2004.

134 Draper, "Beyond Medicine", 312–14. Draper did note distance from Khunde Hospital as a factor for non-use; also some people who had only used Western medicine did not tell him about the illness.

135 Adams, who was researching around the same time, also wrote about continuing use of other medical systems. She carried out her research in Khumjung which was a village that had more contact with tourism and also in Kathmandu where medical choices were different.

136 Interview, Dr Lhakpa Norbu, 2005.

reluctant, therefore, to walk through certain areas along the trails and especially at night. One of these was the small pass on the way to Khunde. As a result, a person who lived in Khunde village and decided to go to the hospital was less at risk than a person travelling from further away and had to go through the pass.

Despite misgivings by many people in Khumbu, the hospital became seen and used as one option in a medical environment where multiple choices of treatments and medical systems were available and regularly used. McKinnon describes how it was not uncommon to visit a house where a triple approach to managing an illness was in progress.[137] People, therefore, did not see a problem in having the religious, the shaman and the Western medical practitioner all present and practising at the same time. Thirty years later these options remained in use, but McKinnon's comment was now unusual. Throughout the intervening period the volunteers' correspondence and annual reports continued to refer to other practitioners in the area, but in the mid-1990s in Khunde the drums of the lhawa were rarely heard at night. In contrast in Phortse, they were. One evening a man was heard coughing continuously and later the lhawa's drum broke the silence of the night. Next morning the man came to see the visiting doctor for medicine.[138] While the business of the lhawa has declined in much of Khumbu, the lama remain busy. The changing fortunes of other practitioners is an important area for consideration in the spread of Western medicine, but many of these changes occurred independently of the encounter with Khunde Hospital and are, therefore, outside the focus of this book.

The Sherpa word for hospital is *menkhang* (medicine house) and provides a clue as to how people could use what may appear to others as incompatible systems.[139] People could come to the hospital and receive medicine while still going to other healers.[140] In Sherpa

137 Personal communication, McKinnon, 12 February 2006.

138 Personal participation.

139 Draper, "Beyond Medicine", 273.

140 Sherry Ortner Paul, "Food for Thought: A Key Symbol in Sherpa Culture", (Ph.D. thesis, University of Chicago, 1970), 166–67. Ortner describes three types of medicine: Western medicine, folk medicine and religious medicine.

healing practices, however, a person ingested little in comparison to the role of medicines at the hospital. People were reluctant to use something when they did not know the ingredients.[141] Western medicine was seen to treat the symptoms rather than the cause and so for people the different systems had varying areas of effectiveness. Martin Gaenszle describes a comparable situation in his study of the Mewahang Rai of East Nepal, in which he examined the interpretation of illness and the respective roles of the shaman and the doctor and health post.[142] Medical knowledge among the Rai, as among the Sherpa, was part of a comprehensive set of beliefs and practices governing all aspects of life. The Rai had incorporated Western medicine into this view by attributing Western medicine to work on the physical level and the shaman on a metaphysical level. The two were not contradictory. "One eats the doctor's pills but still calls the shaman to ensure that the ancestor deity will be pacified."[143]

While a model of multiple therapeutic options offers a way for different systems to exist together, poor utilisation of biomedical facilities continues to exist in Nepal as in many developing countries.[144] Various factors such as staff, clinic times, medicine availability and distance, as well as the more obvious issue of cost, can act as barriers to accessing health care. In Tibet in the early twentieth century, the British had offered medical services free of charge as a deliberate strategy to encourage the use of modern medicine and also as an adjunct to their political aims.[145] Until 1982 the serv-

141 Interview, Dr Lhakpa Norbu, 2005.

142 Martin Gaenszle, "The Shaman and the Doctor: Conflicting Systems of Interpretation and Diagnosis in East Nepal", in *Acculturation and Domination in Traditional Asian Medical Systems*, ed. Dorothea Sich and Waltraud Gottschalk (Stuttgart: Franz Steiner Verlag, 1994), 53–60. The number of non-Sherpa patients has increased throughout the hospital's history and many of these are Rai who have come to live and work in the district, particularly the adjacent and lower area of Pharak.

143 Gaenszle, "The Shaman and the Doctor," 56.

144 See, for example, Dixit, *The Quest for Health*, 30–34.

145 Alex McKay, *Tibet and the British Raj: The Frontier Cadre 1904–1947* (Richmond: Curzon, 1997), 168.

ices at Khunde Hospital were free for Nepalese residents. Although travel and the costs of staying in Khunde for long periods could be problematic for some people, even with a small charge (which was paid for in cash and has approximately equated to the price of a cup of tea bought locally in a lodge or teashop) Western medicine facilities in Khumbu were usually less expensive than other systems.[146]

This perception by those providing health care that the services were free is complicated by the issue of patients giving gifts. Adams describes how the giving of gifts in Sherpa society is important because it enables the giver to establish "a relationship of reciprocity".[147] The assumption of Dr Mingma Gyelgen Sherpa, the district medical officer and medical superintendent of Phaphlu Hospital, was that Sherpa patients offered gifts in order to procure a favourable outcome. When Adams talked to him in 1987 he said he felt he was under enormous pressure. He could do much for a sick person, but many patients could not be cured. The area of Pharak is one thousand metres lower than Khumbu and patients from this area know that they can grow fruit and vegetables that people living in Khumbu cannnot. When such food is scarce, the gift to the doctors at Khunde Hospital of some green vegetables or apples is worth much more than its monetary value.

The nil or low cost of services and medicines at Khunde Hospital could also work against it. During her field research in the late 1960s among Sherpas of the Solu area, Ortner wrote that when she gave out medicines brought back from Khunde Hospital many people insisted on paying for them as otherwise they would not be effective.[148] Nima Yangen, described that when people went to Kathmandu and discovered how expensive such medicine was, they started to use Khunde Hospital and its medicines more. They now knew they cost a lot.[149]

146 See, for example, Adams, "Modes of Production and Medicine". In 1982 a charge for medicines was introduced—see chapter four.

147 Adams, *Tigers of the Snow and Other Virtual Sherpas,* 116–17.

148 Ortner Paul, "Food for Thought", 103–4.

149 Interview, Nima Yangen, 2003.

Many factors, therefore, influenced people's decisions about whether or not to use Khunde Hospital. The experiences with vaccination illustrates the complexity of local responses to the hospital's policies and practices. While much of the hospital's work resulted from a person or their family actively choosing to go to the hospital for treatment, vaccination until the 1980s involved hospital staff going out into the district and sometimes to individual houses. McKinnon's outpatient register for 1967 shows large numbers of people accepting the iodised oil injections to combat iodine deficiency and reduce the disfigurement of large goitres. Going out to people could create pressure for a person to accept, but people were prepared to reject or to avoid having directly to confront hospital staff. In 1974 Dr Paul Silvester followed up on the activities of earlier vaccination campaigns. He wrote that when two student doctors conducted a house-to-house survey in 1970 they found about half the people were away from the house, and about a third of those they did see refused the injection or were on record as refusing it. [150]

Some vaccinations were more popular than others. Smallpox was still endemic in Nepal when the hospital opened and staff continued the earlier policy of Hillary's expeditions and offered smallpox vaccination. [151] The BBC television documentary filmed in late 1969 showed the Khunde doctors giving vaccinations and commenting that whereas people will decline other vaccinations they were keen to have the one for smallpox. [152] When an outbreak of measles spread from Solu into Khumbu in 1973 and caused "significant mortality" many people came to the hospital to be vaccinated as "parents thought that this was smallpox". Unfortunately many people died in the area "without disclosing their illness to the Hospital". [153]

Accepting smallpox vaccination appeared a matter for individual choice. Earlier, even the religious had adopted different strategies. As noted previously, while the young rinpoche was taken on the

150 Dr Paul Silvester to H. K. Kuloy, 5 July 1974, UNICEF representative, Kathmandu, assorted papers [KH].

151 The other vaccination being offered was BCG, to prevent tuberculosis which was common in Khumbu and had a high mortality.

152 *The Sherpas of Everest,* BBC, 1971.

153 [Kunde] Hospital Annual Report for the Year Ending October 31st, 1974.

long journey to Kathmandu in the early 1940s and vaccinated, in 1963 at Thamo the lama and monks who had recently arrived from Tibet declined the offer from Hillary's expedition on the grounds that it would show lack of faith with their own powers to deal with the disease.[154] None of the group died. It is likely that other people in the area would have felt the same way, just as Hillary did. The death of a woman, who had been vaccinated a few days earlier, added to the weight of evidence against vaccination. That she had probably already contracted the disease when she was vaccinated, so the vaccine would not have been effective, was not an appropriate Sherpa explanation. They believed the vaccine had killed her.[155]

The event of death further illustrates how Khumbu Sherpas had their own ideas about the role of the hospital. It also supports the notion of the ongoing nature of the fundamental beliefs underpinning Sherpa society, despite the external image of change, and that people continually engaged with these when deciding whether or not to use the hospital. Unlike the Western world of the volunteers where many people expect to die in hospital, in Sherpa society it was important to die at home. The inpatient register shows that out of 2,079 admissions between January 1974 and December 1997, 50 people (2.4 per cent) have died in hospital.[156] Of the deaths, 12 were stillbirths, 10 other deaths were children under the age of one year and 11 had tuberculosis as a factor. There were 34 Sherpa deaths and two where ethnicity was not listed.

The low number of deaths in the hospital was not because serious illness did not exist, nor that the hospital had been especially successful in its cure rate. Births and deaths did not have to be registered and only a very fragmentary view of the rate and causes of mortality in Khumbu is available from existing records. The evidence suggests continuity in attitudes towards death and the hospital. For example, in 1967 McKinnon wrote that all the people he had seen with acute surgical conditions refused admission "because

154 Gill, *Mountain Midsummer,* 175–77; Hillary, *Schoolhouse in the Clouds,* 47.

155 Gill, *Mountain Midsummer,* 177.

156 The current inpatient registers at the hospital begin from admission number 424 on 28 January 1974. I have not been able to find earlier inpatient records.

of their great fear of dying away from home".[157] Almost twenty years later, of the 52 deaths known to the hospital in Khumbu in the year from August 1985 only one—a newborn with respiratory distress—occurred in hospital.[158] A decade later, in the story used earlier about a woman being seriously injured when she fell off the trail, the family wanted to know whether the hospital staff thought she was going to die before they would allow her to be admitted.[159] People's belief in the importance of dying at home had not changed. This influenced decision-making about what to do when someone was seriously ill, about whether to go to hospital or stay at home and about how people viewed chances of getting better. The concern about dying away from home was increased further if staff at the hospital suggested the patient travel to Kathmandu for investigation or treatment that was beyond the capability of Khunde Hospital. As travel to Kathmandu became easier, affluence increased and health facilities expanded in Kathmandu more people went to Kathmandu and more often. Nevertheless, if the chance of a successful outcome was too low, then a person or their family was likely to decline this option.

The hospital's experience with childbirth again supports the idea and importance of continuing beliefs and practices in the community.[160] People recognised that childbirth was risky for the infant.[161] The newborn needed time to build up its spiritual protec-

157 McKinnon, "Health Problems of Khumbu in Nepal", 143.

158 Khunde Hospital Annual Report, 1 August 1985–31 July 1986.

159 Personal participation.

160 Adams suggests rather the opposite. Adams, *Tigers of the Snow and Other Virtual Sherpas,* 106–7. For a similar view to the one expressed in my analysis, although interpreted within the context of Tibetan identity, see Jennifer Chertow, "Gender, Medicine, and Modernity: Childbirth in Tibet Today: China's Control of Reproductive Choice in Tibet", *Harvard Asia Quarterly* 7, no. 4, 2003, http://www.asiaquarterly.com/content/view/140/40/. Andrea Wiley, however, suggests that in Ladakh the perception of risk from high altitude is seen to be a reason why unlike elsewhere in the Himalayan region most women use biomedical care. Andrea S. Wiley, "Increasing Use of Prenatal Care in Ladakh (India): The Roles of Ecological and Cultural Factors", *Social Science & Medicine* 55, 2002, 1089–102.

161 Adams, *Tigers of the Snow and Other Virtual Sherpas,* 106–7.

tion *(lhungtar)* and make it less vulnerable to attacks from various spirits. The mother and child did not receive visitors for the first few days and the child's naming ceremony occurred several days after the birth. [162] As already noted, sick babies brought to the hospital frequently have a charcoal spot on their nose to prevent the child being seen by ill-intentioned spirits.

There are no midwives in Sherpa society. Traditionally, women delivered their babies at home, either alone or with the assistance of their mother or sister. The important consideration for the person assisting was that it should be someone who had "good thoughts" about the woman, and not someone who might harbour "bad thoughts" which could bring problems. [163] People also liked to keep quiet when a delivery was imminent to avoid attracting the attention of pem or nerpa which could also bring trouble. Today it remains desirable for a woman in labour to avoid being seen by another woman; this, however, does not apply to the female overseas doctors at the hospital but does make travel to the hospital difficult. [164]

Birth is a highly polluting event in which traditionally men were not involved. Today men, either the husband or hospital staff, may be involved both at home and in hospital, even helping with the cleaning up. Paradoxically, male Sherpa hospital staff may be more acceptable than female. Even in the past the husband could be involved if the woman was really in need of help and there was no appropriate close female relative available. [165]

The opening of the hospital presented a new option for women. Adams believed that the Western medical approach to childbirth that women should deliver in hospital "redefined childbirth for Sherpas; the mother now was deemed as much at risk as the infant". [166] She took the example of the episiotomy procedure, referred to by Sherpa women as "the cut", and suggested that "it was clear that

162 This is still the situation.

163 Interview, Ang Rita, 2004.

164 Participant observation of cases of childbirth 1996–98.

165 Interview, Ang Rita, 2004.

166 Adams, *Tigers of the Snow and Other Virtual Sherpas*, 106–7.

contemporary Sherpanis considered an episiotomy a necessary part of a normal delivery". Adams' research in 1987 included women from both Khumjung and Kathmandu, but it is not clear whether she was including both groups in this conclusion. Childbirth experience in a large Kathmandu hospital was different from Khunde Hospital and women had less control over the circumstances. Episiotomies are performed at Khunde Hospital as it is a simpler medical procedure with fewer risks to stitch a clean cut than an uncontrolled tear that may involve a wider area. The hospital's annual report for 1986–87 recorded that Sherpa women seemed to prefer to deliver at home but called the hospital if problems occurred.[167] It is not known how many babies were born in the area during the year, but only nine were born at Khunde Hospital.[168] The doctors noted that as the WHO was promoting home deliveries aided by ancillary workers, they were, therefore, not pushing women to deliver at the hospital if their antenatal history suggested a normal delivery. A demographic survey for the five-year period 1998–2002 recently carried out by the hospital includes the total number of births in the area and shows that over 70 per cent of births still take place at home although this is still a lower level than the national average.[169]

The number of babies born in hospital has increased since McKinnon's time—and particularly from the villages nearest the hospital, but whether the doctor at the hospital was male or female does not appear to have made a significant difference to these patterns. Women were "embarrassed" at being examined.[170] Antenatal consultations rose significantly in the 1990s, but gynaecological problems remain virtually absent from the outpatient register.

Lastly, patterns of resort remain influenced by the Sherpa annual calendar of events and tasks. Mingma Norbu Sherpa, in a short booklet he wrote and published for visitors to the Sagarmatha National Park in 1982, presented the annual cycle as a series of concen-

[167] Kunde Hospital Annual Report, 1 August 1986–31 July 1987.

[168] Inpatient register.

[169] I am grateful to Dr Kami Temba for letting me see the provisional results of his demographic survey carried out for Khumbu and the adjoining area of Pharak. For later analysis, see Epilogue.

[170] Conversation with Ang Tashi Sherpa, Kenzuma, March 2004.

tric circles with each identifying the multiple concerns and activities of Sherpas throughout the year.[171] The calendar is full of festivals and activities in the fields, with the livestock and around the village. More recent additions of mountaineering and trekking feature as well as trading and pilgrimage. The life of a Sherpa in Khumbu is busy and this has affected the way people used the hospital.[172] The outpatient register reveals considerable difference in monthly totals. The winter months of December, January and February, for example, were less busy because many people left and continue to leave the area to go on pilgrimage to Kathmandu and India. Vaccination days held when work in the fields is at its busiest were less well attended. The register totals, however, do not show other practices such as that when festivals occur, people go to the hospital early in the day. Such general observations are reinforced by the practices of the hospital staff who needed time off to attend to their fields or animals and attend religious events.

Staff

While patients formed one aspect of Sherpa encounters with the hospital, a second area was as staff. As there were no Sherpa doctors and limited medical personnel in Nepal, Hillary received permission from the Nepalese government to bring in an overseas doc-

[171] Mingma Norbu Sherpa, *Sherpa Culture: Way of Life, Festivals and Religion of Sherpa People* (Kathmandu: Mingma Norbu Sherpa, 1982) (no page numbers). Mingma Norbu came from Khunde. His story, like that of many Sherpas, began in the village and attending a Hillary school. Later, after tertiary education overseas, he became (in 1980) the first Sherpa warden of the Sagarmatha National Park. He was killed in a helicopter crash in 2006.

[172] McKay notes (p. 150) a medical report from the 1933 visit of a British mission to Bhutan that comments on one reason for the light workload being that the people were "more concerned about their crops than their ailments". Alex McKay, "British-Indian Medical Service Officers in Bhutan, 1905–1947: A Historical Outline", in *The Spider and the Piglet: Proceedings of the First International Seminar on Bhutan Studies,* ed. Karma Ura and Sonam Kinga (Thimphu, Bhutan: Centre for Bhutan Studies, 2004), 137–59, available online at http://www.bhutanstudies.org.bt/publications/spdr-pglt/spdr-pglt.htm

tor to provide the medical services at Khunde Hospital. From the perspective of local Sherpas, having foreign doctors run the hospital was not seen as a problem, because there was no one else to do it.[173] From the beginning, the volunteers employed local staff to assist with the many tasks involved in running the hospital.[174] These staff played a key mediating role in educating both the overseas volunteers about living and working in Sherpa society and the patients about being at the hospital. The small number of staff usually knew the community well and guided the volunteers through their time at the hospital, advising on the myriad issues that affected both the medical and social aspects of being at Khunde. Very few non-Sherpas or Sherpas from outside Khumbu, have been employed at the hospital, and so the volunteers were drawn into a Sherpa world and particularly the Sherpa world of Khumbu.

Khunde Hospital was and remains a small institution. One of the characteristic features of such establishments was that they had few personnel but that they performed a wide range of tasks. The hospital's first employee was Nima Yangen, whose father Khunjo Chumbi was one of the leading men of Khumjung village and supported the hospital. In 1960 he had accompanied Khumjung's yeti scalp around the world as Hillary sought to verify its authenticity. Yangen, as she was more usually known, did not go to the newly established school built by Hillary. Although Sherpas had asked for education, it was not popular with all the community and boys were more likely to go to school than girls. When she was 16 years old, her father took her for the first time to Kathmandu to Shanta Bhawan Hospital which was run by the United Mission to Nepal. On an earlier occasion Khunjo Chumbi had met the American doctor, Bethel Fleming, who ran the hospital as Yangen's mother, Pali, had been treated at the hospital. She developed problems after giving birth along the track while walking to Kathmandu to meet Queen Elizabeth of England who was visiting Nepal.[175] Yangen recalls that

173 Personal communication, Dr Kami Temba, August 2005.

174 Chapter one discussed the increasing administrative functions of the local staff within the hospital and the Trust, while medical issues such as training and qualifications are considered in the next chapter.

175 Hillary, *Schoolhouse in the Clouds,* 101.

her father presented her to Dr Fleming and said "Teach her!" [176] To Yangen, who now lives in Kathmandu like many Khumbu Sherpas, the city contrasted greatly with her home in the mountains. Kathmandu was "very big" and the hospital, where she spent about three years, "very clean". [177] As she had had no schooling, her training was practical rather than a formal nursing course. When Yangen met Hillary in 1966, he said she could go and work at the nearly-finished hospital at Khunde.

In its use of local personnel, the hospital became both an employer and one of the few that offered an alternative to expedition work or tourism which, in the late-1960s, was still in the very early stages of development. There were no independent Sherpa trekking companies. While the overseas medical staff went to Khunde for a variety of reasons and were volunteers for whom financial remuneration was minimal, the local staff throughout regarded working at the hospital as a "job" with expectations about conditions and payment. While Yangen's duties at Khunde were to help the doctor with the patients, people brought food and drink to the hospital and she went with the volunteers to lots of parties. [178] In contrast to the cold houses in the village, the hospital was warm and she and the McKinnons often talked late into the evening. After Yangen married in 1968 she moved to Kathmandu with her husband, but otherwise would have stayed at the hospital. She regarded work at the hospital as "easy", in comparison to the hard work of being a woman in Sherpa society. Sherpa women planted and dug potatoes, weeded the fields, collected firewood and cut grass. Roles and activities differed, but there was almost no segregation of the sexes and unlike the situation for most women in Nepal, Sherpa society was not a "heavily sexist or male-dominant one". [179] The following example illustrates what may appear to outsiders as contradictions.

[176] Interview, Nima Yangen, 2003. Also see Grace Nies Fletcher, *The Fabulous Flemings of Kathmandu: The Story of Two Doctors in Nepal* (London: Quality Book Club, 1964), 187–90.

[177] Interview, Nima Yangen, 2003. This was a comment on the contrast between the hospital and the dirt of Kathmandu and Khumbu.

[178] Ibid.

[179] Ortner, *Life and Death on Mt. Everest,* 232.

In the home, the senior male in the household had the best seat in the house beside the fire, but the women had the right to the seat in front of the fire. With a closed fire and a cold house the seat in front was the warmest.

Throughout most of the period since the hospital opened three staff assisted the volunteers, with the workload dividing into nursing or medical functions, cooking, cleaning and other general and administrative duties. At any time the exact division of duties varied according to the capabilities and ideas of the different personnel. Relations between the volunteers and local staff were mostly harmonious, but from the local staff's point of view, one area of work where there did appear to have been some unhappiness was washing laundry.[180] Yangen pointed out that while she washed the instruments she did not do the hospital laundry. Ang Pasang became cook at the hospital in 1970, replacing Ang Pema who had had an argument about washing patients' clothes and had left. Ang Pasang stayed at the hospital until early 1979. His duties included cooking, washing and helping with the medical work. Laundry appeared to have been less of an issue when there were female staff, but when these staff were away male staff took on this duty and were less happy about doing other people's personal laundry. Washing dishes was not an issue. Local staff and volunteers ate together and in the 1990s all shared in the clearing up after a meal. In Sherpa homes, women did most of the household work, but men were not excluded.

Significant changes in the staffing situation occurred that reflected issues within the hospital and the Trust and the employment situation in Khumbu. Throughout the 1970s staff changed frequently, although Ang Pasang provided continuity for the volunteers. Outside the hospital Hillary's sirdar, Mingma Tsering, played the key support and mediating role. One of the factors influencing recruitment and retention was pay. While Sherpa society is clan-based, money and wealth are also important signs of status in Sherpa society. Before returning to Khunde and employment at the hospital Ang Pasang had worked as a cook at the British Embassy in

[180] I did not ask about this issue, but looking back at my notes I found that people had referred to it directly or indirectly.

Kathmandu. During his nine years at the hospital, in a job that he described as busy, his monthly pay increased nearly five times, but inflation was high in Khumbu.[181] Rising prices also affected staple foods. A tin of potatoes increased in price from NR 2 in 1964, to NR 14 in 1974 and NR 25 in 1988.[182] The amount Ang Pasang earned was still much less than what his friends in the trekking industry earned, although the pay was considerably more than that of the junior and less experienced staff at the hospital. Fisher describes labour shortage when he returned in 1974, which was a reversal of the situation he had observed in 1964.[183] Employment at the hospital offered other advantages. People in the village thought Yangen had a "good job" because it lasted year-round.[184] Employment in the tourist industry revolved around two peak seasons in the spring and autumn.

Since 1981 the local staff situation at the hospital has been stable. One reason for this was that from the 1990s, in particular, key staff regarded themselves as much better off financially. Between 1981 and 1995 only one staff change occurred at the hospital when in 1991 Tsumje replaced Doma Leh. Both these women were from Khunde. The other two members of staff were Kami Temba from Thame and Mingma Temba from Khunde. Kami Temba was first employed as a village health worker in Thame in 1976 before starting work at Khunde Hospital the following year. In 1997 he was accepted to study medicine at the School of Medicine in Fiji, and in 2002 he became the first Sherpa doctor in charge of Khunde Hospital. Mingma Temba has worked at the hospital continuously since early in 1979, both assisting in the clinic and acting as hospital manager when Kami Temba left to go to Fiji.

Each new member of staff, whether local or overseas, had to be inducted into the life and work at the hospital. There were no trained Sherpa health workers. In the beginning the onus was on the volunteers to teach the new local staff member who was often

181 Brower, *Sherpa of Khumbu,* 88–89; Fisher, *Sherpas,* 115–16.

182 Fisher, *Sherpas,* 116.

183 Ibid., 117.

184 Interview, Nima Yangen, 2003.

young. Secular education was a recent introduction to Khumbu and some of the hospital's local staff were still at school during the 1970s when staff turnover was at its highest at the hospital. This stabilised during the 1980s. By the early 1990s the volunteers' Handbook stated that: "It is difficult to characterize Kami and Mingma's jobs as they do so much! They function as interpreters, health workers, nurses and much, much more. They essentially run the hospital. Since early 1991 Kami has also been keeping the accounts." [185] They also assisted patients in what could still be a very unfamiliar situation. The hospital, for example, had electricity from November 1994, but some inpatients came from areas without electricity. They had to be shown how to use electrical equipment, such as the small cooking stove that patients and their families used in the kitchen attached to the long-stay ward. Kami Temba and Mingma Temba were also happier at their improved status rather than being referred to as "the boys". [186] Their knowledge of the local community and advice about issues was valued and their increasing medical expertise, both in the clinical work and as interpreters, made them more valuable to the volunteers. This applied even more as the hospital's medical workload rose during the 1980s with the number of outpatients increasing from 2,722 in 1980 to 6,066 in 1990.

The role of interpreter was a key aspect of the way the hospital operated. The local language was Sherpa, while the first language of the incoming volunteers was English. In Khumbu in the 1960s most of the women only spoke Sherpa, although an increasing number of men also spoke Nepali to varying levels. Those involved with expedition work had more familiarity with Nepali, as well as other languages such as English. Children who went to school started to learn Nepali as this was the language used for teaching. At the beginning parents were more likely to send their sons to school, but in a 1989 household survey hospital volunteer, Dr Marianne Wood, found that female literacy was increasing at a "rapid and steady rate—almost identical, in fact, to that of the male population

[185] The Handbook underwent various revisions. This version in hospital files is undated and unpaginated.

[186] Conversation with Dr Kami Temba, Khunde, April 2004. He knew their jobs depended on how well they got on with volunteers and this varied.

when the schools first opened. Popularity for educating daughters has simply started 20 years later."[187] School attendance between the ages 6–14 years was 69 per cent, but while in Khumjung 78 per cent of girls went to school, in Thame it was only 15 per cent. The greatest imbalance occurred in the higher grades.[188] One result of this has been that there were few girls who had enough education to be accepted for government courses to train health workers.

The volunteers had two choices. They could learn the language, or they could work through an interpreter. In the early years of the hospital, the volunteers often developed good language skills. Frequent changes among local hospital staff, or staff having limited English, encouraged the overseas volunteers to learn either some Sherpa or Nepali. The role of medical interpreter is skilled and requires knowledge of a specialist medical vocabulary. As the local staff developed both their medical and English language skills their relationship with the volunteers changed. They could do more in the hospital and they could converse better with the volunteers and the increasing number of visitors to the hospital. There was also less pressure on the volunteers to learn a language, especially as an increasing level of English was being spoken in the community. English was the mostly widely spoken language in the developing tourism industry and an ability to speak English increased a person's chances of obtaining employment. People wanted the volunteers to help them improve their English.[189]

The local staff's role at the hospital, however, was always more than literal translating. The Sherpa staff learned how to translate between the language and culturally conditioned medical concepts of their own world and that of the outsiders. A patient would relate their symptoms to the local member of staff. Experienced staff would then work out what they thought was the medical problem and ask the appropriate medical questions. This would be relayed to the doctor. The conversation would go to and fro via the interpeter

[187] Dr Marianne Wood, "1989 Survey of Khumbu Region of Nepal" (KH).

[188] Fisher, *Sherpas,* 78–79.

[189] Ortner also noted this while carrying out her research. Ortner, *Life and Death on Mt. Everest,* 15.

until the doctor was clear about the problem, could make a diagnosis and pronounce what was to be done. For example, epigastric pain was one of the commonest reasons for people going to the hospital and patients received antacid or ulcer-healing medicines. The probable cause of the problem, from a biomedical perspective, is due to infection by an organism called *Helicobacter pylori,* but Dr John Heydon was at the hospital for several months in 1996 before he discovered that many patients believed they had been poisoned by a pem. [190] Medical assistant Mingma Temba was negotiating a way through two different sets of beliefs.

Community

The third area of Sherpa contact with Khunde Hospital was at the broader societal level. While the local community petitioned Hillary for different kinds of assistance and, as with other projects, had helped to build Khunde Hospital, their participation in running the hospital was the area where Sherpa involvement appeared less successful. [191] Yet in spite of the limited formal involvement by the community, Khunde Hospital and those living and working there have been closely bound up with the Sherpa world of Khumbu.

Although the prime function of the hospital was to provide health services to the people of the area, the hospital always had a wider role. Firstly, many people had to go to the hospital for reasons other than when they were ill. [192] It was not just a place of fear and sickness or death. For example, teachers went to the hospital to collect extra pay (for working in arduous conditions) while students picked up their scholarships or attended health education talks. Other people received various kinds of financial assistance, such as pensions. Some of the volunteers held lessons in English or craft activities. The kitchen area of the hospital is situated between the clinic room

190 Personal communication. Prior to the early 1980s it was thought that stress and lifestyle caused this problem. Fisher notes a rise among Sherpas in stress-related conditions including ulcers. Fisher, *Sherpas,* 166.

191 This would certainly be the "development" point of view and is considered in chapter four.

192 See chapter one.

and the doctor's flat and was always a space of considerable community business and social activity. While the mail runner was employed for hospital and Trust business, he also carried mail to and from Kathmandu for other people throughout the area. [193] When a telephone service was established in Khumbu in early 1995 and the only line in Khunde given to the hospital, people in the village were able to receive and send faxes and use the telephone. This enabled them to keep in contact with family in Kathmandu or overseas and pursue business arrangements.

While the overall relationship between hospital and community was good, some volunteers were more popular than others and things at times went wrong. The difficulty in interpreting examples of problems from a Sherpa perspective is that most of the sources for these situations are derived from others. Sometimes problems between the hospital and the local community, or parts of it, arose as a result of medical issues, but other examples occurred that related to the hospital's wider role or its existence in Khumbu. Hillary's rule was to keep out of religion and politics. [194] Problems were most likely to occur when the volunteers stepped over an invisible boundary. For example, tensions arose in the early 1990s when Mingma Tsering was reported to the national park authorities for cutting down some trees. [195]

While use of the hospital might be interpreted in terms of Sherpas entering the modern world, this would be only partly true. As Ortner has emphasised, they had their own agendas about what was important for Sherpas. [196] At times people thought that the hospital could assist in what outsiders would consider the "traditional" Sherpa world. For example, periodically monks requested hospital staff for syringes to help in the intricate butter decorations of the *torma* (offering cakes) used in religious ceremonies.

[193] There is a post office in Namche Bazar, but sometimes there were no stamps.

[194] Interview, Hillary, 2002.

[195] Correspondence files at Khunde Hospital.

[196] Ortner, *Life and Death on Mt. Everest.*

Also, not all the changes in Khumbu were about modernisation or the encounter with the West. The development and responses to a new structure of celibate monasticism in Khumbu, which followed the founding of Tengboche monastery in 1916, were about strengthening traditional values of religion and attaining merit. These were central concerns for Sherpa society. Ortner discusses how a number of Hindu influences, such as the worshiping of a Nepalese god, had crept into Sherpa ritual but were removed.[197]

The Sherpas and Khumbu were also being integrated within Nepal.[198] In the 1950s Tenzing described how: "In Solo Khumbu we were remote from the rest of the country. What went on there did not seem to affect us; we had our own customs and ways of life, and knew almost nothing about the nation of which we were politically a part."[199] Sherpas saw the distant Kathmandu Valley as "Nepal". The early patient registers at the hospital contain Sherpa village names, but by the early 1970s most of the villages of the adjacent Pharak area were recorded with Nepalese names. "Sano Gumila", for example, replaced "Gyuphete" and "Rimijung" became "Thulo Gumila".[200]

While this process of Nepalisation occurred throughout the country, the Sherpa as an ethnic group have increased their status within Nepal. This was reflected, for example, in the way Sherpas were recorded in national censuses. Although early censuses asked questions about caste and ethnicity, the information was not published.[201] In 1952/54 questions were introduced and reported on language and religion, but the 1991 census was the first to publish

197 Ibid., 107–10.

198 The expanding Nepalese state is discussed further in chapters three and four.

199 Tenzing Norgay, *Man of Everest,* 145.

200 The Supplement to the *National Geographic,* May 2003 (the 50th anniversary of the ascent of Everest) provides both names, but this is unusual. I would like to thank Mingma Temba for his help with the many village names and their different spellings that appear in the hospital registers. These relate to Khumbu, the wider Solukhumbu district and elsewhere in Nepal.

201 Harka Gurung, *Nepal: Social Demography and Expressions* (Kathmandu: New Era, 2001), 35–36.

the ethnic and caste composition of the Nepalese population.[202] Despite their small numbers of less than 1 per cent of the population, the Sherpa became a separate category.[203] Previously they had been classified with other *Bhote* (ethnically Tibetan) groups who continued to be grouped under this more derogatory term.[204]

Khunde Hospital, with its overseas staff, was not a Sherpa institution and yet to a certain extent was incorporated into Sherpa life. Situated on the edge of Khunde, the volunteers had their closest social relations with this village. While the volunteers respected the local culture and participated in local activities, the position given to them at events was on Sherpa terms. The Khunde doctor was treated with respect, but at a party was of lesser status than the senior male member of the household and other senior men in the village or, if female, the senior women in the village.[205] Ortner in 1970 discussed seating arrangements at parties and how this was an important part of ritual and an expression of hierarchy within Sherpa society.[206] Local staff also had their own individual position within Sherpa society. It was important, therefore, for the hospital's acceptance in the community that staff were suitable socially and, since home visits invariably involved cups of tea, could participate in Sherpa hospitality. Not all were permitted to share a communal cup. In 1997, when the hospital was looking to employ a new medical assistant, this issue was a key factor in deciding on the suitability of applicants.[207]

Participation within village life had obligations. If staff wished to go to parties held at *Losar* (New Year), then it was expected that the

202 Following the success of the "People's Movement" in 1990, different ethnicity became more acceptable.

203 Central Bureau of Statistics, *Statistical Year Book of Nepal 2001*, 12 and 52. The 1991 population census recorded 110,358 Sherpa and a total Nepalese population of 18,491,097. Fisher, however, notes that the Sherpa Cultural Centre at Tengboche lists 30,000 Sherpas. Fisher, *Sherpas,* 187.

204 Bista, *People of Nepal*, 159. Also see Kunwar, *Fire of Himal,* 121–22.

205 Personal participation.

206 Ortner Paul, "Food for Thought", 316–21.

207 Personal participation.

hospital would also take its turn and hold a party.[208] The situation was the same at *Phangni* (summer festival). If staff wished to join in, then they too paid a sum of money into the kitty for the supply of food and drink for what was often a party lasting for about five days. At Dumje, however, the volunteers could attend, but the hospital was not expected to take on the onerous financial responsibility of becoming a sponsor. Dumje was a festival for the whole community to celebrate the anniversary of the death of the founder of Khumbu's first gompa, Lama Sanga Dorje, and to request the gods "to subdue demonic enemies of the village".[209] Houseowners took it in turn to meet the costs of this most important village religious event and von Fürer-Haimendorf believed that recent immigrants to the area gained social recognition by assuming responsibility in the discharge of public duties.[210]

Sherpa involvement with Khunde Hospital, therefore, operated in three spheres: they were patients, staff or community. I have discussed issues specifically in relation to Khunde Hospital, but what was happening regarding Sherpas and Khunde Hospital was an integral part of the events of the broader Sherpa world of Khumbu since the 1960s. Khunde Hospital both contributed to what occurred around it and in turn was influenced by the process. In the last part of this chapter I use examples from some of the limited, although slowly increasing, amount of written work by Sherpas to consider their views of change and the place of Khunde Hospital in the transformation of Khumbu.

Sherpa Views of Change and the Place of Khunde Hospital

From the early 1950s to the present, visitors from outside Nepal have placed the Sherpas and Khumbu in a discourse of change. Although little has been written from a Sherpa perspective, unlike the opinions expressed by the area's increasing number of visitors, Sherpas also considered and debated over change. Tenzing Norgay

208 The Trust acknowledges this is an important function of the hospital and pays.

209 Mingma Norbu, *Sherpa Culture,* no page numbers.

210 Von Fürer-Haimendorf, *The Sherpas of Nepal,* 101.

referred to change in his first autobiography published in 1955. Unlike most Western writers who considered change in response to the West's entry into the Everest area, Tenzing reflected on Sherpas who had moved to Darjeeling and had begun a new way of life as "town people".[211] Tenzing contrasted these to the "country people" of Solukhumbu. He saw Sherpas as being able to adapt to new ideas and ways of doing things. He was positive about the concept of change, and even though he was less happy about some of the younger people knowing little of Sherpa customs and the language he concluded that "at least it is better to learn and grow and make mistakes than always to go on the same".[212] Even though this book was written with the American author James Ramsey Ullman, this last idea was quite different to other Western writers who tended to view the old ways with a rosy hue.

His second autobiography, which was told to Malcolm Barnes, was published in 1977. It recounted his life after Everest and was much more gloomy, both in discussing his personal life and Solukhumbu. While he did not blame Sherpas for wanting economic development, he was pessimistic about the effects on Sherpa culture.[213] He praised much of Hillary's work in education, but believed the school "in the end is certain to destroy the traditional way of life, at least as I know it".[214] He was positive about Khunde Hospital which he visited for the first time in 1969.

In his introduction to *Tenzing and the Sherpas of Everest,* Tenzing's grandson, Tashi Tenzing, wrote that the aim of the book was

> to give all Sherpas the recognition and credit they have so long deserved. It is written to remove the veil of anonymity which they have worn for most of the past one hundred years. It is written to expose their weak-

[211] Tenzing Norgay, *Man of Everest,* 126–27.

[212] Ibid., 134.

[213] Tenzing Norgay Sherpa (as told to Malcolm Barnes), *After Everest: An Autobiography* (London: George Allen & Unwin, 1977), 41–43. An inherent sadness with his life existed underneath Tenzing's smiling face and is clear throughout the book.

[214] Tenzing Norgay, *After Everest*, 139.

> nesses and problems and explain the challenges they have faced and still encounter.[215]

Tashi reflected on their rapidly changing world and believed the impact had been both positive and negative. The early isolated, subsistence life was tough and the opportunities through climbing brought increasing affluence. On the other hand:

> Where once we lost our people to illness and poor harvests we now have wonderful medical facilities, schools and food aplenty. However, that which we held so true before this change—a deeply ingrained sense of tradition, cultural strength, and a family and social structure which bound us all together—is now being weakened and slowly dismantled by the intrusion of a new world which offers comparatively so much more excitement, comfort and variety to our young people.[216]

Yet, like his grandfather forty years earlier, he viewed Sherpas as able to "adapt well and quickly". Consequently he felt confident that they "will survive this transformation with our culture and our ancient values intact".

Although he came from Darjeeling, the Sherpa world that Tashi Tenzing described was that of the Everest area. As Nepal became the centre for much of the climbing in the Himalaya, the focus for mountaineering expeditions had shifted away from Darjeeling. Most Sherpas lived in Solukhumbu and "this community holds the key to the future of the Sherpa culture and way of life".[217] Hillary's work had given many Sherpas a basic education before the advent of mass tourism "giving them a measure of 'breathing space' in which to prepare mentally and culturally for the ways of the West". The way Hillary worked by responding to Sherpa requests, involving them in the process and ultimately devolving responsibility to them had "empowered" them.

In *Triumph on Everest: A Tribute from the Sherpas of Nepal*, produced to celebrate the fiftieth anniversary of the first ascent of Everest, Khumbu Sherpas have written several short contributions that refer

215 Judy and Tashi Tenzing, *Tenzing and the Sherpas of Everest,* xxi–xxii.

216 Ibid., xx.

217 Ibid., 190.

to development and change in their region.[218] For example, Ang Tsering Sherpa, President of the Nepal Mountaineering Association, acknowledges Hillary's support and contribution and names three key projects—Khumjung School, Lukla airport and Khunde Hospital.[219] Throughout this small book emerge the different strands in Sherpa views of their changing world: the harshness of life in the 1950s that nobody wished to return to; the opportunities presented by education for individual lives and the ability of the community to cope with the tourism that has underpinned the economic development of the region; the development of an infrastructure of which health care was an integral part and the services offered at Khunde Hospital were modern medicine; and the important role of Sherpas in shaping their own future. They wished to enjoy this development but within a strong Sherpa culture, which for them emphasised the "inside" values rather than "outside" trappings which, though important, have less meaning. People's use of Khunde Hospital reflected this view of the wider Sherpa world of Khumbu.

Conclusion

Hillary built Khunde Hospital to provide Western style medical services for the people of the area, but although the new medical system brought changes that increased over time it did not displace the old. Khunde Hospital became incorporated into a plural medical environment that Sherpas saw in terms of options rather than conflicting systems.

Most historical studies about the introduction and spread of Western medicine among different cultures portray an earlier period than the second half of the twentieth century, when the distance of time may make it easier to acknowledge the existence of harmful and benevolent spirits. It is much harder to dismiss such beliefs as mere superstition when, despite all the changes that have occurred

[218] Ang Rita Sherpa and Susan Höivik, eds, *Sherpas on Everest: A Tribute from the Sherpas of Nepal* (Kathmandu: Mandala Book Point, 2003). This Ang Rita is the son of Mingma Tsering and his wife Ang Dooli.

[219] Ang Rita and Höivik, *Sherpas on Everest*, 82.

for Sherpas in the past fifty years, the resilience of their spirit-suffused belief system was clearly evident in the late 1990s and not just among the predominantly rural population that by definition Khunde Hospital treats. Each day people came to the hospital or were seen in the community who were well educated and with some having trained overseas, or were people who travelled to and from Kathmandu or overseas, or people who worked with the thousands of visitors who annually visit the area.

While ethnographic studies of Sherpas acknowledge to varying degrees that people adopt a plural approach to dealing with sickness, this chapter has explored Sherpa encounters with Khunde Hospital from a historical perspective to see whether or how people have incorporated Khunde Hospital and its biomedical practice into their lives between the mid-1960s and the late-1990s. It is not an ethnographic study of who are the Sherpa at the end of the twentieth century. Nor have my sources allowed me to analyse how categories such as class or status influence patient use and non-use of the hospital.

While many people in Khumbu would have heard of the type of medicine offered by Khunde Hospital in 1966 and some, such as those employed by the expeditions or those living on an expedition route, may have used it, Sherpa beliefs and practices about sickness at the time the hospital opened revolved around a different system to that of the overseas volunteers who came from New Zealand to work at the hospital. The Sherpa world of gods, spirits, ghosts and pollution, and the healing practices of lama and lhawa were the key to understanding Sherpa responses to sickness, both in terms of traditional practices and also their engagement with other medical systems, which included being a patient at Khunde Hospital. Thirty years later a Sherpa world of sickness was still the key to understanding people's use of the hospital.

Within this broad picture, however, multiple strands exist of people's multiple, ongoing and varying encounters with the hospital, its staff and biomedicine over time. Every Sherpa and his or family has their own story or stories. Nevertheless, in examining the broad encounter of Khumbu Sherpas with Khunde Hospital the conclusion that emerges is that a mixture of continuity and change has occurred since the hospital opened in 1966. As such, this study concurs with the findings of others regarding the introduction and spread of biomedicine in the Himalayan region, but projects these responses to a more recent period of time. The degree of change was considerable and must not be overlooked, but what may be surprising to outsiders if not Sherpas, was the extent of continuity in their beliefs and practices about sickness and that these informed people's responses to Khunde Hospital and the provision of Western medicine.

The findings of this chapter suggest that Adams has overemphasised the degree of modernisation that has occurred. Sherpas in Khumbu were curious about the hospital but not overawed, and despite Draper's concern about their lack of control of biomedical knowledge, they showed considerable agency in their use and non-use of the hospital's services. While the number of patients at the hospital has risen considerably, people used the hospital selectively and pragmatically, primarily based around their perception of the efficacy of an intervention. Going to the doctor and taking the hospital's medicines could treat symptoms but did not prevent people from consulting a lama or lhawa who would deal with the root cause of a problem. These other practitioners also had to deal with the changing Khumbu environment and experienced varying fortunes that are both beyond the scope of this book and often about issues other than choices between different or conflicting medical systems.

Khunde Hospital also had a wider role in Sherpa society than just as a place to go when sick as it was embedded in a network of different relationships with people in the community. Furthermore, it was a part of Hillary's overall programme. Khunde Hospital was also an employer, and although only small it was important because unlike the tourism industry it offered long-term work. The local staff played an important role in the introduction and acceptance of the hospital and Western medical practice, because they educated the overseas staff about living and working in a Sherpa community and particularly through their role of interpreter they mediated between hospital and community. Staff stability since the early 1980s, and their increasing medical and language skills, contributed to senior local staff taking on more important roles in the medical work and the running of both the hospital and Hillary's other projects in the area.

Khunde Hospital was, however, just one of many changes occurring in Sherpa lives throughout this period. It was a force for change and was in turn influenced by what was occurring around it. Sherpa written accounts viewed the hospital as an integral part of necessary modernisation, but saw that there were both positive and negative sides to a process that has led to major political, economic and social changes for the people and the place. This chapter's examination of sickness and people's use of Khunde Hospital provides a way of examining how people dealt with something new and shows the constant and piecemeal negotiation that has occurred since the hospital opened in 1966. After more than thirty years Khunde Hospital was used widely and was the main provider of biomedical services, yet it remained for many reasons embedded in a Sherpa world where Sherpa beliefs in sickness causation still prevailed and where Sherpas considered Western medicine to be an option rather than an automatic choice and an option that could be used in conjunction with other practices. By the late 1990s hospital and community were used to and allowed for each other's different ways. The next chapter explores the hospital's side of the encounter.

3

Khunde Hospital as a Western Medicine Project

> There is great need for a small hospital in the Khumbu region; one doctor and a dozen beds would probably be enough initially. It would then be possible for really sick people to come from the surrounding villages for treatment and stay in the hospital without depleting their small store of money in paying for accommodation. It would also be feasible to initiate and supervise health schemes such as the introduction of iodine, regular vaccinations and so on. I can think of no more satisfying task for a doctor than a couple of years spent working among these fine mountain people.
>
> Sir Edmund Hillary, *Schoolhouse in the Clouds,* 112

This vision of Sir Edmund Hillary for health services in Khumbu not only served as a blueprint for the project at the beginning, but also continued to frame the structure and functioning of Khunde Hospital. Hillary's unwritten assumption here was that the hospital would provide modern, Western style biomedical services which the area lacked and which he believed could do much to improve the health of the local population. The extreme physical environment of Khumbu and its isolation provided many challenges for the provision of services, but Khunde Hospital quickly became the main source of medical services in Khumbu and has functioned ever since as the main face of Western medicine for the local population.

The aim of this chapter is to examine the medical work of Khunde Hospital. Many factors affect the provision of health care services, but I argue that the task of those providing these services was challenged by the physical environment, the health problems that existed and also by how the mainly Sherpa inhabitants of the area regarded Western medicine. (From this perspective, the chapter should be read not as a continuation of the previous one, but instead be seen as considering the other side of the sickness encounter. Some evidence, therefore, is relevant for both.) Khumbu contained a small population in a remote, rugged, cold and high-altitude area of a poor country and the health issues dealt with by staff at the hospital reflected this environment. At the same time, as discussed in the last chapter, local Sherpas regarded Khunde Hospital as one of a range of options available when sick and used its services on a pragmatic and selective basis. While complementary or alternative medical practices have gained in popularity at the expense of allopathic medicine in Western countries, the overseas staff of Khunde Hospital were aware that the position was reversed in Khumbu. Local Sherpas viewed Western medicine, even if modern, as alternative and complementary.

A key concern of this chapter is the way in which the staff engaged in an ongoing dialogue with Sherpa beliefs and practices; it records the overseas volunteers' responses and how they adapted their practice of Western medicine to the plural medical environment that existed in Khumbu. Although patient responses and the mediating role of local staff have been discussed in the literature, similar attention has not been given to the Western practitioners—although doctors are the people most likely to have written accounts of their life and work.[1] Despite local people's increasing use of the hospital, providing health services at Khunde Hospital has involved a process of accommodation between Sherpa beliefs and practices and those of Western medicine, which has resulted in a coexistence of difference rather than the transformation of either.

[1] For one of the few articles that does consider a dialogue between medical practice and cultural beliefs and practices, see David Gordon, "A Sword of Empire? Medicine and Colonialism at King William's Town, Xhosaland, 1856–91", in *Medicine and Colonial Identity,* ed. Mary P. Sutphen and Bridie Andrews (London: Routledge, 2003), 41–60. Gordon discusses how one colonial doctor in rural nineteenth century South Africa at times changed his practice due to local pressures or colonial policy. For discussion of a twentieth century practitioner in the Canadian Arctic, also a colonial context, see Frank James Tester and Paule McNicoll, "'Why Don't They Get It?' Talk of Medicine as Science: St Luke's Hospital, Panniqtuuq, Baffin Island", *Social History of Medicine* 19, no. 1, 2006, 87–106.

Each acknowledged and could incorporate aspects of the other's beliefs and practices when dealing with a person's sickness, and yet remained separate systems.

While the main focus of the hospital's work was the local population, the rise of tourism in the region brought an increasing number of visitors to Khumbu. Sickness was common and tourists became patients at Khunde Hospital. Some of the health problems were the same as those experienced by the local residents, but the most important hazard for visitors was, and despite increasing knowledge continues to be, the effects of high altitude. Some aspects of tourist or trekker health created difficulties for the staff at the hospital as visitor needs and wants often differed from those of the local population.

The first part of the chapter considers Khumbu's health issues from a biomedical perspective. It examines what and how information was gained about the health problems of Sherpas and then looks at the introduction and limited development of Western medicine in Nepal by the 1960s. The second and major part of the chapter discusses practising medicine at Khunde Hospital. It begins by looking at the work of the first doctor, John McKinnon, and his acknowledgement that he was providing health care in a plural medical environment. Many of these early issues remained important. Despite increasing use of the hospital, staff were engaged in an ongoing encounter with Sherpa beliefs and practices in their efforts to provide both curative and preventive health services. Overseas staff considered that the region's iodine deficiency was the major public health problem and a case study of the hospital's policies and practices, together with discussions about research and health education highlight the complexity and array of issues involved in medical practice at Khunde Hospital. The section concludes with a discussion about a very different group of patients—tourists. Visitors to the Everest area struggled to cope with the challenges of the high-altitude environment and also have had a wider influence on medical practice in the area. The final part of the chapter examines the development of village-based services so that some health care could be provided close to where people lived.

A Western Medical View of Health Problems Among Khumbu Sherpas

Until the early 1960s scant information from a biomedical perspective was available about health and disease patterns among Khumbu Sherpas. The Nepalese government was the main health service provider, but no permanent services existed in Khumbu until this period.[2] Although Western doctors came into contact with Khumbu Sherpas earlier, particularly through the latter's employment on expeditions during the first half of the twentieth century, these encounters occurred away from their high-altitude home areas. Similarly, the British Army examined Gurkha recruits from the central hill areas of Nepal, but this revealed little about disease patterns in their home communities.[3] The growth in biomedical knowledge about Sherpas and health problems in Nepal coincided with the opening up of the country during the 1950s. It also came at a time when the dependency on Western knowledge, as Randall Packard has written, "was the first principle of all development schemes"[4], development was becoming internationalised and an international health focus was increasingly on an Asia that was decolonising and emerging as a region of nation-states.[5] Against this background, the Nepalese government increased its influence and knowledge, medical visitors from other countries observed, treated and wrote about their experiences and, as will be discussed further in the next chapter, international aid agencies and secular and religious non-

[2] Some smallpox vaccination was carried out "by a United Nations doctor at approximately 5-yearly intervals". M. B. Gill, "The Sherpas: A Survey of an Isolated Mountain Community" (Department of Preventive and Social Medicine diss., University of Otago, 1961), 16. As noted in chapter one, in 1963 Hillary refers to the presence of a medical orderly at the checkpost at Namche Bazar. Hillary, *Schoolhouse in the Clouds,* 48.

[3] Frederick L. Dunn, "Medical-Geographical Observations in Central Nepal", *Milbank Memorial Fund Quarterly* 40, 1962, 125–48.

[4] Packard, "Visions of Postwar Health and Development", in Cooper and Packard, *International Development and the Social Sciences,* 101.

[5] Cooper and Packard, "Introduction", in Cooper and Packard, *International Development and the Social Sciences,* 8–9.

government organisations (NGOs) arrived in Nepal to promote and assist with the development of the country.

As there were no government officials based in the area and few outside visitors, the earliest medical references to the health status of Khumbu residents may be those gathered secretly by Indian explorer Hari Ram for the Survey of India in 1885.[6] Hari Ram was disguised as a "*baid* (physician)" and carried with him "a stock of European and native medicines".[7] His plans to travel to Tibet received a temporary setback when the Governor of the district refused to allow him to continue.

> The explorer had therefore to make a lengthened stay at this place, during which time he endeavoured to ingratiate himself with the inhabitants by treating their sick. One of the commonest diseases in the locality was goitre, and as he succeeded in curing the Governor's daughter-in-law of this he was naturally taken into favour.[8]

We do not know Hari Ram's method of treatment or which medical system he employed, but it is known that in the nineteenth century iodine was used in the South Asia region for the treatment of goitre, was known about by the British and that iodine-bearing remedies

[6] Report on Routes by Explorer Hari Ram, *Records of the Survey of India*, 8 (2): 383–99. For an account of the Indian explorers, see Indra Singh Rawat, *Indian Explorers of the Nineteenth Century: An Account of Indian Explorers in the Himalayas, Tibet, Mongolia and Central Asia* (Delhi: Publications Division, Ministry of Information and Broadcasting, Government of India, 1973).

[7] Report on Routes by Explorer Hari Ram, *Records of the Survey of India,* 8 (2): 383. This was the usual practice. "I have always made my explorers take a supply of medicines with them, mostly of native kinds, with only a few ordinary European sorts to present to people on their journeys." Memorandum on the Trans-Himalayan Explorations for 1871, by Major T. G. Montgomerie, R. E., Deputy Superintendent G. T. Survey, in charge of the Trans-Himalayan Exploring Parties, in *Records of the Survey of India: Exploration in Tibet and Neighbouring Regions, 1865–1879* (Dehra Dun: Survey of India, 1915), 8 (1): 116–20. In 1871 Hari Ram carried with him a Hindi translation of a medical treatise on the use of such drugs.

[8] Report on Routes by Explorer Hari Ram, *Records of the Survey of India,* 8 (2): 386. A goitre is a swelling of the thyroid gland at the front of the neck.

were stocked by Indian bazaar druggists.[9] Hari Ram's information about health problems was also an incidental part of his report about the route he was exploring. Hari Ram spent six weeks in the area, and apart from mentioning goitre and an earlier smallpox epidemic he made no other references to such issues.

The first biomedical article about ill health in Khumbu appeared in 1952 when *The Lancet* published a short account by Dr Michael Ward, who had been the main instigator of the 1951 Mount Everest Reconnaissance Expedition.[10] Other early Western visitors into the area in the 1950s also wrote about their travels and made passing references to health and disease issues. Ward mentioned several people in Namche Bazar with gonorrhoea, who said they had contracted the disease in Tibet, but how prevalent it was in Tibet is difficult to judge from the limited sources available.[11] Ward also reported that a variety of eye complaints, such as chronic conjunctivitis and cataracts, were "fairly common" and that he had heard of an epidemic in Pharak where abdominal pain and nose-bleeds were the common symptoms.[12]

As Ward journeyed through Nepal he had noted "for the purposes of record" diseases he encountered.[13] Little was known in other countries about Nepal's health problems and medical travellers began writing about disease issues they observed. Carl Taylor, a physician with a Chicago Natural History Museum expedition to central Nepal in 1949–50, considered that "to the scientist of today" Nepal "presents a field almost as untouched as Central Africa did to

[9] M. Miles, "Goitre, Cretinism and Iodine in South Asia: Historical Perspectives on a Continuing Scourge", *Medical History* 42, 1998, 47–67.

[10] Michael Ward, "In Eastern Nepal", *Lancet* 263, no. 2, July–December 1952, 238–39.

[11] McKay, *Their Footprints Remain*, 147–53. For a vivid account of apparent Tibetan enthusiasm for injections to combat syphilis during a 1950 journey in south-eastern Tibet, see George N. Patterson, *Tibetan Journey* (London: Faber and Faber, 1954), 95–103.

[12] Ward, "In Eastern Nepal", 238.

[13] Michael Ward, *In This Short Span: A Mountaineering Memoir* (London: Victor Gollancz, 1972), 88.

Livingstone a century ago".[14] Not until the mid-1960s, when a national health survey was carried out, was there a more comprehensive understanding, both inside and outside the country, of Nepal's health problems.[15]

Information about sickness in high-altitude mountainous areas such as Khumbu remained scarce, as practical difficulties in carrying out research led to sample villages above 2,900 metres not being included in the national survey.[16] The term "high altitude" does not have a precise medical definition because of the variation in an individual person's susceptibility to the effects of the hypoxia (lack of oxygen) that occurs with increasing altitude, but it is commonly used to refer to areas around and over 3,000 metres above sea level. The permanent villages of Khumbu are situated between 3,400 metres and 4,000 metres; Khunde is at 3,840 metres. Knowledge about the effect of altitude on these resident high-altitude populations has come from studies of various groups of people around the world. Sherpas have been the most frequently cited example from the Himalayan region.[17]

The main focus on Sherpas as research subjects has been in terms of their adaptation to the hypoxic environment when compared with populations from lowland areas or other high-altitude regions. So effectively were these high-altitude residents able to cope with their environment that the concept of a distinctive biological "high-altitude man" developed.[18] Little was known, however, about high-altitude populations outside the Andes in South America. In the

[14] Carl E. Taylor, "A Medical Survey of the Kali Gandak and Pokhara Valleys of Central Nepal", *Geographical Review* 41, 1951, 421–37.

[15] Robert M. Worth and Narayan K. Shah, *Nepal Health Survey, 1965–1966* (Honolulu: University of Hawaii Press, 1969), 1–4 and 8–9.

[16] Worth and Shah, *Nepal Health Survey*, 3–4.

[17] For example, see Michael P. Ward, James S. Milledge and John B. West, *High Altitude Medicine and Physiology,* 3rd ed. (London: Arnold, 2000), chapter 17, High altitude populations, and passim.

[18] Donald Heath and David Reid Williams, *High-Altitude Medicine and Pathology* (London: Butterworths, 1989), 332–33. Also see Jorge Lossio, "Altitude Medicine and Physiology", *Wellcome History* 29, summer 2005, 9. Lossio discusses how this concept emerged as a reaction by scientists in South America to the images of inferiority presented by Western physiologists.

1960s Sherpas were included in such research. Since Tibet was inaccessible to Western researchers and the Cultural Revolution resulted in a lack of Chinese research in the region until the 1980s, studies carried out in the Everest area made a significant contribution to scientific advances.[19] Although similarities existed, points of contrast emerged between the various groups, such as Sherpas having lower haemoglobin levels than groups in the Andes. It is thought that Sherpas have to some extent adapted more to their hypoxic environment than the inhabitants of the Andes, and that this is related to the greater length of time that Sherpas have lived at high altitude and to genetic isolation.[20] Adjustment to life at high altitude is a complex process, involving most systems of the body. The more general view is that there is no generic "high-altitude man", only different groups of people whose characteristics are the result of the interaction between genetic and various environmental influences.[21]

Many studies of high-altitude groups around the world were done during the decade following the International Council of Scientific Unions' establishment in 1964 of the International Biologi-

[19] Shu-Tsu Hu, "Hypoxia Research in China: An Overview", in *Hypoxia, Exercise, and Altitude: Proceedings of the Third Banff International Hypoxia Symposium,* ed. John R. Sutton, Charles S. Houston and Norman L. Jones (New York: A. R. Liss, 1983), 157–71.

[20] Susan Niermeyer, Stacy Zamudio and Lorna G. Moore, "The People", in *High Altitude: An Exploration of Human Adaptation,* ed. Thomas F. Hornbein and Robert B. Schoene (New York and Basel: Marcel Dekker, 2001), 43–100. See also I. G. Pawson, "Growth and Development in High Altitude Populations: A Review of Ethiopian, Peruvian, and Nepalese Studies", *Proceedings of the Royal Society of London* B. 194, 1976, 83–98; and Amitabha Basu, Ranjan Gupta and Sanat K. Bhattacharya, "Altitude and Biology in the Sherpa: An Alternative Approach to the Study of High Altitude Biology in the Context of the Eastern Himalayan Situation", *Journal of the Indian Anthropological Society* (Calcutta) 14, 1979, 139–48.

[21] Conclusions are tentative. It is extremely difficult, when interpreting research results, to decide whether any difference can be attributed to the high-altitude environment or to racial, nutritional or economic factors. The effects of poor nutrition and chronic hypoxia, for example, are similar on growth and development. Ward, Milledge and West, *High Altitude Medicine and Physiology,* 203.

cal Programme. It was believed that the world's rapidly expanding human population required a better scientific understanding of the environment in order to more effectively manage natural resources. Part of the programme was concerned with the adaptability of human populations in different conditions. High altitude was one environment for study.[22] One problem of researching Sherpas was their considerable mobility, which could affect interpretation of research results.[23] Sherpas travelled widely within and between areas of high and low altitude.

Some scientific work was carried out in association with Hillary's expeditions. While Sherpas were better able to cope with hard physical work at high altitude than people who lived in lower regions, Hillary also began to learn about health issues in the area, such as childhood and maternal mortality. The influence of high altitude on these problems was more limited. He also saw the successes and potential for biomedical treatment. A young couple had an eighteen-month old child with tuberculosis of the spine. "I can still see the father's large, sad eyes filling with hopelessness as he was told that the only chance was a hospital—how could he spare the time and money for this?"[24]

These experiences, as the quotation at the beginning of this chapter demonstrates, not only fuelled Hillary's desire to provide health care but also significantly influenced the way he conceived of such help. Hillary's expeditions had doctors. In the Western medical system the doctor was the pivotal person in health care and the hospital the focal institution. Hillary's vision for Khunde Hospital was formulated at a time when the top-down, doctor-hospital model of health services predominated.[25] Improving people's health was about providing access to health services. Until 1963 the medical experience of his expedition doctors was hospital-based, and in the case of the young New Zealand climbing doctors, Gill and

[22] See P. T. Baker, ed., *The Biology of High-Altitude Peoples* (Cambridge: Cambridge University Press, 1978).

[23] Ward considered the possibility of doing research among Sherpas, but instead went to the more isolated Bhutan. Ward, *In This Short Span,* 218–19.

[24] Hillary, *Schoolhouse in the Clouds*, 102.

[25] See chapter four of this book.

Houghton, in 1963 it was also limited. In contrast, the doctor for the 1964 Himalayan Schoolhouse Expedition was Max Pearl, an experienced general practitioner from Auckland. He became Hillary's medical advisor. The facilities and access to specialist services to be found in a large urban area such as Auckland were very different from rural, remote Khumbu, but Pearl infused Hillary's medical programme with a broader primary care approach to health issues which combined well with Hillary's own grassroots way of working with Sherpas.

As Hillary's expeditions spent more time in the area they learned an increasing amount about health issues, which they then wrote about. In 1960–61 Michael Gill, then a medical student, spent nine months as a climber with Hillary's Himalayan Scientific and Mountaineering Expedition and helping "as best I could with any medical problems that arose" when he was travelling or staying in a village.[26] On his return to medical school he wrote a dissertation about Sherpas and their health problems. In 1965 Pearl had an article published in the *New Zealand Medical Journal* about his experiences with Hillary's 1964 expedition.[27]

Gill, in his longer account, discussed Sherpa life more broadly than Pearl. He attributed the relative absence of the infectious diseases that wrought havoc at lower altitudes to the lack of contaminated water, few flies and cold temperatures.[28] It was too cold for the carrier mosquito in malaria to become established. Although Gill considered that personal hygiene was generally poor, the dry system for the disposal of sewage was effective. Smallpox was present, but while he saw "many pock-marked Tibetans" there were "very few affected Sherpas".[29] Children suffered widely from chronic upper respiratory infections, with smoke and the cold suggested as causes. Respiratory infections were also present in older age groups and he also saw cases of tuberculosis. The high childhood mortality

[26] Gill, "The Sherpas", 6–7.

[27] Pearl, "Kiwi in the Khumbu", 584–88.

[28] Gill assumed the water was not contaminated, but in reality this would depend on the source of the supply and the location of human habitation and grazing animals.

[29] Gill, "The Sherpas", 16.

contributed to the small size of families. Common but less severe problems were a mild conjunctivitis and dental caries. He heard that venereal disease was common, although he did not know how and when it became established in the area or which type was commonest. The Sherpa diet seemed adequate, but goitre was very common and cretinism "not uncommon".[30] He also saw evidence of past minor injuries, but surmised that serious injury probably resulted in death.

Gill wrote that he wanted to describe a "stable healthy and self-sufficient" community.[31] Pearl also considered the "Sherpa's general health was good".[32] To Gill and Pearl the idea of a healthy people or healthy environment was not the same as saying that there was no medical work to be done. Pearl reported "there was plenty of work offering" with the commonest complaints being respiratory tract infections, impetigo and other skin problems, gastritis and eye infections.[33] He thought that the perinatal mortality rate was "probably high", but for Pearl the greatest public health problem confronting the area was goitre.[34]

Vincanne Adams, in discussing the Sherpa, has situated this apparently paradoxical situation of the need for medical services in a healthy population around the "continued fulfillment of Western desires for exotic Otherness".[35] Sherpas were in need of help, but they also deserved help. The medical accounts, however, were more concerned with the absence of tropical diseases, the physical environment and the medical conditions they did encounter.[36] Romantic

[30] Ibid., 17.

[31] Ibid., 20.

[32] Pearl, "Kiwi in the Khumbu", 586.

[33] Ibid.

[34] Ibid. The perinatal mortality rate includes stillbirths plus deaths in the first week per 1,000 total births.

[35] Adams, *Tigers of the Snow and Other Virtual Sherpas,* 90–92.

[36] The two ideas are linked. Issues of climate, environment, health and disease have a much longer association, however, than the recognition of their key role, both as science and ideology, in European imperial expansion. In an article about nineteenth century representations of India in British medical topography, Mark Harrison argues that such dichotomies are too rigid and

stories from travellers in the Himalaya told of health, longevity and wealth, but little concrete evidence existed to support claims for extreme old age.[37] (In comparison to the local people, the travellers often struggled in this new environment.) The epidemiological explanation is that the Sherpa were a survivor population. Hillary observed of the harsh mountain life that Khumbu was "A Land without Convalescents".[38] When people became sick, they either got better or they died. As a result, when outsiders walked through an area they saw healthy people.[39]

Information about Khumbu's health problems was being gathered by foreign medical practitioners and appeared in foreign general and medical literature.[40] These outsider accounts of the country's medical needs emphasised the lack of health services—by which they meant Western medicine. Although Khunde Hospital's origins lay outside Nepal, biomedicine was expanding within its borders. Hillary's 1964 expedition members were unaware that the Nepalese government had opened a clinic in Namche Bazar, and so perhaps outside accounts could have overestimated the lack of biomedical services. Nevertheless, the country's first health survey confirmed the bleak situation, as few of the residents in the sample villages had easy access to such health services.

---

simplistic. Essential difference and potential for improvement could exist together and Indians could be active agents rather than passive recipients of Western knowledge. Mark Harrison, "Differences of Degree: Representations of India in British Medical Topography, 1820–c.1870", in *Medical Geography in Historical Perspective,* ed. Nicolaas A. Rupke (London: *Medical History* Supplement no. 20, Wellcome Trust Centre for the History of Medicine at UCL, 2000), 51–69. Harrison rightly points to the need to be aware of changing European perceptions over time, although articles on Nepal in the 1950s also reflect the persistence of such ideas.

[37] Ward, Milledge and West, *High Altitude Medicine and Physiology,* 203.

[38] Hillary, *Schoolhouse in the Clouds,* 107.

[39] Some sick and the elderly, however, probably remained out of sight inside their houses and so escaped the gaze of passing travellers.

[40] The Nepalese government was unhappy about this. See chapter four of this book.

The Spread of Western Medicine in Nepal

Despite the presence of a British Residency from the early nineteenth century and generally friendly relations between the Nepalese and British governments, Nepal guarded its political independence.[41] Nepalese sovereignty was a cornerstone of Nepalese policy. The government also prohibited Christian missionary activity to further protect its purity as the world's only Hindu kingdom. Missionaries were active near Nepal's border and some provided medical as well as evangelical services, occasionally crossing into Nepal.[42] Little has been written about the limited development of Western medical services in Nepal in the nineteenth and early twentieth century, but, although more work needs to be done, sources suggest that the Nepalese government pursued its own path of development even with British support.

Hemang Dixit's account of Nepal's early health services focuses on the building of hospitals.[43] Despite Nepal's relative isolation from Western countries associated with the rise of scientific medicine, the development of such services was also occurring in Nepal at a similar time and in a similar way to other countries. The late nineteenth and early twentieth century was the key period internationally in the transition that led to the hospital becoming the

[41] Michael H. Fisher, *Indirect Rule in India: Residents and the Residency System, 1764–1858* (Delhi: Oxford University Press, 1991), 414–22 and Asad Husain, *British India's Relations with the Kingdom of Nepal, 1857–1947: A Diplomatic History of Nepal* (London: George Allen and Unwin, 1970). Husain discusses how the Gurkha soldiers were the main reason for friendly relations being cultivated by the Government of India. Also see Richard Burghart, "The Formation of the Concept of Nation-State in Nepal", *Journal of Asian Studies* 14, no. 1, 1984, 101–25, and Graham E. Clarke, "Blood, Territory and National Identity in Himalayan States", in *Asian Forms of the Nation,* ed. Stein Tønnesson and Hans Antlöv (Richmond: Curzon, 1996), 205–36.

[42] Jan Minderhoud, "The Christian Presence in Nepal before 1951", *Indian Church History Review,* December 1990, 144–64; Dixit, *The Quest for Health*.

[43] Dixit, *The Quest for Health,* 21–29. Also see B. R. Marasini, "Health and Hospital Development in Nepal", *Journal of Nepal Medical Association* 42, 2003, 306–11.

focal point for treating the sick rather than a place of shelter.[44] The rulers of Nepal built a number of health facilities as a form of personal charity to the poor.[45] The first, Prithvi Bir Hospital, was established by Maharaja Bir Shamsher in Kathmandu in 1890 with 30 beds and looked after both male and female patients.[46] Facilities in other parts of the country were added during the rule of his brother, Maharaja Chandra Shamsher. The government brought in doctors from Bengal to staff these institutions. Perceval Landon, in his two-volume account *Nepal* which was first published in 1928, enthusiastically described Chandra's personal benevolence, but Ludwig Stiller suggests viewing development such as in health services also in terms of expediency.[47] Chandra's main concern was the administration of Nepal, but he believed that the younger generations of the Rana families were returning from their travels in India wanting to see their country develop.[48]

A key question for the development of Western medicine in Nepal centres on the influence of the British medical personnel and hospital at the British Residency.[49] Alex McKay's work highlights the importance of British imperial policies and personnel in biomedicine's spread in the wider Himalayan region, but he also shows how local circumstances affected the process in each area.[50] Further

[44] See, for example, Charles E. Rosenberg, *The Care of Strangers: The Rise of America's Hospital System* (New York: Basic Books, 1987). See also Susan Heydon, "Parochialism or a Fair Deal? A History of the South Otago Hospital Board 1921–1989", M.A. thesis, University of Otago, 1996, 28. In New Zealand between 1913–14 and 1920–22 the proportion of patients treated in hospital per 1,000 population rose from 26.8 to 42.6.

[45] See chapter four regarding hospitals and philanthropy in Nepal.

[46] Dixit, *The Quest for Health,* 21.

[47] Perceval Landon, *Nepal* (New Delhi: Asian Educational Services, 1993 [1928]), 2: 183; Stiller, *Nepal: Growth of a Nation,* 156.

[48] Dane Kennedy notes that in India in the British hill station of Mussoorie the largest house in the early twentieth century, Fairlawn Palace, belonged to the Maharaja of Nepal. Dane Kennedy, *The Magic Mountains: Hill Stations and the British Raj* (Berkeley: University of California Press, 1996), 208.

[49] In 1920 its status was upgraded to a Legation.

[50] See bibliography but particularly McKay, *Their Footprints Remain*. Nepal is not included in McKay's research except for incidental references.

research is again needed, but while the annual medical reports appeared little different from British medical reports elsewhere in the region, other sources suggest a more limited degree of influence and an increasingly active Nepalese role. It appears that biomedicine in Nepal, both in practice and ideologically, developed outside the colonial framework.

Dr Henry Ambrose Oldfield, who had begun his career in India as assistant-surgeon in the Bengal Army, was appointed surgeon to the British Residency in 1850 but the two volumes of his *Sketches from Nipal* provide little medical information either about his own work or health problems in Nepal.[51] Oldfield mentions in passing a small hospital attached to the Residency, but his medical duties in such a small station were light and so left him plenty of time to pursue other interests until he left Kathmandu in 1863.[52] He was, however, on good terms with the Maharaja, Jung Bahadur, who called him on occasions to visit members of his family. Jung Bahadur also supported vaccination and Oldfield vaccinated his eldest son while the Maharaja was in England in 1850.[53]

Providing medical attention to members of leading families was consistent with British policy elsewhere in the Himalayan region, but G. H. D. Gimlette's account of his time as Residency Surgeon from 1883–87 highlighted the Residency's physical isolation within the country, its lack of influence and the Nepalese government's intention to preserve their independence.[54] Landon provided a list of "about" 153 Europeans who had been allowed to visit Nepal between 1881 and 1925, a few of whom were either doctors or dentists brought in to visit senior Nepalese personnel or their wives.[55]

51 Henry Ambrose Oldfield, *Sketches from Nipal,* 2 vols. (London: W. H. Allen, 1880).

52 Oldfield, *Sketches from Nipal,* 1: iv and 191.

53 In this period although Nepal had a king the Maharaja as prime minister was ruler. The Maharaja was a member of the Rana family. Succession passed between brothers.

54 G. H. D. Gimlette, *Nepal and the Nepalese* (London: H. F. & G. Witherby, 1928), 87–89.

55 Landon, *Nepal,* 2: Appendix 24, 298–305. This total excluded the residents, envoys and official surgeons. The Residency/Legation had the services of an Escort and most of the small number of visitors came from the military.

The list, which was given to Landon by the Nepalese government, demonstrated the strict control on access pursued by the Nepalese authorities.

The Residency's medical work was similarly constrained. Gimlette described a serious cholera epidemic in 1885: "From the commencement of the epidemic, urgent representations were made to the Durbar from the Residency, of the desirability of erecting some temporary hospitals for the reception and treatment of cholera cases; they were entirely disregarded, as might have been expected."[56] As the Nepalese government developed its own medical services, the British medical personnel became even more marginal. In 1939 the Envoy, Lieutenant-Colonel Geoffrey Betham, wrote to the Government of India that outside the Legation the medical services of the surgeon were "rarely called for" and that: "Within recent years the Nepalese Government have organised and improved their Medical Department greatly. Now there are several Indian doctors in the Nepalese government's employ with high medical qualifications."[57]

Further independence was also shown through the position adopted by the Nepalese government towards Ayurvedic medicine.[58] Biomedicine had a part to play in health care, but—as occurred with Sherpas—it neither arrived into a vacuum nor necessar-

[56] Gimlette, *Nepal and the Nepalese,* 195. Gimlette (pp 174–75) admitted that he was not particularly liked after he complained about the due lack of ceremony on some of his professional visits.

[57] Lieutenant-Colonel G. L. Betham to the Secretary to the Government of India in the External Affairs Department, New Delhi, 27 March 1939 OIOC L/P&S 12/3073/21/60, Nepal: British Legation at Katmandu: Legation Surgeon [British Library, London]. P&S refers to the Political and Secret Department.

[58] Ayurvedic medicine was the principal medical system of Hindu India. Although it is primarily associated with India, it was practised elsewhere too. For a recent collection of essays that examines national and transnational tensions in the way medical systems are conceptualised, see Joseph S. Alter, ed., *Asian Medicine and Globalization* (Philadelphia, Pennsylvania: University of Pennsylvania Press, 2005).

ily displaced other systems.[59] Jung Bahadur was enthusiastic about European surgery and Oldfield wrote that "I have often found it exceedingly convenient to be able to borrow some of his instruments when our hospital was deficient in them."[60] Nevertheless "In medical cases, Jang says his own country doctors understand their treatment better than Europeans do. When he himself is indisposed he never consults me medically, but does invariably in everything surgical."[61]

This government support of Ayurvedic medicine continued alongside modern medicine.[62] In 1933 the Nepalese government included both systems when it established the Department of Health Services, which was to be responsible for the promotion, regulation and management of government facilities. The following year the government established training institutions for both systems, although in each case the numbers trained were small.[63] When the country's first five-year development plan began in 1956 there were 63 government Ayurvedic dispensaries and 34 biomedical hospitals and 24 dispensaries.[64] For a population of over 8 million people the facilities and services were inadequate. The number of dispensaries in both systems was small and the total number of hospital beds

59 See Charles Leslie, "Interpretation of Illness: Syncretism in Modern Ayurveda", in *Paths to Asian Medical Knowledge,* ed. C. Leslie and A. Young (Berkeley, California: University of California Press, 1992), 177–208.

60 Oldfield, *Sketches from Nipal,* 1: 252–53. For advances in surgery in the nineteenth century and the rise of the "cult of the surgeon", see W. F. Bynum, *Science and the Practice of Medicine in the Nineteenth Century* (Cambridge: Cambridge University Press, 1994), 137.

61 Oldfield, *Sketches from Nipal,* 1: 252.

62 In India and Sri Lanka (Ceylon) the indigenous medical system became associated with cultural revival and nationalist politics. Margaret Jones, *Health Policy in Britain's Model Colony: Ceylon, 1900–1948* (New Delhi: Orient Longman, 2004), 99.

63 Dixit, *The Quest for Health*, 138–39. Between 1934 and the establishment in 1972 of the Institute of Medicine, 512 Ayurvedic personnel of various grades were trained while 238 compounders and 213 dressers graduated from the Civil Medical School.

64 Dixit, *The Quest for Health*, 45 and 27.

throughout the country was just 625.[65] In practice, most Nepalese had no choice but to use a variety of indigenous healers that functioned outside both the Western and Ayurvedic systems.

It is tempting, but arguable, to divide the history of Western medical services within Nepal into the situation before and after the opening of the country's borders to Western visitors. Considerable expansion occurred in the 1950s following the entry of foreign aid into health programmes, but within government there was less of a break because of the continuing dominance of high-caste elite families in national and regional affairs.[66] Also, the Nepalese government, albeit in a limited way, had promoted some development of biomedicine before the relaxation of its policy of exclusion to Western countries and afterwards continued to direct its advance within Nepal. Western medicine developed in Nepal as a government service and outside the colonisation/decolonisation/nationalism framework that underpinned its development in much of South Asia. After 1950, the development of such services continued and intensified with the injection of foreign aid.[67] As Packard has written, "The postwar vision of health and development was much more pervasive and encompassing" and national and international health policies "reflected a new realization of the need to extend the provision of health care to entire populations".[68] Nevertheless, most Nepalese still had significant problems in accessing any health facility at all given the difficulties of travel within this country of few roads, large rivers and rugged terrain.

[65] In contrast, Sri Lanka had developed extensive primary care services. Jones, *Health Policy in Britain's Model Colony.*

[66] Leo E. Rose, "The National Political Culture and Institutions in Nepal", in *The Post-Colonial States of South Asia: Democracy, Development and Identity,* ed. Amita Shastri and A. Jeyaratnam Wilson (New York: Palgrave, 2001), 114–38; Saul J. Weiner, "'Source Force' and the Nepal Medical Profession", *Social Science & Medicine* 29, no. 5, 1989, 669–75. Marasini acknowledges the importance of the post-1951 development, but regards the Rana period as "the important era" in health and hospital development. Marasini, "Health and Hospital Development in Nepal", 308.

[67] See chapter four. Although he provides no details for Nepal, see Amrith, *Decolonizing International Health* for the wider context in the region.

[68] Packard, "Visions of Postwar Health and Development", 96.

By the mid-1960s, when Hillary was beginning his health programmes in Khumbu, expansion of Nepal's biomedical services had occurred in three main directions.[69] Western medicine had strengthened its base in urban centres with the Government building more hospitals and clinics, the formation of professional associations, the establishment of a nurse training school and in 1956 the formation of the Ministry of Health. Non-government organisations (NGOs), both domestic and foreign, also established their presence as health care providers.[70] The second area involved the expansion of health services into rural areas through the provision of family planning and maternal and child health services in selected areas and then gradually beginning to build health posts throughout Nepal. The health clinic in Namche Bazar was one of nine developed in 1964.[71] The third type of activity involved the introduction of vertical programmes for the control of communicable disease, beginning with malaria eradication in 1958. Programmes for smallpox, tuberculosis and leprosy followed in the 1960s. The development of new technologies made the cost of disease control more affordable and contributed to this "expanding vision" of international health policies and programmes.[72] In practice, however, lack of finance and personnel hampered such efforts in a poor, rural country such as Nepal that had an inadequate infrastructure to support the implementation of policies.

Hillary's experiences during the early 1960s and his building of the hospital at Khunde, therefore, need to be set against this broad scenario of on the one hand health service development but on the other hand the lack of services throughout most of this predominantly rural country. The situation was one where the government was the main provider, but had begun to allow some non-government activity. It recognised plural medical systems, but promoted a mainly biomedical model for the development of the country's health

[69] Streefland, "The Frontier of Modern Western Medicine in Nepal".

[70] Foreign NGOs in Nepal are now referred to as INGOs.

[71] Dixit, *The Quest for Health,* 46. By the time of the national health survey in 1965 there were 102 health posts throughout the country.

[72] Packard, "Visions of Postwar Health and Development", 99.

services. In Khumbu, however, other than the information that was being gathered mainly by Hillary's own expedition personnel, little more was known. The area lacked Western medical services, and during the 1963 smallpox epidemic Hillary responded and vaccinated people throughout the region. Although this was well received in Kathmandu, Hillary's position in Nepal was in fact problematic.[73] Despite facing difficulties with Nepalese bureaucracy at times, Hillary's experiences with the sick people his expeditions encountered provided the basis for his health plans for the area. The limited presence of Western medicine both in the immediate area and throughout the country had implications for the hospital's work that form the basis of the next section. Hospital policy was medical, but its implementation faced considerable environmental and cultural challenges.

Practising Medicine at Khunde Hospital

Hillary knew that Sherpas had their own ideas about sickness. "Despite this acceptance of the supernatural in health matters", he wrote "the Sherpas are now firm supporters of Western medicine and take full advantage of the treatment offered".[74] He had received Sherpa gratitude for the widespread smallpox vaccination carried out during the 1963 epidemic, he saw the doctors busy with patients when his expeditions passed through the country and he had seen the results of successful medical treatment. As he left Khunde in December 1966, he knew that such services could be provided permanently. Dr John McKinnon had been on his 1964 expedition while he was still a medical student at the University of Otago and so was already familiar with the people, the area and its health issues and filled with the enthusiasm of a young and recently qualified doctor. Louise Hillary wrote how McKinnon and his wife Diane looked "cheerful and carefree at the thought of being on their own among the Sherpas for a year".[75]

[73] See chapter four.

[74] Hillary, *Schoolhouse in the Clouds,* 112.

[75] Louise Hillary, *A Yak for Christmas,* 157.

The first part of this section focuses on McKinnon's work. His time at Khunde Hospital has provided the foundation for the way the hospital has since operated. During the first three months of 1967 McKinnon saw 722 patients.[76] He was optimistic for the future of the hospital. Over a full year he expected to treat a daily average of 20 to 30 patients rather than the eight he saw during these three months. In the cold winter months many people left the area, and heavy snowfall had hindered travel so that he only saw 20 people in 11 days. Six months later, when McKinnon reviewed Khunde Hospital's first nine months of working in the area, he wrote of the mixed response to "modern medicine".[77] He did not give a patient total in this review, but his earlier anticipated daily average of patients at the hospital had not occurred. Although he also treated patients when he visited villages, a smaller than expected total of 1,924 people went to the hospital for treatment.[78] He remained optimistic, believing that attitudes towards using the hospital had begun to change. He thought that "the passage of several years, with exposure to modern medical practice and local publication of therapeutic successes will lead to even greater acceptance."[79]

McKinnon wrote these views about the acceptance of Western medicine as the first point in his discussion of the area's health problems and further comments were interspersed when discussing particular medical issues. It showed that he was considering how local Sherpas responded to the hospital as an integral part of his thinking and practice. McKinnon, as he recounted later, saw Sherpas as always interested in new ideas, adapting quickly and not constrained by customs or social structure.[80] In his review he proceeded to describe his scheme for the area to deal with the major issue of tuberculosis and referred to the research and trial to control

76 "Outline of Patients seen from 1/1/67 until 31/3/67". Annual Reports 1967–1983 [KH].

77 McKinnon, "Health Problems of Khumbu." This report was later published as "Health Problems of Khumbu in Nepal: The Work at the Kunde Hospital", *New Zealand Medical Journal* 67, no. 140, January 1968, 140–43.

78 Outpatient register.

79 McKinnon, "Health Problems of Khumbu", 2.

80 Interview with Dr John McKinnon, Khunde, March 1997.

the effects of the lack of iodine in Khumbu. He believed malnutrition was uncommon. He encouraged women to attend for antenatal care, but still "despite encouragement, not one woman has been delivered at the hospital".[81] In his brief earlier summary of cases, he had written that he had carried out four forceps deliveries, but these had all occurred away from the medical environment of the hospital. Here he had also written that he thought family planning would increase as the "glad news" spread.[82] In the review he recorded that 27 women had received intra-uterine contraceptive devices (IUCDs). Cases of leprosy were "sporadic" and he was treating five cases of lepromatous and one case of tuberculoid leprosy at home. Most of his medical practice concerned respiratory infections, with "acute bronchitis" the most common diagnosis.[83] Other medical problems were eye complaints, worms, impetigo, chronic otitis media and dental extractions, but he had not seen cases of measles, chickenpox, mumps or whooping cough. He had carried out a number of minor surgical procedures, such as skin grafting for burns, but while he had seen acute surgical cases, "all patients have refused hospitalisation when seriously ill because of their great fear of dying away from home".[84]

McKinnon used words such as "medically unsophisticated" to describe Sherpas, "modern medical practice" for the work at Khunde Hospital and "propaganda" regarding the benefits of village visits.[85] Such language fitted easily into the discourse of the 1960s of the continuing superiority of Western medicine and also supports the notion of unequal power relations between the Western outsiders and indigenous Sherpas. Inequality also existed within the Nepalese social structure. In his study of the Mewahang Rai of East Nepal, Martin Gaenszle found that the representative of the health post was often from another ethnic group or even a high-caste Hindu

[81] McKinnon, "Health Problems of Khumbu", 5.

[82] "Outline of Patients".

[83] In the "Outline of patients", 10 per cent of patients were diagnosed as having respiratory complaints, and these were the most common presenting conditions.

[84] McKinnon, "Health Problems of Khumbu", 6.

[85] Ibid., 2.

whose rules for social interaction were different.[86] In an informative aside, Hemang Dixit mentions that international researchers have carried out most of the studies into socio-cultural aspects of health "about which we ourselves have not cared very much".[87] Such language and attitudes fit less easily with Hillary's description of the community farewell for the McKinnons in August 1968. The speeches, thanks and gifts may not have been surprising, but "more than anything it was the tears from these rugged people—floods of tears. I wonder how many of us will have a whole community weep in sorrow at our departure?"[88]

So what did these seemingly contradictory images of use and non-use, arrogance and affection mean, and how did the overseas staff respond? McKinnon's task, as the quote at the start of this chapter outlines, was to treat sick people from the community on either an outpatient or inpatient basis. Chapter two discussed how Western medicine did not enter a vacuum but encountered a world where Sherpas had their own beliefs and practices about sickness. Gaenszle concluded by expressing the view that if problems of affordability and accessiblity for using health posts were minimised, and trust and respect existed between villagers and health post, then "a certain harmony can be achieved".[89]

Western medical practitioners in the 1960s were extremely optimistic about what could be done to improve the level of people's health. Major advances over the previous twenty years, particularly in the treatment of infectious disease, led, for example, Sir MacFarlane Burnet in the third edition of *Natural History of Infectious Disease* to proclaim: "In 1961 it is hardly an exaggeration to say that no previously healthy child or adult need die of any bacterial or protozoal

[86] Gaenszle, "The Shaman and the Doctor", 58–59.

[87] Dixit, *The Quest for Health*, 30. Dixit is a professor in child health.

[88] Hillary, *Nothing Venture, Nothing Win,* 272. Nima Yangen, the McKinnons' nurse-assistant, also described the tears on their departure. Interview, Nima Yangen, 2003.

[89] Gaenszle, "The Shaman and the Doctor", 59.

infection if he can reach an adequately equipped hospital before the infection has irreparably damaged his tissues."[90]

In a country such as Nepal where most people lacked access to biomedical health services, the first aim was to provide them so as to be able then to effect an improvement in health status. Accordingly, the hospital opened its doors in the anticipation that people would start using its services. People could go to the hospital to be examined and treated for their different health problems. Clinics were held daily. The main hospital building contained a one-room "surgery/dispensary", which became the centre of hospital activities. The hospital had X-ray facilities and staff could also carry out simple laboratory tests. In addition, inpatients could be looked after in the adjoining three-bed ward for acute cases and a separate building with a further eight beds.

Patients who went to the hospital initiated the contact. McKinnon believed that families whose members had been involved with expeditions in the past were "in general, enthusiastic believers of modern medicine and come readily to the hospital", but he was aware that he saw little or nothing of some families although he did not sense antagonism.[91] The longer the McKinnons spent in the community the more they learned about its needs and could develop and refine the hospital's services. The classification of diseases given at the beginning of the hospital's first outpatient register, and recorded throughout the book, confirms not surprisingly, his Western medicine approach. Gill had noted few elderly people, but McKinnon had such patients. Among this group were several patients with congestive heart failure or cataracts. McKinnon responded to this newly discovered medical need by sending back to New Zealand a request for ophthalmic equipment that would enable him to remove cataracts. As the case-mix of patients became

[90] Sir Macfarlane Burnet, *Natural History of Infectious Disease,* 3rd ed. (Cambridge: Cambridge University Press, 1962), 3. Burnet was a Nobel Laureate and Director of the Walter and Eliza Hall Institute, Melbourne, Australia. Sunil Amrith, however, discusses a growing pessimism by the early 1960s of the potential for success of the mass public health campaigns for disease control. Amrith, *Decolonizing International Health.*

[91] McKinnon, "Health Problems of Khumbu", 2.

clearer, he adapted his medicine order. Some, mainly of Indian origin, were bought in Kathmandu, but at this time most medicines and equipment were brought from New Zealand.

The McKinnons had two local staff to assist them at the hospital. These were the volunteers' principal link with the community. As Vincanne Adams has noted, being a successful doctor at Khunde Hospital was both about the medicine and about how the volunteers fitted into a Sherpa world.[92] The hospital was quiet at times, and so the McKinnons became very involved with the social life of the local community. As McKinnon reflected much later, "That was where the action was."[93] Nima Yangen helped with medical duties, but she was also friend and guide to the McKinnons on living in a Sherpa village. Volunteers and patients came to know each other outside the hospital and the context of sickness. Through staff, such as Nima Yangen, each set of volunteers built up a knowledge of the local community and their beliefs that also placed their patients in a network of relations. A diagnosis according to Western medicine principles was usually different from the patient's perception of the cause of the problem, but the volunteers came to know their patients, their circumstances and understand how people approached problems. This knowledge underpinned the medical encounter.

McKinnon also knew that the hospital was regarded as optional when people were sick. He thought the hospital had a "harmonious" relationship with other medical systems and made a point of visiting the various monasteries.[94] The lhawa were active and he did not believe they talked against the hospital. Ang Pema was the hospital cook and helped with general duties, but he was also an interpreter for a lhawa.[95] McKinnon believed people were covering their options. It was not unusual for him to visit a house and find doctor, lama and lhawa all present at the same time.

[92] Adams, *Tigers of the Snow and Other Virtual Sherpas,* 117–18.

[93] Interview, McKinnon, 1997.

[94] Ibid.

[95] Ibid. A lhawa in a trance speaks the language of the spirits that have possessed him/her which requires someone to interpret for those present.

McKinnon's work and medical practice at Khunde Hospital, therefore, was influenced not only by the health problems encountered, but also by how the Sherpa inhabitants of the area regarded the hospital as one of a range of options available to consult (or not) when sick. Despite local people's increasing use of the hospital and the volunteers' own beliefs in the value of Western medicine, staff had to respond on an ongoing basis to the encounter between Western medicine and Sherpa beliefs and practices. This, above all, has shaped medical practice at Khunde Hospital. Western medicine's position was limited and McKinnon was both reactive and proactive in his response. Five years later Dr Lindsay Strang wrote in the hospital's annual report that "Western medicine continues to be accepted only slowly and still traditional forms are often resorted to initially especially for serious conditions." [96] The overseas staff became used to offering Western medicine in this plural setting of coexistence between different systems of dealing with sickness where the local population might use all, any or none of them. This, although use of the hospital's services steadily increased, remained; and such views continued to pervade the writing of annual reports, correspondence and published articles in popular or scholarly literature. Simon Maclaurin and Marianne Wood, who were both doctors, wrote at the end of their two years in the area in 1989 that "We believe that the Sherpas' ambivalence to our medicine is because they have a fundamentally different belief in the causation of disease." [97]

Even without such challenges to their medicine, inexperienced doctors could feel their "isolation" strongly in Khunde Hospital. After being appointed, volunteers learned about the hospital's work from medical personnel within the Himalayan Trust and particularly from former doctors at Khunde. The McKinnons left in August 1968 and were replaced by Dr Richard and Lesley Evans. Some of the early couples, such as the Evans and their successors Drs Selwyn and Ann Lang, had little time to prepare. In the 1970s the "Dear Successor" letters from the current volunteers and the Hospital

[96] Kunde Hospital Report for the Year Ending 31 October 1972.

[97] Kunde Hospital Annual Report, August 1988 to June 1989.

Handbook provided further information both about the medical work and life at Khunde.

Although personnel changed, the system for providing medical services at Khunde Hospital continued to be based around the early model of a doctor who was based at the hospital but supported village-based services.[98] Medical work was a mixture of curative and preventive services. Serious or unusual cases, such as a man being attacked by a bear or being asked to treat a sick yak, interspersed the common respiratory, gastro-intestinal and skin conditions. Trauma was common in the rugged terrain. The doctor saw and treated most people at the hospital as outpatients, but also had a small number of inpatients. He or she also visited people in their homes and made trips to outlying villages. Different Khunde volunteers organised the precise working of these arrangements. For example, when both were doctors one could make a village trip, while the other looked after patients at the hospital. The question arose whether Khunde Hospital needed one or two doctors, particularly as the workload increased. When there was only one doctor, the immediacy of the clinical situation tended to prevail, as did work at the hospital over work in the community. In the 1980s and 1990s two-doctor volunteer couples were more usual.[99] There were always a number of issues at any one time for the hospital staff to deal with, but the small size of the organisation meant, probably inevitably, that individual volunteers were not able to deal with everything simultaneously. It was also not always possible to delegate. Volunteers changed approximately every two years, but while there was insufficient time for each volunteer to build and develop systems or programmes the familiar structure and way of working provided an internal continuity. Both volunteers and community became used to each other.

As discussed in chapter two, the idea of efficacy is a central debate among scholars and provides a useful analytical device for examining the hospital's work. The doctors at Khunde were soon aware that their most valuable tool for persuading people to use Western

[98] See chapter four about changing ideas of appropriate ways to provide health services for poor countries such as Nepal.

[99] Only the Himalayan Trust in New Zealand appointed couples with a single doctor. See Appendix 1.

medicine was the provision of quick, effective treatment. They observed that people used the hospital for acute conditions that were treated successfully and speedily, but much less so for chronic conditions that were harder to cure with medicines or other treatment. Many bacterial infections and trauma responded well to treatment at the hospital. A dental extraction made people pain-free, initially often after years of discomfort because people had had no opportunity for treatment in the district before the hospital opened. Injections of iodised oil reduced the size of the large disfiguring goitres caused by the severe iodine deficiency in the area. McKinnon presented the idea of family planning for women in the area as "baby no come" medicine.[100] Smallpox vaccinations reduced the risk of contracting and dying from the disease that was endemic in Nepal until the early 1970s.[101]

Although the volunteers knew that their patients often interpreted success and failure differently from themselves, both the overseas and local staff were very conscious that success would encourage use of the hospital, but that failure would lead to criticism and discourage attendance. This placed considerable pressure on the staff. Such situations occurred not only when the hospital had just opened but also when its position in the local health infrastructure seemed well established. The Evans expressed excitement and relief in a letter home in November 1968:

> The greatest news is that we have had our first delivery in the hospital! Till now it has been impossible to get expectant mothers to come to the hospital to deliver, but at last it has happened. . . . We hope that more will come now that this one has been successful. . . . A lot depended on this one to set a good precedent. If it had been a difficult or abnormal birth, or the baby was a cretin or something, nobody would have ever come again.[102]

[100] Evans letters, 26 August 1968.

[101] The volunteers were aware that people already associated the procedure of smallpox vaccination with preventing the disease, but that this was not the case with vaccination against tuberculosis. BCG also had varying degrees of effectiveness. Tuberculosis "TB" was a disease learned from the hospital.

[102] Evans letters, 11 November 1968.

The baby was a boy. As sons are important in Sherpa society, hospital staff and family were even happier. Almost thirty years later, hospital staff were providing terminal care at home for a seriously ill patient. Not long before the man died he was offered an injection, but it was declined. The family said that people in the village would say that the injection had caused his death and so would blame the hospital.[103] Such a comment also illustrated the open relationship that could occur between hospital staff, both local and overseas, and patients.

Providing obstetric care for women presented a number of challenges for staff at the hospital and gave rise to some of the most demanding medical practice for individual doctors at different times during their stay at Khunde. Successful obstetrics was concerned with two lives—the mother and the child. Good obstetric practice involved the care of the mother and foetus before birth, the delivery, and immediate care of the mother and child in the postnatal period. The challenges arose from a combination of factors that included the volunteer's own level of skill and experience, specific obstetric problems and good practice, the isolation of the hospital, and how local women regarded the hospital in matters of childbirth. It is clear from hospital records and personal correspondence that these issues were ongoing. While shifts in people's use of the hospital have occurred, the basic tension between these four areas continues.

The doctors viewed it as good medical practice to encourage women to attend for antenatal care and have their babies in hospital. Nepal had, and like much of the developing world continues to have, high maternal and infant mortality rates.[104] So what were the doctors going to do when they found that women acted differ-

[103] Personal participation. The comment was made to our medical assistant, Gayse Nuru Sherpa.

[104] Various attempts have been made to estimate these rates for Nepal. For infant mortality rates, which are considered to be an important indicator of overall health conditions, see *Population of Nepal,* ESCAP Country Monograph Series No. 6 (Bangkok: United Nations, 1980), 50–51. Less information is available for maternal mortality rates. Even in the mid-1990s the rates vary considerably according to which source is used, ranging between 515 and 1,500 per 100,000 births. Dixit, *The Quest for Health,* 2nd ed. (Kathmandu: Educational Enterprise, 1999), 129 and 142.

ently? In their analysis of the first five years of the hospital's work, the Langs reported that of 74 women who came in for antenatal care only nine subsequently were delivered by the doctor.[105] The total number of births in the area was not known, but during this period the hospital staff were involved in 25 deliveries, of which 11 were in hospital and 14 at home. Distance was one factor in the decision to have a baby at home, as six of the domiciliary births were in the more distant village of Thame. It was hard to walk when in labour, uncomfortable to be carried and the risk existed of having the baby along the way. Five deliveries, however, were in Namche Bazar which was only one hour's walk away and two in Khunde itself. Staff also knew that Sherpa women did not want to be seen while in labour. Whatever explanations may be offered, babies are notoriously unpredictable in announcing their impending arrival, which makes planning difficult.

The response from the volunteers was another example that demonstrated the ongoing nature of the encounter between Sherpa beliefs and practices and those of Western medical practice. To achieve safer deliveries, the hospital staff tried to encourage women to have their babies in hospital, especially when problems were picked up antenatally. Although in New Zealand in the 1970s the home birth movement was beginning, doctors were trained to deliver babies in the medicalised environment of hospitals where specialist help was available for complications.[106] As most women in Khumbu continued to deliver at home, the volunteers responded to requests for

[105] Khunde Hospital Annual Report for the Year Ending 31 October 1971: Including an Analysis of Cases for the First Five Years (1967–1971).

[106] For a contemporary short article that argued for the presence of husbands at a hospital delivery "if some sections of the profession were not actively discouraging", see A Medical Student's Wife, "In Support of Husbands in a Delivery Theatre", *Digest* 6, no. 2, October 1965, 29–30. *Digest* was published by the Medical Students' Association of the University of Otago, which was then New Zealand's only medical school. For the medicalisation of childbirth in New Zealand, see Charlotte M. Parkes, "The Impact of the Medicalisation of New Zealand's Maternity Services on Women's Experience of Childbirth, 1904–1937", in *A Healthy Country: Essays on the Social History of Medicine in New Zealand,* ed. Linda Bryder (Wellington: Bridget Williams Books, 1991), 165–80.

assistance and went out to the women, even though they knew that they could face some of their most difficult medical experiences at Khunde Hospital. The doctors were more likely to be called out for cases of prolonged labour and these were at greater risk of being problematic. Of the fourteen home deliveries between 1967–71, the doctors considered eight to be complicated.[107]

While the number of babies born in hospital increased, particularly from the villages nearest the hospital, this pattern of hospital response to requests for assistance at home continued. A recent demographic survey carried out by the hospital for the five-year period 1998–2002 included the total number of births in the area and showed that over 70 per cent of births in Khumbu still occurred at home, which was a slightly lower level than the national average.[108]

Another aspect of medical practice at Khunde that was keenly felt by the volunteers was the death of a patient. In many cases this evoked a sense of failure. "I felt grossly inadequate" wrote Dr Marianne Wood as she left a bottle of medicine for a sick child that she and the mother knew would soon be dead.[109] "Walking back to Kunde after that experience my mind was completely a whirl with the meaning of it all." Volunteers also felt frustration when they heard of someone dying who had not come to the hospital when treatment could have helped.

Most deaths occurred in the community and the volunteers learned that it was important for Sherpas to die at home. This challenged the volunteers as well as the patient and the family. In the volunteers' medical world, the doctor was expected to do as much as possible for the sick person, even if the eventual outcome was the death of the patient. What happened if the patient and/or the family wanted to leave the hospital to ensure that death was at home, but before the doctor felt he or she could give no more treatment? As people came to know the hospital and as hospital staff came to

[107] Khunde Hospital Annual Report for the Year Ending 31 October 1971: Including an Analysis of Cases for the First Five Years (1967–1971).

[108] Draft Survey Summary Report, June 2003.

[109] Kunde Hospital Annual Report, August 1988 to June 1989.

know their patients an accommodation could occur between the two sets of beliefs, although the volunteers also knew they were in the weaker negotiating position and had to take any opportunities they were given. In the story used in chapter two about the woman falling off the trail, I promised her husband that I would tell him if we thought his wife was not going to respond to treatment and die. Fortunately she recovered after a few weeks. This family lived in Khunde and it was easy to take her home. Unfortunately in another case where the patient lived several hours walk away, the family took the man home with medicines, but staff at the hospital heard that he died three weeks later.[110]

Death in hospital was uncommon, but when it did occur the family would organise the after-death arrangements. In a very unusual occurrence, two deaths occurred within 36 hours in 1989 during the handover between two sets of volunteers.[111] Neither patient lived in Khumbu, but both had family members staying with them. One family was Sherpa and the body was cremated, while the other was Rai; her body was buried.

A different situation occurred when a patient who lived a long way from the hospital died and if he had had no family members or friends to look after him while in hospital or to attend to arrangements after death. One result of the increasing economic development of the area was that people from other areas came to Khumbu in search of employment. Large numbers of porters from low-altitude areas worked on trekking and climbing expeditions. In most cases, however, somebody accompanied the sick person if they needed admitting as an inpatient. Other patients came to Khunde when seriously sick because they had limited health services in their home area. They walked or were carried for several days before reaching Khunde, but again usually someone stayed with them while they were in hospital. The problem for the hospital came particularly when death occurred and the patient was alone. Then the volunteers found themselves involved in the practical arrange-

110 Personal participation.

111 Kunde Hospital Annual Report, August 1988 to June 1989.

ments afterwards with the patient's body being buried outside the village.[112]

Although being near a dead body is polluting, the presence of ghosts in the hospital from people who have died there created further issues for the hospital staff. People were and remain reluctant to be admitted. They also do not like being on their own. A woman in late pregnancy was admitted with very high blood pressure for bedrest.[113] The next morning, after being regaled by another patient with stories of the hospital ghosts, her blood pressure was even higher. She went home. At times monks have been invited by hospital staff to come to the hospital and exorcise the ghosts.

What such actions and responses indicate is awareness on the volunteers' part of their patients' conceptual world and their own willingness to try and practise Western medicine within this environment. The volunteers learned what was acceptable and what was less so, what was possible and what had little chance of success. They also realised that there were many things going on in the community that the outsider doctor would never know. The doctors adapted their practice and adopted different strategies. Sometimes the process was gradual, but in other cases the approach has been similar throughout the whole period. For example, few blood tests are carried out. The hospital only has limited laboratory facilities, but from the beginning hospital staff knew of local reluctance. Some medicines are supposed to be taken four times a day, but are rarely prescribed in this way because patients are unlikely to comply with this. A different kind of accommodation occurred when a hole was made in the wall between the clinic and the inpatient ward and a door was put in, so that women could go through without being seen by other women outside the hospital.[114]

The following story illustrates how the strategy for a whole area of medical practice for one doctor was changed as a result of a trau-

112 Personal participation.

113 Ibid.

114 Letter from Dr Marianne Wood to Mike Gill and Trust friends, 25 February 1988 [Wilson papers].

matic experience shortly after arrival at Khunde Hospital.[115] The case involved the death of a baby and the outcome for the doctor's subsequent practice was the message that "all babies are good babies" and that even if the doctor was worried, he or she should not convey this fear. The baby boy was born after a difficult delivery at home which was attended by hospital staff, and resuscitation was carried out. The baby began to respond, was visited at home again, but over the next day had difficulty feeding, and at the hospital staff's request, was admitted. The baby would not suck but his mother was able to express milk. I later wrote "The baby seemed quite alert, clutched my finger and looked around." The following morning the mother decided to go home. The baby was cocooned against the monsoon rain, and tucked against his head were two pictures of the Dalai Lama whom Sherpas revered. The mother said she would return the following day if difficulties occurred. The baby died. We had thought the baby could be saved, but had not conveyed this clearly to the family, who thought the baby was "sickly" and so preferred to have the baby die at home.

Another area for the doctors to deal with was their relationship with other local practitioners. Their responses ranged from the passive (of knowing that there were other healers practising in the community) to the active (of directly engaging with them). The Langs wrote in their 1970–71 annual report that: "It is difficult to assess what proportion of patients there are whose care we share with the lamas. However we have seldom known rituals to conflict with western medicine, and can claim an amicable relationship with most of our 'professional' colleagues."[116] The hospital's annual reports convey the ongoing pluralism existing in the area and the regular letters from the volunteers to the Trust medical subcommittee also describe many individual cases. In contrast to other annual reports, doctors Penny Dawson and Jamie Uhrig began their 1981–82 report with a series of cases to illustrate the variety of prac-

[115] Diary, Dr John Heydon, and my notes, 7–11 August 1996. Throughout our two years at Khunde Hospital I kept notes on consecutive obstetric cases.

[116] Kunde Hospital Annual Report for the Year Ending 31 October 1971: Including an Analysis of Cases for the First Five Years (1967–1971).

tice at the hospital. One of these referred to their dealings with one of the lhawa:

> We made a home visit to [patient] at Pungitenga as her neighbour said she was about to die of a breast problem. She was advised to come to Kunde for incision and drainage of her breast abscess, but was hesitant to do so because one of the spirit mediums told her that she would meet a bad spirit on the trail. We then visited the spirit medium's house with a gift of chung (local beer) and asked him if the trail was now free of bad spirits. He declared the trail safe so [patient] came to hospital and recovered very quickly from her operation. When later asked to see a Kunde woman with a breast abscess, the spirit medium gave her a spiritual prescription and then advised her to go to hospital. [117]

This degree of engagement was unusual, but illustrates the awareness among different practitioners of each other's role and particularly the volunteers' acceptance of their importance to the patient.

As a generalisation, although the volunteers' individual responses varied in degree, they did not mind these other practitioners except when they delayed a seriously ill patient from being seen by the doctor. Later in their report Dawson and Uhrig wrote that: "The hospital and health workers maintain close relationships with and receive excellent cooperation from all the lamas and Tibetan physicians. The Kunde doctors have also exchanged visits with some of the spirit mediums to develop closer ties and obtain earlier medical referrals." [118] In their report the following year they commented that "doctors disparagement of the work of the lhawas simply damages hospital credibility". [119] Nevertheless, their successors were less enthusiastic and reported the example of a lhawa "agreeing with us that a patient needed to come to the hospital for a drip, but at the same time was telling the family that the last patient dripped at the hospital, died." [120]

117 Kunde Hospital Annual Report, September 1981 to August 1982.

118 Ibid.

119 Kunde Hospital Annual Report, September 1982 to August 1983.

120 Kunde Hospital Annual Report, 1 September1984 to 31 July 1985.

Concern about the lateness of referrals from lhawa was common and a number, as in the following story a few years later, related to suspected tuberculosis:

> Yesterday a couple from Pangboche brought a 3-year-old girl who we are certain had TB. We had seen them initially in Pangboche 2 months ago, again at their home 3 weeks ago and on both occasions said we thought the baby might have TB and that they had to come to the hospital for investigation and treatment. Finally, at 7 yesterday morning, they arrived. The little girl was in a frightful state—severely wasted, dehydrated and with neck stiffness. We did an X-ray but when presented with the possibility of a blood test the parents refused. They also refused any treatment with injections, saying that the baby was too weak to have injections and they would only use oral therapy. We tried to reason with them, but it was hopeless, and they left. We found out later that they had come to us from [name], one of the Khumjung Hlawas (the real reason for them coming down this way). During the night he had done a trance and told them that the cause of the illness was pem (poison). They had come to the hospital so we would look into the stomach and see the snakes that were in there and give the appropriate (oral) medicine. In lieu of our treatment they will probably go to the Du Rimpoche who is supposed to have good poison medicine. For us it was very upsetting and frustrating, as we don't think it was too late to reverse the disease. [121]

This problem occurred even when the same lhawa, like many of the other practitioners, used the hospital themselves. [122]

Preventive health: A case study of iodine deficiency

The discussion so far has concentrated on the treatment aspect of the hospital's work and on the health problems of the individual

121 Drs Elly Kroef and Keith Buswell to Mike Gill, family and friends, 24 June 1985. Khunde Hospital, 1984–1989, Doctors' Reports, Correspondence, etc. Book 1 [SEHF, Toronto].

122 The early registers include patients seen outside the hospital. As with the lay community, using the hospital appeared to be a matter of individual choice and therefore not a conflict between different homogenous groups. From the beginning the patient registers show that many of the monks (but not all) were treated as patients both at the hospital and when visited in the monasteries.

patient. An important part of the volunteers' work revolved around the preventive health programmes aimed at improving the overall health of the community, mainly those of family planning, immunisation and dealing with the effects of the region's iodine deficiency. Draper criticised the hospital for not being sufficiently proactive in public health issues.[123]

This section provides a case study of iodine deficiency in Khumbu and looks at how initially Hillary and Pearl, and then the hospital staff, responded to the problem. By examining one issue over a period of time, the complexity of medical practice at Khunde Hospital becomes clearer, as do the ebbs and flows of policies with changing personnel, different knowledge, other people's ideas and other organisations being involved. It illuminates how despite there being a technical solution available, as M. Miles concludes, caution should be exercised against "simplistic thinking".[124] Such an approach, however, has been at the heart of development discourse, both theory and practice. Lastly, it should be remembered that although Pearl and Hillary may have considered iodine deficiency as the most important public health issue, it was still only one among many health problems to be dealt with by the hospital staff at any one time.

The popular image of Sherpas was of a strong, hardy, fit people, but this "impression of vitality is misleading" wrote Dr H. Kaye Ibbertson who undertook research on the problem of iodine deficiency among Sherpas while Hillary was building Khunde Hospital.[125]

123 Draper, "Beyond Medicine", 390. Although acknowledging that Draper's thesis is unfinished, his work on development, I believe, reflects the complex relationship between anthropology and development, theory and practice. See James Ferguson, "Anthropology and Its Evil Twin: 'Development' in the Constitution of a Discipline", in Cooper and Packard, *International Development and the Social Sciences*, 150–75.

124 Miles, "Goitre, Cretinism and Iodine in South Asia", 67.

125 H. K. Ibbertson, "Himalayan Goitre", in *Abbottempo,* Book 3, ed. Robert G. Richardson (Amsterdam: Abbott Universal, 1969), 30–33. I would like to thank Dr (now Professor) Ibbertson for a copy of this publication. For a well-known early survey in the Himalayan region, see R. McCarrison, "Observations on Endemic Cretinism in the Chitral and Gilgit Valleys", *Lancet*, 31 October 1908, 1275–80. "Endemic cretinism" describes a spec-

Iodine is a trace element that the body requires for the production of the thyroid hormones that are needed for normal growth and development.[126] Its lack in the human diet can lead to various medical problems that include the formation of a goitre (enlargement of the thyroid gland), cretinism (congenital hypothyroidism), and an increase in foetal and infant deaths.[127] Where the problem is severe the overall functioning of a whole community may be impaired.[128] Iodine deficiency is widespread in mountainous regions, such as Khumbu, where the soil lacks iodine, although the problem is neither confined to these areas nor to the Third World.[129] In the late 1980s nearly a fifth of the world's population was at risk from IDD. The principal method for supplementing iodine in the human body is through the iodisation of salt, but iodised salt was not available in Nepal in the 1960s. Sherpas used rock salt from Tibet and still prefer it, for example, in making tea.

---

trum of congenital defects in a community (all associated with iodine deficiency) ranging from people with mental deficiency or deaf mutism of varying degrees, varying severity of paralysis of the arms and legs, to people whose problem is a coordination defect. Basil S. Hetzel, *The Story of Iodine Deficiency: An International Challenge in Nutrition* (Oxford: Oxford University Press, 1989), 36.

126 Hetzel, *The Story of Iodine Deficiency,* 21.

127 Ibid., 84. Various problems can cause goitres, but in Khumbu the main cause is iodine deficiency.

128 John B. Stanbury, "Commentary on Dr. Hetzel's Review of the Global Problem of Iodine Deficiency Disorders", in "The Prevention and Control of Iodine Deficiency Disorders", by Basil S. Hetzel (Rome: Administrative Committee on Coordination – Sub-Committee on Nutrition (ACC/SCN) State-of-the-Art Series, Nutrition Policy discussion Paper No. 3, March 1988, 116–9. In 1987 the United Nations developed a ten-year programme through its ACC/SCN for the prevention and control of IDD. Hetzel, an Australian, was Executive Director of the International Council for Control of Iodine Deficiency Disorders (ICCIDD) that was established in Kathmandu in March 1986.

129 Hetzel, *The Story of Iodine Deficiency,* 147. It is also found in areas prone to high rainfall and flooding. For a discussion of goitre in New Zealand between 1920 and 1950, see Diana Brown, "'Stepping-stone to Cretinism': Goitre in New Zealand, 1920-1950", B.A. Hons diss., University of Otago, 2000.

In his 1964 article Pearl wrote that he regarded iodine deficiency as the biggest public health problem in Khumbu.[130] Pearl's photos caught the interest of Ibbertson, who in 1961 had become the physician in charge of the Radioisotope Unit at Auckland Hospital.[131] Much was still unknown about the role of iodine. Hillary, Pearl and Ibbertson worked out a programme that was "based on wanting to solve everything".[132] When Ibbertson arrived in 1966 he was able to see the positive effects of the potassium iodate tablets that were given weekly to each child at Khumjung School since Hillary's visit the previous year.[133] Ibbertson's team, which included Gill and the very practical physicist Jack Tait from Christchurch, was attached to the main expedition organised by Hillary, which meant that Ibbertson could concentrate on the research, but leave the enormous amount of work associated with running and being on an expedition in a remote area to others. Having scientists who could work in challenging conditions in the field was important, but even more significantly the researchers were able to benefit from the support Hillary's work enjoyed in Khumbu and use Hillary's links with local communities to gain participants for the research.

The research team's results confirmed the initial impressions of the severe problem in Khumbu.[134] The team examined 1,294 Sherpas and found a prevalence of goitre of 92 per cent; in 63 per cent the enlargement of the thyroid gland was clearly visible. A group of 475 were examined in more detail, of which 30 per cent were considered clinically hypothyroid (underactive thyroid gland) with

[130] Pearl, "Kiwi in Khumbu", 586.

[131] Professor H. Kaye Ibbertson, personal communication, 11 June 1998. The Unit incorporated a thyroid clinic and gradually served as the basis of a Department of Endocrinology.

[132] Interview with Professor H. Kaye Ibbertson, Auckland, May 2002. The research was funded by the Atomic Energy Agency and the Wellcome Trust.

[133] H. K. Ibbertson, "Goitre and Cretinism in the High Himalayas", *New Zealand Medical Journal* 80, no. 529, 11 December 1974, 484–88.

[134] H. K. Ibbertson, J. M. Tait, M. Pearl, T. Lim, J. McKinnon, M. B. Gill, "Endemic Cretinism in Nepal", in *Endemic Cretinism,* Monograph Series No. 2, ed. B. S. Hetzel and O. D. Pharoah (Papua New Guinea: Institute of Human Biology, 1971), 71–88. "Prevalence" is the number of cases of a disease that are present in a particular population at a given time.

facial pallor and puffiness, slowness of thought and movement, and evident cold intolerance. The prevalence of cretinism was 5.9 per cent and deaf-mutism 4.7 per cent, the combined rate being higher than that described in most other studies elsewhere in the world. The village of Phortse was the most severely affected with 93.5 per cent of its 215 inhabitants having goitres, almost 40 per cent being clinically hypothyroid, a cretinism rate of 10.2 per cent and deaf-mutism rate of 3.1 per cent. While the research participants were to some extent self-selected, the team had examined 95 per cent of the population in Phortse, 75 per cent in Khunde where the team was based and 40 per cent in Khumjung.

The last few weeks of the research team's stay in Khumbu was spent initiating a treatment programme which would use an injection of iodised oil (lipiodol).[135] This was to be under the supervision of McKinnon at the newly constructed hospital. A 600-person double-blind therapy trial was begun in the villages surveyed using injections of either iodised oil or saline or thyroxine or placebo tablets.[136] Another group of 600 people received iodised oil only. Goitres shrank dramatically which provided good publicity for the new hospital.[137] Ibbertson described how cretin children lost weight and became more active.[138] In his 1975 autobiography Hillary told the story of one young man who "had responded so positively to iodine that he speeded up his normal shambling gait beyond his sense of balance and ended up with a broken collarbone".[139]

Injections for goitre prophylaxis had first been used in remote, rugged New Guinea in the late 1950s.[140] By the early 1970s the injection of iodised oil had been widely accepted in the medical lit-

135 Ibbertson, "Himalayan Goitre", 30 and 33; Ibbertson, "Goitre and Cretinism in the High Himalayas".

136 McKinnon, "Health Problems of Khumbu", 4.

137 Interview, McKinnon, 1997.

138 Ibbertson, "Himalayan Goitre", 33.

139 Hillary, *Nothing Venture, Nothing Win*, 270.

140 Hetzel, *The Story of Iodine Deficiency*, 58–62; Ibbertson, "Goitre and Cretinism in the High Himalayas", 488; S. F. McCullagh, "The Huon Peninsula Endemic: I. The Effectiveness of an Intramuscular Depot of Iodized Oil in the Control of Endemic Goitre", *Medical Journal of Australia,* 25 May 1963,

erature as an effective form of treatment and prophylaxis of goitre in remote areas of severe endemic iodine deficiency where iodised salt was not available. Goitre was widespread throughout Nepal. In 1973 the Government of Nepal established a Goitre Control Project that was to be responsible for the purchase and distribution of iodised salt from India.[141] The project was unsuccessful in its early years, and when one hundred samples were tested in 1979 not one was found to be adequately iodised. That year the Government gave the Goitre and Cretinism Eradication Project, as it came to be called, responsibility for a mass iodised oil injection campaign, mainly in the hills and mountains. The project was linked with the Ministry of Health's Expanded Programme of Immunisation (EPI), with support from WHO and UNICEF. It began in 1980 with four target districts each year and with the aim of covering 90 per cent of the total population, especially women of childbearing age and children. By the mid-1980s some progress had been made with what were now referred to as iodine deficiency disorders (IDD).[142] Nearly two-and-a-half million injections had been given by 1986 in twenty-eight of the country's seventy-five districts; twenty of these were in the mountains.[143] As was repeatedly found in Nepal, and this cannot be overemphasised, the rugged topography, limited infrastructure and lack of financial and human resources made implementation of any such projects difficult. The government continued its salt iodisation programme, but 50 per cent of samples tested in 1985 were still inadequately iodised. There were also delays in transportation, problems with packaging, storage and delivery to remote areas. With the unsatisfactory situation regarding

---

769–77. McCullagh, however, had raised concerns about the risk of iodism and felt that the injections should not be given to people with goitres.

141 Hetzel, *The Story of Iodine Deficiency,* 198–99. The Goitre Control Project was bilateral cooperation between the governments of Nepal and India. India also had a major iodine deficiency problem, and its own salt iodisation programme was inadequate (pp. 87–88).

142 Hetzel suggested the term iodine deficiency disorders (IDD) in 1983 to denote the wide spectrum of problems. Hetzel, *The Story of Iodine Deficiency,* 84–85.

143 Ibid., 141–43 and 198.

the importation of salt from India, the Goverment began to plan its own iodisation plants in a bilateral project with the Government of India.

In the early 1990s Khunde Hospital doctors, David Murdoch and Elizabeth Harding, studied various groups of Khumbu Sherpas and tested salt supplies to assess the current situation regarding the prevalence of goitre and cretinism. [144] With rates of goitre of 21 per cent, deaf-mutism 1.3 per cent and cretinism 0.5 per cent, IDD were much less than in 1966, but Harding and Murdoch believed iodine deficiency continued to be a major problem for Khumbu requiring "a clear control strategy, combining ongoing iodine supplementation and education". [145] Khumbu was classified as a region of mild to moderate iodine deficiency. One of their criticisms was that since the iodised oil injections were given initially, although it is recommended they should be repeated every three to five years, "further supplementation by iodised oil has been sporadic at best". [146] They criticised the hospital for not having a maintenance iodine suppplementation programme. They were also particularly surprised that there had been no cretins born since 1966. [147]

What had happened? The early phase of dealing with Khumbu's iodine deficiency described a very proactive approach from Hillary, his medical adviser, Pearl, and McKinnon, the doctor at Khunde Hospital. A problem had been identified, research carried out and action taken. Although Ibbertson made follow-up visits in 1968 and

[144] David R. Murdoch, Elizabeth G. Harding and John T. Dunn, "Persistence of Iodine Deficiency 25 Years After Initial Correction Efforts in the Khumbu Region of Nepal", *New Zealand Medical Journal* 112, 23 July 1999, 266–68.

[145] Murdoch, Harding and Dunn, "Persistence of Iodine Deficiency 25 Years After", 266.

[146] Ibid., 268.

[147] The level of cretinism is a sensitive indicator for iodine deficiency and the low level could perhaps suggest that Murdoch and Harding were being overly harsh in their criticism of the hospital's performance. I am grateful to Professor Ibbertson for his comments regarding cretinism and iodine deficiency. Interview, Ibbertson, May 2002. In fact, one cretin was born, but to a mother who had refused the injection.

1972, management of iodine deficiency in Khumbu after 1966 was from Khunde Hospital.[148]

Early hospital records show many people being given the injections, but written sources currently stored at the hospital provide little and only periodic information about ongoing policies and practices.[149] Iodine injections were available at the hospital throughout the period and were given when people requested them or as part of other vaccination campaigns. Medical knowledge, especially initially, about the length of time before another injection was needed was imprecise. In the early 1970s Lindsay Strang believed that research suggested the period between injections could be more than five years and perhaps up to seven.[150] In 1973 the hospital received a large donation of the injections from UNICEF.[151] Monitoring of the iodine programme does appear to have been limited. A letter in 1974 to the UNICEF representative in Kathmandu by Khunde doctor Paul Silvester referred to both inadequate and misleading records in that he believed not all recipients had been recorded.[152] Silvester thought that the 500 iodine injections he had given "would seem to reflect maintenance of the initial energetic programme". He had in stock a further 840 ampoules. The hospital had also received gifts of iodised salt. In the early 1980s, Canadian doctors,

148 Ibbertson, personal communication, 11 June 1998; H. K. Ibbertson, P. D. Gluckman, M. S. Croxson, L. J. W. Strang, "Goiter and Cretinism in the Himalayas: A Reassessment", in *Endemic Goiter and Cretinism: Continuing Threats to World Health,* ed. J. T. Dunn and G. A. Medeiros-Neto (Pan-American Health Organization Scientific Publication No. 292, 1974), 129–34.

149 Apart from the patient registers, many other hospital records have been retained only on an ad hoc basis.

150 Kunde Hospital Report for the Year Ending 31 October 1972. Recommendations following a government survey in 1985 in six districts suggested four years. S. Acharya, "Monitoring and Evaluation of an IDD Control Program in Nepal", in *The Prevention and Control of Iodine Deficiency Disorders,* ed. Basil S. Hetzel, John T. Dunn and John B. Stanbury (Amsterdam: Elsevier, 1987), 213–16.

151 Kunde Hospital Annual Report for the Year Ending 31 October 1973.

152 Paul Silvester to H. K. Kuloy, UNICEF Representative, Kathmandu, 5 July 1974, assorted papers [KH].

Penny Dawson and Jamie Uhrig, referred in their annual reports to the injections being offered to all residents at the same time as BCG vaccinations, being available on demand year round and being offered to all women who brought their children to the annual vaccination clinics. [153] No mention about the iodine issue subsequently was made in the annual reports until the early 1990s. [154]

Hospital records are variable, both in respect to the iodine deficiency issue and other programmes, and some practical considerations do need to be taken into consideration. The number of hospital staff was small, and while it would be possible to focus on any one programme the demands on the time of the staff were many. Clinical work was immediate, village visits could take days, and, as has been discussed in chapter one, staff were also involved in non-medical roles. As each set of volunteers changed, there would be a period of settling into the work of the hospital at the beginning. The tendency was for the volunteers to concentrate on particular problems at a given time. For example, recruiting and training hospital staff was more of an issue in the 1970s, when there was considerable turnover, than in the 1980s and 90s. Prioritising work was further influenced by the interests and training of the different staff. Early volunteers, for instance, had less public health training or experience. Also, part of the apparent decreasing activity by the hospital regarding iodine deficiency probably also related to increasing activity by the Nepalese government programme for giving iodised oil injections. The Solukhumbu district was covered in 1984–85, 1989–90 and in 1995. [155] Coverage varied, but the earlier mass campaigns by the hospital were no longer necessary. In 1997, the policy was to offer injections to all pregnant women who had not received one in 1995 and who were not taking iodised salt. [156]

153 Kunde Hospital Annual Report, September 1981–August 1982 and Kunde Hospital Annual Report, September 1982 to August 1983.

154 Kunde Hospital Annual Report, 1 June 1991 to 31 May 1992.

155 Marjatta Tolvanen, Project Officer, Nutrition, UNICEF to Elizabeth Harding, 20 December 1994 [KH]. The expanding presence of government health services in the region and Khunde Hospital's decreasing isolation is discussed in chapter four.

156 Kunde Hospital and Village Clinics Annual Report 1997.

Research, monitoring and evaluation

The question of iodine deficiency also raised some concerns surrounding the issue of research and this further complicates discussion of the question of a proactive or more reactive policy on the part of the hospital. The government health authorities in Nepal expressed concern at the apparent delay in producing a report on the 1966 research, and criticism also appeared in the local press and in the *Journal of Nepal Medical Association* that suggested foreign research was being carried out in Nepal but that the Nepalese would not benefit.[157] This was never the intention. In his report to the Director of Health on the health problems of Khumbu and the work of Khunde Hospital during its first nine months, McKinnon commented on the worth of the research believing that: "Before studies are completed, it is not possible to recommend definitive treatment but it is hoped that this research project will demonstrate an easy, cheap and effective method of controlling the widespread and economically damaging effects of iodine lack."[158] Ibbertson's research aimed to find out about goitre and cretinism in Khumbu, initiate a treatment and prevention programme and would also contribute to the international research debate that was occurring in this period about how to deal with the problem in areas around the world such as Khumbu.

Carrying out research and providing health care services, however, have separate concerns. The research process had involved a detailed history, examination, anthropometric measurements and tests.[159] Dr Mike Gill, who was assisting Ibbertson and who had been to Khumbu several times, later recalled that the people were very co-operative "with laughter and witty comments to the fore" during the measurement process.[160] People were more reluctant about the tests, but the team eventually obtained about 350 blood

[157] McKinnon to Dr Joshi, Director of Health, 6 October 1967. Also see *Journal of Nepal Medical Association* 5, no. 1, January 1967, 60–62 and 6, no. 1, January 1968, 31–33.

[158] McKinnon, "Health Problems of Khumbu", 4.

[159] Ibbertson, "Himalayan Goitre", 30–33.

[160] Gill, email to author, 8 January 1998.

and urine samples. [161] Hillary's sirdar Mingma Tsering played a key role in persuading people to give blood samples. When the treatment programme and trial began, the village of Phortse was used as a control. Ibbertson recalled that when he visited Nepal in 1968 to carry out follow-up work Phortse villagers were unhappy. [162] It was the only time he felt unwelcome. Ibbertson was due to return while Selwyn and Ann Lang were the Khunde doctors, but when delays occurred and they did not hear from him they gave iodine injections to Phortse villagers who were "distressed" that they had not yet been able to get them. [163] Difficulties created by the distance between Nepal and New Zealand and the poor and slow means of communication contributed to the uncomfortable situation that the doctors at Khunde found themselves in. The giving of the injections ended the controlled trial in Khumbu, but this research issue was in any case coming to a close. By this time the iodised oil injection was being incorporated into international public health practice, and an investigation in New Guinea that was published in *The Lancet* in 1971 confirmed the link with cretinism and was accepted as definitive. [164]

Research continued to arise periodically as an issue. One type of situation occurred when outsiders wanted to take advantage of the hospital's facilities and its close relationship with the community. Both Adams and Draper had access to the hospital's records and Adams described scenes in the hospital's clinic. [165] In the early 1990s a researcher working in the area claimed she was associated with the hospital when she was not, but a directive from the Himalayan Trust's medical sub-committee in New Zealand allowed the doctors at the hospital to decline access to the hospital's records. [166] Other researchers were more supportive. For example, in Septem-

161 Ibbertson, "Himalayan Goitre", 32.

162 Interview, Ibbertson, 2002.

163 Interview, Drs Selwyn and Ann Lang, 2002.

164 Hetzel, *The Story of Iodine Deficiency,* 65.

165 Adams, *Tigers of the Snow and Other Virtual Sherpas,* 96–98. The volunteers at Khunde Hospital were unhappy when they found out how they had been portrayed in the book.

166 Personal communication, Professor David Murdoch, November 2005.

ber 1991 a Japanese team investigated fifty people in Namche and Khumjung with symptoms of dyspepsia which was one of the commonest presenting symptoms at the hospital. Staff were only able to carry out a limited range of tests and procedures at the hospital, and so the opportunity to investigate a common problem further was welcome. Twenty of these people were found to have "obvious upper GI pathology, including 9 with peptic ulceration".[167] Doctors Murdoch and Cook continued in their annual report that they took anyone presenting with dyspeptic symptoms "seriously".

Yet another scenario was when the volunteers wanted to undertake some investigation themselves. For example, in 1989 one of the doctors was keen to investigate a local syndrome. When she referred the issue back to the Trust in New Zealand, the latter's response was cautious urging her to "consider the broader implications, in particular as it relates to community attitudes towards the hospital".[168] The importance of the hospital's relationship with the community and the trust that can be bestowed was reinforced in 1997 when, during a study to look at the prevalence of hepatitis, the headmaster of Khumjung School said he was happy for the school to participate, but only the Khunde doctor and local hospital staff were allowed to carry out the testing.[169] The visiting medical student was excluded.

Research, surveys, monitoring and evaluation were proactive tools that helped the doctors to deal with health issues in the area, but much research undertaken in Nepal bemoans the lack of accurate data. Censuses have been undertaken in Nepal since 1911, but collecting reliable information in the mountains was and remains difficult. In June and July 1970 the Langs visited each house in Khumbu and carried out a demographic survey.[170] They recorded a

167 Kunde Hospital Annual Report 1 June 1991 to 31 May 1992. "GI" refers to gastro-intestinal.

168 McKinnon to Drs Ian Schokking and Catherine Hagen, 10 October 1989, Correspondence 89–91 (Ian & Catherine) [KH].

169 Personal communication, Dr John Heydon, 1997.

170 Kunde Hospital Annual Report 1 November 1969 to 31 October 1970 + Demographic Survey of the Upper Khumbu East No. 3 Nepal. This was published as S. D. R. Lang and Ann Lang, "The Kunde Hospital and a

total population for Khumbu of 2,761.[171] The study revealed a neonatal (first month of life) mortality rate of 51 per 1,000 live births, an infant (first year of life) mortality rate of 158 per 1,000 live births and a childhood (1 to 12 years) mortality rate of 130 per 1,000 live births. As the Langs starkly summarised "Over one-quarter of children born alive fail to live into their teens".[172]

The information gained from this study could have provided the baseline information for the hospital to monitor health programmes in the area, but paradoxically it has been used most by other researchers.[173] In 1989 hospital staff undertook a follow-up survey for most of the area, but the analysis and write-up was not finished.[174] Without such data it was impossible to monitor the effectiveness of the hospital's work in statistical terms. Harding and Murdoch's later criticism of a lack of a maintenance programme to deal with iodine deficiency was symptomatic of a wider lack of policy planning and direction. Before she undertook her survey, Dr Marianne Wood had written back to New Zealand that she believed

> very strongly that the Trust should have some proper figures on things like infant mortality and literacy. It's easy to assume that simply because we are all doing our best that things must be improving. It will also give a concrete point with which to compare things in another 20 years![175]

Demographic Survey of the Upper Khumbu, Nepal", *New Zealand Medical Journal* 74, 1971, 1–8.

171 The 1971 government census total for the equivalent area of the Namche and Khumjung panchayat was 2,578.

172 Lang and Lang, "The Kunde Hospital and a demographic survey", 4.

173 Charles A. Weitz, Ivan G. Pawson, M. Velma Weitz, Selwyn D. R. Lang and Ann Lang, "Cultural Factors Affecting the Demographic Structure of a High Altitude Nepalese Population", *Social Biology* 25, Fall 1978, 179–95; Pawson, Stanford and Adams, "Effects of Modernization on the Khumbu Region of Nepal." The Langs' article in the *NZMJ* is widely cited in a range of literature about both Khumbu and the wider Himalayan region. For example, see Andrea S. Wiley, *An Ecology of High-Altitude Infancy: A Biocultural Perspective* (Cambridge: Cambridge University Press, 2004).

174 Wood, "1989 Survey of Khumbu Region of Nepal".

175 Marianne Wood to Mike Gill and friends, 27 February 1989 [Wilson papers].

However, collecting reliable data takes a lot of time.[176]

Health education

Despite the importance of having useful information to monitor and evaluate, the hospital's main aim was to encourage the local population to use biomedicine. The Khunde volunteers were guests in the local community and in Nepal. They had no means of coercion; however seriously they viewed a medical problem, they had no method of compelling someone to accept their treatment.

The volunteers have had to be patient, but this should not be viewed as indifference. Local Sherpas and hospital staff have gone about their business, sometimes together and sometimes along different paths. Usually the relationship was harmonious. Frustration felt by the staff often led to an attitude of resignation about what to do, but on a few occasions there has been considerable anger. One of these times was in 1984 and concerned the destruction of a large number of doses of measles vaccine by children in the village. The vaccine had arrived from UNICEF in Kathmandu months too early for the following year's vaccination programme and in the monsoon presented considerable cold storage problems. Doctors Keith Buswell and Elly Kroef found the only place cold enough was in the bucket in the water pipe intake. When they went to check it a few days later they were "horrified" to find only 18 of the 50 vials were there.[177] "We were furious and started going around the village looking for it." They found several smashed vials on the hillside behind the hospital. Hillary's sirdar, Mingma Tsering, "decided that it would be best if he took over and did so." The culprits were found. "They all ended up in the hospital kitchen, with the rest of Kunde crowding at the windows seeing what would happen and probably hoping for a beating." The volunteers, not surprisingly, felt "pretty upset about the whole thing, firstly because we didn't

[176] In 2003 Dr Kami Temba Sherpa and Khunde Hospital assistants Mingma Temba Sherpa and Gayse Nuru Sherpa carried out a demographic survey of both Khumbu and Pharak.

[177] Drs Keith Buswell and Elly Kroef to Gill, 22 June 1984, Elly & Keith's letters and replies, [KH].

want the vaccine sent in the first place, and secondly because the kids here would wantonly destroy the vaccine, while surely knowing it belonged to the hospital."

While success was the best means for promoting Western medicine, the volunteers also used health education to promote a biomedical model of health issues and to encourage people to use the hospital. Much of the education was done on an individual basis, either in the clinic or when out visiting a patient. The other approach was to target groups. Schoolchildren were seen as the key to bringing about changes. The idea was that they would take what they learned in school and spread the message at home. From May 1970 the hospital had its own classroom and children and teachers from five of the six schools in the area attended regular talks and demonstrations on "basic anatomy, physiology, hygiene, and first-aid".[178] Senior students also learned about reproduction and contraception. As the Trust's role in the schools changed, so did the hospital's position with regard to the formal teaching of health education, especially as health became part of the Nepalese school curriculum.

The effectiveness of health education and health promotion in developing countries is unproven. Although few rigorous studies have been carried out, one of these was undertaken at a hospital in Kathmandu.[179] Despite individual health education being given by trained female health workers, it was found that there was no significant impact on maternal knowledge and practices of child-care or on infant health outcomes, although there was a small improvement in the uptake of family planning. In the case of iodine deficiency in Khumbu, Murdoch and Harding found a low level of knowledge about the problem in the early 1990s. They looked at lo-

[178] Lang and Lang, "The Kunde Hospital and a Demographic Survey", 4. The other school, in Namche Bazar, was run by the government and was always "too busy" to attend.

[179] Alison Bolam, Dharma S. Manandhar, Purna Shrestha, Matthew Ellis, Anthony M. de L. Costello, "The Effects of Postnatal Health Education for Mothers on Infant Care and Family Planning Practices in Nepal: A Randomised Controlled Trial", *British Medical Journal* 316, 1998, 805–11. The role of the mother-in-law in social relationships had been ignored.

cal understanding of iodine deficiency. Two Sherpa health workers questioned a group of 201 consecutive Sherpas attending Khunde Hospital or the village health clinics.[180] Of the people surveyed, only 11 per cent understood that goitre was related to the lack of iodine.

This finding puzzled Ibbertson who believed that they had put a lot of effort into educating people about the issue.[181] Health education pursues a course that promotes knowledge as the basis upon which to encourage a change in attitudes and so produce a change in behaviour. While those people who did associate goitre with the lack of iodine had a much higher level of schooling than those who did not, it would seem that many of those who had received health education lessons had either forgotten what they had been taught or perhaps did not believe the reason.[182] Nevertheless, many more of those questioned, 54 per cent, knew about methods of treatment with many mentioning the injections. Even if knowledge amongst Khumbu villagers appears deficient, changed behaviour by having an iodised oil injection or using iodised salt has decreased, if not eradicated, the problem of iodine deficiency disorders in Khumbu.[183]

Another key topic for health education was hygiene. In Western medical terms, hygiene for the volunteer doctors at Khunde Hospital concerned personal cleanliness and preventing the spread of disease. Teaching about the importance of hygiene was one thing, but implementing hygienic practices was quite another. Khumbu is

[180] Murdoch, Harding and Dunn, "Persistence of Iodine Deficiency 25 Years and After," 267–68. They assumed all Sherpas had seen cretins and people with goitre. There are Sherpa words for both, and even separate words for male and female cretins.

[181] Interview, Ibbertson, May 2002.

[182] Murdoch, Harding and Dunn, "Persistence of Iodine Deficiency 25 Years and After," 268. A mean value of 8 years of schooling as compared with 1.6 years. The age range was 11 to 86 years, but 69 per cent were female who probably had less schooling. Other sources of information were the hospital or the village clinics.

[183] The most recent survey of iodine status, based on a community study, records a further decline. Emma Heydon, "A survey of iodine status in a Sherpa community", B.Med.Sci. thesis, University of Otago, 2006.

dusty, with the fine dust penetrating everywhere. The air is cold or freezing much of the year and the water is also cold. Water has to be collected from springs or tanks and carried to a person's house, but in Khumjung in the dry spring months the spring dried up. Khunde Hospital had a year-round supply of running water, but at times during winter the pipe froze when there was no sunshine and the hospital had to rely on a tank in the kitchen until the pipe thawed. Keeping oneself clean in such an environment is difficult and without hot water is uncomfortable. Traditionally, people washed themselves and their clothes very infrequently, but one of the big changes that long-term hospital employees note has been the improvement in the personal hygiene of Khumbu people.[184] It did not occur as a result of a short-term project to educate people, but was a gradual process over decades. Soap, which people can afford to buy, is available at the weekly market and the increasing number of small shops around the district. One of the perks for people working at the hospital is the access to a hot shower and water to wash clothes.

Hygiene was also taught to help prevent the spread of disease, but this has probably had less effect. While the hospital's water supply in the mid-1990s was clean, others, for example in Namche Bazar where the houses are situated above the source, were contaminated.[185] Less than a quarter of the rural population of Nepal in the mid-1980s had access to safe drinking water.[186] The spread of disease, however, is not connected to the quality of water alone. What happens afterwards, such as whether people wash their hands, is no less important. In 1971 the Langs noted that "Self-limiting diarrhoeas are extremely prevalent at the time of Sherpa festivals when

184 Conversations with Kami Temba and Mingma Temba, Khunde, 1996–98.

185 The water supply at the hospital and in Namche Bazar was tested while we were there. Namche Bazar now has an improved water supply. See Epilogue, note 14.

186 Almas Ali, *Status of Health in Nepal* (Resource Centre for Primary Health Care Nepal and South-South Solidarity, India, July 1991), 16. Source of Data: International Drinking Water Supply and Sanitation Decade, Nepal Resource Mobilisation Profile, 1986.

the convivial glass of chang passes freely from hand to hand."[187] Diarrhoeal disease remains common. In 1997 diarrhoea was the fourth commonest presenting problem at the hospital with 491 (6.78 per cent of the total) outpatient consultations.[188] The risk of disease is heightened with the large number of visitors each trekking season and especially when the weather is warmer. The dry sanitation system of Sherpa toilets works well for much of the year, but the need to cope with thousands of visitors in a small area over a short period presents serious challenges. The disposal of rubbish is also a problem and is again exacerbated by the large number of tourists.[189]

Tourists and Khunde Hospital

The health need of the local people was the reason for the hospital's existence and was why the volunteers went to Khunde Hospital. The last part of this discussion on practising medicine examines sickness among the increasing number of overseas visitors to the area. Dealing with tourists became an integral part of the medical work of Khunde Hospital and the lives of the overseas volunteers while they were at Khunde. That less than 4 per cent of the hospital's outpatient consultations in 1996 were for tourists in no way reflected the considerable amount of time expended on this group of patients.[190]

While many people, both inhabitants and visitors, become sick for various reasons associated with the cold, rugged physical environment or poor hygiene, the most pervasive factor influencing the health of travellers in the Everest region was the lack of oxygen

[187] Kunde Hospital Annual report for the Year Ending 31 October 1971: Including an Analysis of Cases for the First Five Years (1967–1971), 19.

[188] Kunde Hospital and Village Clinics Annual Report 1997. The hospital acts as the village clinic for the immediate area. People in other villages would use their village clinic and so the total would be higher.

[189] See, for example, Paul Rogers and John Aitchison, *Towards Sustainable Tourism in the Everest Region of Nepal* (Kathmandu: IUCN – The World Conservation Union and ICPL, 1998).

[190] Kunde Hospital and Village Clinics Annual Report 1996.

due to the very high altitude. It was not an area of medicine considered important in the medical school training of the volunteer doctors and in New Zealand nobody lived at high altitude. The Trust's medical members advised new appointees to learn about health problems at high altitude before they left for Khunde, but experience was gained on the job. All the villages of Khumbu were above 3,000 metres and the popular tourist destinations were over 5,000 metres.

Most visitors experienced some form of sickness, ranging from the relatively minor inconvenience of the common cold to conditions resulting in death. [191] When sick, tourists self-treated, were treated by their group or another visitor, or sought help from a health facility. An increasing number of outpatient consultations at Khunde Hospital reflected the rising number of tourists in the area. In 1967 there were just three tourist consultations, but by 1996 the number had increased to 265 (3.7 per cent of total consultations). [192] Consultation was sought for a wide range of problems, and not just for conditions such as diarrhoea that are commonly associated with travel. Inpatient figures presented another profile. Of the 178 tourist admissions between October 1970 and December 1997, 72 (8 per cent of the total hospital admissions) were for altitude sickness. [193]

Research on travellers in Khumbu has contributed to advancing knowledge about the effects of high altitude on non-resident populations and has shown the extent of the problem for the Everest area. The severity of the altitude hazard was realised by Evans. He wrote that during the 16 months in 1968–69 that he was at Khunde, 800 tourists had visited the area, of which eight had had severe altitude

[191] See, for example, David R. Murdoch, "Symptoms of Infection and Altitude Illness Among Hikers in the Mount Everest Region of Nepal", *Aviation, Space, and Environmental Medicine,* February 1995, 148–51. Out of 283 hikers (trekkers) surveyed, Murdoch found that 87 per cent had symptoms of infection.

[192] Kunde Hospital and Village Clinics Annual Report 1996.

[193] Other categories were: respiratory problems—26; gastro-intestinal complaints—24; trauma—21 and other causes—35.

sickness and two had died distanced from any help.[194] The seminal paper in *The Lancet* in 1976 described a study based on the Himalayan Rescue Association's post at Pheriche at 4,243 metres.[195] This health post was set up in the early 1970s to help sick tourists and to carry out research. The study found that 53 per cent of those investigated had symptoms of altitude sickness.

The higher people go and the faster the rate of ascent, the more likely they are to develop altitude sickness, with problems ranging from a mild headache to death. Patients at Khunde Hospital who were normally resident at low altitude, whether they were visitors from overseas or from within Nepal such as most porters and government officials, have shown the range of symptoms that constitute altitude sickness.[196] Those that have been admitted to hospital represented the serious end of the spectrum, but the rate of severe altitude sickness in the region has declined since the 1960s.[197]

Evans' report emphasised the importance of warning people about the effects of high altitude and what to do if someone became severely sick.[198] The present emphasis on prevention was a more recent development from the later 1970s.[199] Severe altitude sickness is largely avoidable. The prevention approach indicated that

194 Hillary Hospital Report, [August] to 12 December 1969. The top of the page is torn, obscuring the date.

195 P. H. Hackett, D. Rennie and H. D. Levine, "The Incidence, Importance, and Prophylaxis of Acute Mountain Sickness", *Lancet,* 1976, 1149–54.

196 David Murdoch and Lynley Cook, "Altitude Illness in Nepalis", *Journal of Nepal Medical Association* 31, July–September 1993, 288–92. This paper was presented at the International Conference on the Role of General Practitioners in Developing Countries, Kathmandu, 1–4 February, 1993.

197 Personal communication, Professor David Murdoch, June 2004. See also John B. West, *High Life: A History of High-Altitude Physiology and Medicine* (New York: Oxford University Press for the American Physiological Society, 1998), 384–85 and Charles S. Houston, *Going High: The Story of Man and Altitude,* 3rd ed. (Boston: Little, Brown, 1987), 179. West describes an overall reduction in altitude sickness, while Murdoch emphasises the decline in severe altitude sickness.

198 Hillary Hospital Report [August] to 12 December 1969.

199 Personal communication, Murdoch, 2004. The education promoted by the Himalayan Rescue Association began this development.

the best way to cope with the high altitude conditions of the Everest area was to employ a conservative rate of ascent, to stop climbing if one was feeling unwell and descend if one's condition did not improve. The problem with the Everest area is that it remains difficult to descend quickly to a safe altitude. Treatment with oxygen, or a portable pressure bag (in the 1990s), and medication then assumed greater importance.

Lastly, the high-altitude tourist, whether trekker or climber, had an impact on the provision of health services for the local population. The growth of tourism worldwide since the 1960s resulted in rising numbers of people visiting high-altitude areas. The first issue concerned what the doctors at Khunde called "trekker medicine". By the 1960s, Himalayan expeditions had built a tradition of providing medical care to local populations in areas through which they travelled. At that stage there were often no biomedical services, but the increasing number of expeditions and trekkers to the Everest area continued to provide medicines and treatment to local people.[200] This was given and used in good faith, but created some problems. Doctors at the hospital were concerned about various issues such as continuity of care, particularly for chronic problems, people not using the permanent services and the lack of medical knowledge of the trekkers and indeed some of the tourist doctors.[201] From the hospital's perspective, the peak period of concern was the mid-1970s through to the early 1980s. This was the period in which the Sagarmatha National Park was established, the World Bank undertook a regional tourism study, and there were often several other doctors in the area.[202] Although these mainly researched high-altitude issues, their treatment of local patients was seen by the overseas staff at the hospital to further fragment care. The area had a lot of cases of tuberculosis, for example, and monitoring completion of treatment was difficult at the best of times.

[200] Such assistance peaks in the spring and autumn when most visitors come to the area.

[201] This is well documented in the correspondence files at Khunde Hospital.

[202] See, for example, Dr Rob Riley's "Report of Khumbu Medical Services Meeting" which was held at the Everest View Hotel on 4 May 1977, assorted papers [KH].

Another concern for hospital staff involved rising expectations. Khunde Hospital was generally well equipped and supplied, but remained oriented towards providing basic health care services.[203] Visiting doctors sometimes saw a patient and then referred them to the hospital with a note requesting a test or medicine that the hospital did not have, thus risking a lowering of the standing of the hospital to the patient.[204] A related dilemma was that local people knew that visitors carried medicines for their personal use. The WHO recommends, and not only for a country with limited resources such as Nepal, the use of oral fluids for rehydration in cases of uncomplicated diarrhoea, which is very common among both local people and visitors. Visitors, however, carry medicines, including potent antibiotics, which can considerably speed up recovery from an unpleasant condition; not surprisingly, local people also want these.

Behind the statistics and the policies was another set of stories for the volunteers that they wrote about in reports, correspondence with the Trust or the SEHF, and letters home to family and friends. The details of each case were in sharp contrast to the stories they wrote about local Sherpas and further demonstrated the complexity of medical practice at Khunde Hospital. At any given time, a doctor at Khunde Hospital had to be able to deal with a local Sherpa patient who believed that spirits had caused their problem or a visitor who was used to the best medical facilities of a city. At Khunde Hospital the two patients probably shared the same room.

The Development of Village Health Services

In Nepal in 1961 only 3.6 per cent of the population lived in towns with five thousand or more people.[205] Access to health services for those living in rural areas was a problem. While the volunteers at Khunde Hospital did not think that cost was a particular barrier to people using the hospital because services were free, they did

203 Kunde Hospital Handbook, revised by Drs Elly Kroef and Keith Buswell, February 1985, 1: no page numbers.

204 Personal communication, Dr John Heydon, June 2004.

205 ESCAP, *Population of Nepal*, 20–21.

have concerns about access in terms of distance.[206] Khunde Hospital was situated at the centre of a triangle of which the apex was Namche Bazar, and the sides extended up the river valleys of the Bhote Kosi in one direction and the Imja Khola in the other. Most patients walked or were carried to the hospital. McKinnon believed that there was a need for making services more accessible in relation to where people lived. While a third of Khumbu's population lived in Khunde and Khumjung, two-thirds lived further away. The greater the distance, the more major an excursion was a visit to the hospital.[207]

From the start, McKinnon went out to the villages of the area. He visited the villages further away approximately once a month and more frequently visited Namche Bazar. Going out from the hospital to where people lived allowed him the opportunity to reach those who perhaps would not go to the hospital. Successful treatment enabled people to see the benefits of the medicine he believed in and he was able to keep in contact with patients "too old, or too sick, to make the journey to the hospital".[208]

The first attempt at providing a service based in the community arose as a result of the need to continue tuberculosis treatment.[209] Evidence from the national health survey of 1965–66 showed that tuberculosis was widespread in Nepal, but most serious in Kathmandu.[210] Limited treatment was available in some parts of Nepal, and in 1965 the government established the Tuberculosis Control Project with the help of the WHO and UNICEF.[211] The project's

206 See chapter two for an alternative discussion. In the case of tuberculosis, McKinnon did see that there were financial implications.

207 Hillary was aware of this, as the initial quote shows, because unlike government health posts he provided inpatient facilities so that people did not have to use their limited resources.

208 McKinnon, "Health Problems of Khumbu", 2.

209 Ibid., 3. The hospital followed the recommendations of the WHO Tuberculosis Research Centre in Madras, India. See Amrith, "In Search of a 'Magic Bullet' for Tuberculosis".

210 Worth and Shah, *Nepal Health Survey,* 69.

211 Dirgh Singh Bam and Ian Smith, "Principles of Effective Tuberculosis Control in Nepal", *Journal of Nepal Medical Association* 34, 1996, 3–7.

primary aim was to give BCG vaccinations to the whole population. Treatment with a standard chemotherapy was also introduced the same year. The western and central mountain regions were thought to be relatively free of the disease, but based on the experience of his earlier expeditions, Hillary considered tuberculosis to be a major health problem in Khumbu.[212]

After three months of daily treatment at the hospital tuberculosis patients returned home to their villages, but still required twice weekly streptomycin injections and isoniazid tablets for eighteen months to two years. McKinnon realised that this requirement to come to the hospital for treatment so frequently, and over a long period, seriously disrupted people's lives. People were poor and could not afford to spend long periods of time away from their homes or work. Some villages in Khumbu were up to five hours walk from the hospital, and the journey could take much longer when a person was sick.[213] McKinnon decided to train a young man from each of the main villages to provide the treatment at home.[214] In the three-month training course at the hospital, McKinnon also taught a basic knowledge of health and disease. By October 1967 the scheme had ten patients in two villages.[215] These "village nurses" were also helpful contact people during the doctor's village visits. The scheme expanded as the numbers on tuberculosis treatment increased, and by May 1968 there were 43 patients receiving their treatment in their home village.[216]

The second phase in the development of village-based services in Khumbu came in 1970 through the use of teachers as health assistants in those villages that had Hillary schools—that is Thame,

212 As already noted, Khumbu was not included in the national survey.

213 Temporary settlements, such as those in the higher summer pasture areas, were even further away.

214 Boys were more likely to have had some education. See chapter two of this book.

215 McKinnon, "Health Problems of Khumbu", 3.

216 McKinnon to Dr Das, Director, Department of Health, Kunde Hospital: Six Monthly Report Dec. 1967/May 1968.

Phortse, Pangboche and the monastic school at Tengboche.[217] Namche Bazar was excluded as it had a Government health post, which for a short time (from November 1970) had a doctor. The teachers went to Khunde Hospital for fortnightly lectures and demonstrations and were taught to administer the necessary drugs prescribed to those receiving tuberculosis treatment. In their village they had a simple medical kit to treat patients who came to them with minor health complaints, but they were to refer to the hospital or to the doctor's monthly clinic the people who had more serious problems. They were also to keep in contact with villagers who had chronic illnesses. The health assistant also had an important role to promote health education in the village. In 1970–71 the health assistants saw between them approximately two thousand outpatients throughout the district during the year—as many as at Khunde Hospital.[218]

The third stage in the development of the village health system occurred in the mid-1970s and was one that the hospital continued to use. In many countries during this period various schemes based on the "barefoot doctor" concept were set up. They aimed to bring a basic level of health services to as many people as possible, particularly in rural areas of Third World countries. The most famous example was in China, which in 1973 became a member of the WHO.[219] The new scheme at Khunde Hospital, nevertheless, was a continuation of its earlier policy to provide health services nearer to where people lived and the way the scheme developed was in response to specific local conditions.

217 Kunde Hospital Report for the Year Ending 31 October, 1971: Including an Analysis of Cases for the First Five Years (1967–1971).

218 Ibid.

219 For a nationalist interpretation of China's influence on the WHO, see Sung Lee, "WHO and the Developing World: The Contest for Ideology", in Cunningham and Andrews, *Western Medicine as Contested Knowledge,* 24–45. For more balanced discussion see Marcos Cueto, "The Origins of Primary Health Care and Selective Primary Health Care", *American Journal of Public Health* 94, no. 11, 2004, 1864–74, and Socrates Litsios, "The Christian Medical Commission and the Development of the World Health Organization's Primary Health Care Approach", *American Journal of Public Health* 94, no. 11, 2004, 1884–93.

Khunde Hospital's village health service scheme was based on the village health worker, who was a resident of the area in which he or she worked, and whose role was intended to be both educative as well as curative.[220] It was introduced after changes in the government's national education system resulted in teacher turnover during 1974 and 1975 and made the provision of village services based on teachers difficult. In 1976 Dr Rob Riley wrote in his annual report that he had been concentrating on re-establishing the health assistant scheme which had ceased to function over the previous eighteen months.[221] By the middle of the year he had trained three assistants for Thame, Deboche (near Tengboche) and Chaurikharka (in Pharak) and he hoped to establish a further post at Gomila (in Pharak) and Phortse. The role of these assistants was similar to the earlier system; the emphasis was on simple treatment, advice, education and referral at an early stage to Khunde Hospital of the more seriously sick. Riley concentrated on tuberculosis, goitre and cretinism, family planning, nutrition and general hygiene, and hoped that the health worker would be able to provide health education to local schoolchildren.

The village health workers initially practised from their own homes. In 1976 Kami Temba was employed to be the village health worker in Thame. He saw about four or five patients daily, made a few house calls and once or twice a year accompanied the doctor visiting every house to give BCG vaccinations and iodised oil injections.[222] Gradually clinics were built in most of the villages where health workers were based. The first was built in Thame in 1979, followed shortly afterwards by clinics in Chaurikharka and Gomila.

The numbers of patients seen by the village health workers fluctuated, and over the years the doctors at Khunde found various problem areas relating to the provision of village health services. These were distance, personnel and training. As Hillary's work expanded, the question of distance from Khunde increasingly became

220 Kunde Hospital Village Health Worker Manual, 1980 [KH].

221 Kunde Hospital Annual Report for the Year Ending 30 June 1976.

222 Interview with Kami Temba, Khunde, June 1997.

an issue. Providing a clinic locally helped patients with minor problems, but it was difficult for village health workers and patients with serious problems to get to the hospital and for hospital staff to visit the clinic or patients in the area.

The two areas particularly affected were the Rolwaling Valley and Solu which were both outside Khumbu. During 1970–71 Dr Selwyn Lang made a number of medical trips into the Rolwaling Valley, but he considered these to be more of a public relations exercise.[223] Although the Trust built a school in the main village of Beding in 1972, and while he was there Lang's successor, Dr Lindsay Strang, gave smallpox and BCG vaccinations, communication with Khunde was very difficult as the route crossed the high and difficult Tesi Lapsa pass.[224] During the early 1970s the teacher health assistant scheme had expanded into the more populous Solu part of the district, where although the route was easier the journey to and from Khunde still took several days. The opening of another hospital at Phaphlu in January 1976, however, allowed the Khunde doctor to refocus on medical work in Khumbu and Pharak.

The issue of distance resurfaced in the mid-1980s when Hillary built a clinic at Bung, a Rai village at an altitude of 1,680 metres and four days walk from Khunde. Bung had a large, poor population and no one in the Trust denied its need for health services. The project of a clinic at Bung began with a request to Hillary.[225] Mingma Tsering and his wife Ang Dooli had a Rai servant from the Bung area who also helped with the Trust working parties. In 1981 he approached Hillary regarding the possibility of a clinic for Bung. After consulting with the doctors at Khunde, Hillary declined the request. Bung was too far away. In 1984 Hillary received another petition and again consulted with the doctors at Khunde. There was a different volunteer couple and they agreed to the project. Both volunteers were doctors and they did not believe that Bung would be a problem to look after. Bung was a busy clinic. Between Au-

223 Kunde Hospital Report for the Year Ending 31 October, 1971: Including an Analysis of Cases for the First Five Years (1967–1971).

224 Kunde Hospital Report for the Year Ending 31 October 1972.

225 Interview, Kami Temba, June 1997.

gust and December 1985 it saw 3,284 patients.[226] It continued to see more patients than all the other village clinics combined, and for a time more than Khunde Hospital itself. During 1996 the estimated total of 5,400 patients were seen.[227] The patient workload at Khunde increased considerably after the 1980s, making it more difficult to spend up to two weeks away especially when there was only one doctor. In 1996 at a Himalayan Trust meeting held in Phaphlu Dr Mingma Gyelgen, the District Health Officer and senior medical officer at Phaphlu Hospital, announced the government's intention of taking over the clinic at Bung, with some continuing Trust support.[228] After a period of uncertainty, which also saw one of the health workers, Shri Doze Rai, go for formal health worker training in Kathmandu, the Nepalese government assumed responsibility for Bung on 1 September 1997.

The problems of personnel and training were closely linked and occupied a considerable amount of the volunteers' time.[229] The village health workers were part-time and employed by the volunteers at Khunde. Nepal had few trained health workers, and the Khunde doctors often found it difficult to find someone whom they could train to work in the village clinics or to replace people who had left. The hospital also faced competition from the trekking industry. The job of village health worker was year-round, but less lucrative and tied people to the village. Despite these problems, within Khumbu the village health worker situation was fairly stable. Pharak was less settled, with health posts opening and closing and politics playing a much greater role than in Khumbu.

The issue of training was complicated. One problem related to how the government regarded health workers trained at Khunde Hospital and is discussed in the next chapter on aid projects, but a second was of more immediate concern to the volunteers trying to deal with health problems and provide services. The village health

226 Health Workers [KH]. The records of the patients seen at village clinics are incomplete.

227 Kunde Hospital and Village Clinics Annual Report 1996.

228 Ibid.

229 Information for this section is drawn from the annual reports and the Health Workers file at Khunde Hospital.

workers had variable ability and variable education that limited in practice what they could do or were willing to do. In the early 1980s, Khunde Hospital doctors, Dawson and Uhrig, believed they had overcome the problems related to the training of two illiterate women as village health workers and saw benefits in having women who could relate to other women in the village who were also illiterate.[230] Later annual reports, however, often commented on the difficulties and limited service that such village health workers could provide, but the volunteers' options were limited when there were no more suitable replacements. As was the case with the hospital, providing village health services was subject to many varied factors that separately and together influenced policy and practice throughout the period and at some times and in some places more than others.

The following story provides a fitting conclusion in that it summarises the nature of the relationship between services provided at or by the hospital and those provided in or by community level health workers and illustrates both changing and ongoing features of medical encounters in the area. In July 1997 the Khunde doctor was called to help a woman in obstructed labour. Neither he nor the village health worker knew the woman had been in labour for a few days, because even though the woman had received some antenatal care at Khunde and an ultrasound examination in Kathmandu childbirth remained for the most part a family affair at home. The doctor had just finished a clinic in a village, where he had seen and treated a variety of patients who had turned up as the doctor was visiting, or who had been brought in by the village health worker for the doctor's opinion and treatment. The village was a day's walk from the hospital at Khunde. After several hours of waiting at the woman's house nothing had happened and the doctor wrote in his diary how it was "very worrying for all concerned".[231] He continued:

> There is a monk here. He is reading the texts with incredible speed. When he finished he went and prayed over the woman then Mingma

[230] Undated, typed document, four pages, found in Khunde Hospital, 1984–1989, Doctors' Reports, Correspondence, etc. Book 1 (SEHF, Toronto).

[231] Dr John Heydon, diary, 29 and 30 July 1997 [Heydon papers].

> [hospital health worker] asked him to pray over him and he did and for . . . [the patient] and Emma and I. We need all the help we can get and I mean that sincerely.

The day wore on. A porter arrived with the obstetric equipment from the hospital. It was dark and wet and so there was no means of transferring the woman by air to a major hospital in Kathmandu. The doctor called Khunde Hospital on the only phone in the area. In a very public conversation he listened, as (trying to make myself heard above the sound of heavy rain on a tin roof) I yelled over the telephone instructions for an operation we hoped he would not have to carry out. When he returned to his patient the situation had begun to improve. "Relief" he wrote. The night slowly passed. At 1.40 am a live baby girl was born and mother and child were well.

Although the particular circumstances differed, all the doctors who have spent time at Khunde Hospital have found themselves in such situations and experienced the strong emotions, both positive and negative, of practising Western medicine in this region. The telephone was a recent addition, but there were still no roads to ease travel either within or outside the area, and flying conditions in the mountains remained difficult and often impossible in the monsoon. Families sought help from the hospital when complications during childbirth arose, but away from the hospital the doctors lacked its facilities and equipment or the help of other staff. Such problems were beyond the level of skill of the village health workers and it was fortuitous in this case, particularly in view of the distance from Khunde, that the doctor was in the village. In most of Nepal no such help would have been available. Finally, the delivery had occurred in a plural medical encounter where both doctor and monk carried out their respective duties in the same house. The doctor was neither surprised nor uncomfortable with the monk's presence. As in the last chapter's conclusion, Khunde Hospital as a Western medicine project operated in an environment where staff, as well as patients, became used to each other's ideas and practices.

Conclusion

Hillary built the small hospital at Khunde at a time when Western medicine's presence in Nepal was limited, especially in rural areas where most people lived. More than thirty years later it remains so, because services for a variety of reasons are limited. The new approaches in international health in the 1960s promoting the expansion of basic health services, both curative and preventive, to more people and particularly those living in rural areas required, as Judith Justice has written, "close, long-term relationships between health care providers and rural communities".[232] Slowly, the Government as the main provider has extended services, built health facilities and trained and appointed staff, but getting everything together, all of the time and supplied with the ongoing resources needed to provide health services is an enormous, difficult and expensive challenge. The task was even greater for a country such as Nepal that started with so little. Rural health facilities often continue to be, as Justice had found in the late 1970s, "generally understaffed, undersupplied, and underutilized."[233]

Seen in this context, Khunde Hospital's achievement is considerable. In a close and long-term relationship with the community, the overseas volunteer doctors at Khunde and the hospital, with its outpatient and inpatient facilities, were at the centre of a Western style system of health care that has provided both curative and preventive services continuously for more than thirty years.[234] Staff at the hospital treated a wide range of conditions and an increasing number of patients, both people living in the area and others who travelled from further afield, including tourists from other countries. Most patients at the hospital were people from nearby villages, but from the beginning the doctor sought to extend the hospital's influence and improve access by first developing services and then building clinics close to where people lived.

A number of points arise out of this discussion that are pertinent to continuing issues facing the provision of health services in rural areas. Firstly, as befits an institution serving a small population, Khunde Hospital is small in size and only has a few personnel, who have to carry out a wide range of often demanding and

232 Justice, *Policies, Plans, & People,* 1–2.

233 Ibid., 9.

234 Now over forty years. See Epilogue.

competing tasks. In practice it was not possible to devote the same amount of energy to each issue all of the time. Also, the same staff could not both be in the hospital and out in the community. When both volunteers were doctors, the medical workload could be divided. Nevertheless, however important public health issues were, treating patients with acute conditions came first and a seriously ill person at the hospital, probably inevitably, occupied the attentions of the staff before a person with a lesser or chronic problem in the community. A serious case at the hospital could involve all the staff for many hours. In any case, neglecting the sick person who had sought hospital treatment would have damaged the hospital's standing within the community.

A second issue that emerges is the question of time; it is an important and often overlooked factor and relevant to issues of both curative and preventive health services. Changes have occurred, but more slowly and a little at a time, taking longer than anticipated. Over the period considered, patient numbers have risen and more people used the hospital for more conditions, but staff remained aware that people used the hospital pragmatically and selectively. The case study of the hospital's response to the major public health problem of iodine deficiency reveals not only the complexity of medical practice but also the ebbs and flows of a policy over time. Also, and this is particularly important in terms of health policy, curative and preventive services went hand in hand, with successful treatment of illness laying the foundation for messages about prevention. Again, this took time.

Lastly, the opening of the hospital should be seen in terms of the introduction and spread of the Western medical system. While extending services was a proactive measure, this chapter has argued that the overseas medical staff not only responded to the challenges of the environment and the diseases and health issues encountered, but also to how people regarded Western medicine and how they used the hospital and its services. In other words, medical practice was also reactive. As discussed in the last chapter, the encounter was negotiated and ongoing. Just as Sherpas were expected to learn new ideas, so a doctor's preconceived biomedical world was often equally challenged as doctors discovered that people used the hospital selectively and did not necessarily accept explanations and treatment of their illnesses, since these were based on a different medical system. The continuing relevance of alternative ideas and practices regarding sickness is well-known, but this point is of more than academic interest as it influences what a biomedical practitioner can do, how and what can be expected. This chapter's focus on the role and the agency of the doctor has a significance beyond the region, in view of its neglect in the literature. The information provided by a series of doctors, not just one practitioner, who have practised medicine over more than thirty years at Khunde Hospital emphasises how important this is. That may have been less surprising in 1966, but such patient responses remained significant and have continued to influence the ongoing dialogue on how the different doctors provided Western medical services. Again this is important for international health policy, because even if the facilities and services are present and are provided in a culturally sensitive manner it does not necessarily mean they will be taken up or will lead to change in attitudes and behaviour. The underlying assumption to the aid and development approach is therefore challenged.

4

Khunde Hospital as an Aid Project

Khunde Hospital is the visible expression of aid.

Interview, Ibbertson, 2002

We should not expect people to be continuously grateful for what is being done for them—the giver-receiver relationship is always a tricky and dangerous one, and most aid is strongly flavoured with self-interest.

Sir Edmund Hillary, *Schoolhouse in the Clouds,* 5

In *Schoolhouse in the Clouds* Hillary discussed his views on aid, but instead of focusing on aid as the "gift", such as the actual hospital or school, he raised the issue of the relationship between the provider (or, as in the above quotation, the "giver") and the receiver. Chapter one discussed how Hillary's ideas of friendship and partnership, of listening to and working with people, suffused his aid programme. His own relationship with Sherpas acted as a mantle that enveloped all his projects and those who worked with him. Hillary was the first foreigner to provide such ongoing assistance to the people of the Everest area and Khunde Hospital was one of his early projects. It was a visible expression of what he was doing and how and as a building it was also something tangible. Hillary's work relied on other people seeing value in what he did and then giving money, supplies, or time to enable him to continue. Hillary needed this support both to enable him to build Khunde Hospital but also to sustain the hospital's ongoing medical work.

The hospital also became something more than a symbol of Hillary's personal involvement because the giving of aid created a bond with expectations and obligations.[1] The hospital's shiny roof, that

[1] Marcel Mauss, *The Gift: Forms and Functions of Exchange in Archaic Societies* (London: Cohen & West, 1970 [1925]). For a study of gift-giving in a South Asian context, the creation of auspiciousness and inter-caste relationships,

was visible to all on reaching the small pass before descending into Khunde village, pronounced that "development" had arrived. Aid was the mechanism that helped people and communities to "develop", which in the 1960s was seen in terms of a linear transition from "tradition" to "modernity". Just as Western medicine was an expression of modernity in healing practices, the hospital was its embodiment.[2] Even if Khunde Hospital was physically little more than an outpatient clinic with a few beds for inpatients, it was always called a hospital. The presence of the hospital signified that the area had modern health services, since development to most Nepalese was not an abstract idea but something material.[3] Hillary's aid, therefore, brought development to Sherpas in Khumbu through building the hospital and providing health services.

The aim of this chapter is to explore the question: "What has being an aid project meant for Khunde Hospital?" I adopt a broad approach to examining the concept of "aid". The hospital has attracted international support from a diverse array of sources, ranging from individuals, commercial companies, non-governmental organisations to the official aid of governments. Through examining this support to the hospital I argue that multiple and multi-layered aid relationships, with a host of expectations and obligations, were established between the giver and the receiver. These relationships were grounded in the specific local and national contexts of Khunde Hospital's situation in the Everest region of Nepal but were also influenced by changing international aid and development discourses over this period.

By 1998 Khunde Hospital had been providing medical services as an aid project for more than thirty years. In that time changing ideas (across the world) about the role of health in development, the type of health services and ways of working with the "receivers" profoundly influenced the wider aid environment in which

see Gloria Goodwin Raheja, *The Poison in the Gift: Ritual, Prestation, and the Dominant Caste in a North Indian Village* (Chicago: University of Chicago Press, 1988).

2 Connor, "Healing Powers in Contemporary Asia".

3 Pigg, "Unintended Consequences".

Khunde Hospital functioned.[4] While this chapter is not primarily about development, aid was a means of funding it. The two are entwined. Shifting views on ways to achieve development in turn affected projects because such ideas directed funding pathways. At different points in its history, Khunde Hospital was considered both suitable and unsuitable as an official aid project. Throughout the period though, the overseas popular perception was of a project that was doing a good job for a worthy cause.

The chapter begins by exploring the wider context in which the hospital operated and examines why a hospital at Khunde was set up as a foreign-funded and administered private aid project and then considers why Khunde Hospital remained one. Nepal was a poor country where most of the biomedical health services were provided through the government, but these were limited. Throughout the period the gradual expansion of infrastructure, strategic policies and programmes was heavily supported by foreign aid and influenced by donors and changing ideas about the place and type of health services to be supported. An analysis of the failed Hospital Advisory Committee provides a case study of one of the key concepts of development—community participation. The final part of the chapter discusses how staff at Khunde negotiated the hospital's position within this aid framework. It examines its relationships with different organisations and mechanisms of control, the influence of visitors, and the hospital's increasing engagement with government health programmes.

Why Was Khunde Hospital an Aid Project?

The political events of 1950–51, which led to the overthrow of the Rana regime that had ruled Nepal since 1846, ushered in a new

[4] Ideas about givers and receivers and the nature of the relationship between them have evolved from an initial focus on the giver, then to the receiver, to the idea of partnership and currently to the participation and transformation of both. Sheila A. Robinson, "Development and Philanthropy in the Context of South Asia: Moving Toward Transformation", in *Philanthropy and Cultural Context: Western Philanthropy in South, East, and Southeast Asia in the Twentieth Century,* ed. Soma Hewa and Philo Hove (Lanham: University Press of America, 1997), 295–314. Robinson discusses her work in Nepal.

set of political leaders whose overt aim was to bring about social change and modernise the country. This coincided with a new era in international politics following the end of the Second World War that saw the expansion of international development through the mechanism of foreign aid. The confluence of these two forces, as Sudhindra Sharma has discussed, "were to shape Nepal for the rest of the century".[5] Foreign aid would fund the modernisation that the Nepalese sought.

The provision of Western medical services was an important element for the Nepalese in this modernising process. Sunil Amrith highlights how health became "part of a broader promise that gripped large parts of the world after 1945", although in Nepal's case the promise did not coincide with anti-colonial struggles that occurred in many places.[6] During the 1950s and early 1960s the Nepalese government sought to expand the country's very limited Western medical services. Although the few facilities available meant that most of the population did not have access to this type of medicine and used a range of other systems and practices when sick, knowledge of its existence was widespread. Western medicine was modern medicine. It was a system from the outside and the paradigm for the new international health programmes. These were funded through foreign aid budgets of wealthier countries and would have considerable influence on how poorer nations provided health care for their citizens. Policies were formulated at an international agency level, adopted in aid-recipient countries and as Judith Justice has shown in her study of primary health care and foreign aid in Nepal might eventually be implemented in remote villages.[7] On the one hand, the provision of services for people in areas that lacked them was beneficial. On the other hand, the fact that these services were being provided, what was provided and how it was done, were each heavily influenced by the funders who wished to direct what happened to their aid money. The situation in Nepal, however, differed to some extent from much of the South Asian

5 Sharma, "Half a Century of Foreign Aid", xxvi.

6 Amrith, *Decolonizing International Health,* 2.

7 Justice, *Policies, Plans, & People.*

region, because in Nepal the use of Western medicine, although part of a modernisation discourse, was not bound up with a former colonial process. [8]

Since the government provided most Western medicine services in Nepal, why was the hospital at Khunde a private overseas aid project and not a government facility? Chapter three discussed how in the 1950s and early 1960s the government expanded its curative services and infrastructure and concentrated on urban rather than rural areas. In many countries Christian missionaries provided health services, particularly in remote regions but in Nepal there were none. In the early 1950s, however, the Nepalese government changed its stance to allow some non-proselytising activities by mission organisations previously barred from working inside the country. In 1952 it accepted the Nepal Evangelistic Band's offer to build a hospital at Pokhara. [9] In May 1953 it gave permission to the United Mission to Nepal to build a hospital at Tansen and start a series of Maternity Welfare Centres in Kathmandu. [10] Despite the government concentrating on health services in the main urban areas, in 1964 it opened a clinic in Namche Bazar, the small administrative centre of Khumbu where government presence was only just beginning to develop. As the clinic was under the authority of the Home Ministry rather than the Ministry of Health, its establishment was probably related to its position near the border rather than the general expansion of health services into rural areas. Further expansion of health facilities in Khumbu was not part of government planning. [11]

[8] That foreign aid and development might be "imperial" is a separate discussion. For an introduction to continuities with colonial medicine, see Randall M. Packard, "Post-Colonial Medicine", in *Medicine in the Twentieth Century,* ed. Roger Cooter and John Pickstone (Amsterdam: Harwood Academic Publishers, 2000), 97–112.

[9] Lindell, *Nepal and the Gospel of God*, 130.

[10] Ibid., 142.

[11] Beginning in 1956, Nepal had a series of five-year plans. These combined details of the government's projected expenditure on development projects, general guidelines for the private sector and targets that the economy was to meet as a whole. John Whelpton, *A History of Nepal* (Cambridge: Cambridge University Press, 2005), 125. For a study of Nepal's planning experience

Another avenue for the establishment of a hospital was the possibility of Nepalese philanthropy.[12] In a country where foreign donors have occupied the dominant role, the literature on the history and practice of philanthropy in Nepal, as Marc Sidel has noted, is very limited.[13] During Rana rule, health facilities were introduced as a form of charity to the poor and supported through the *guthi* (a form of land tenure) system of endowed land. Mahesh Regmi, in his study of landownership in Nepal, pointed out that this was the only guaranteed protection from arbitrary government action.[14] At the end of the Rana regime approximately 4 per cent of the total cultivated land in Nepal was under guthi tenure. These endowments were primarily made to earn religious merit but most, as well as the richest, were to be found in the Kathmandu Valley and the eastern and central Terai.[15]

Nepal was a Hindu kingdom, but people, such as the Sherpa, living near the northern border of Nepal were mostly Buddhist and were considered unimportant to the country's social and political

---

from 1951 to 1976, see Ludwig F. Stiller and Ram Prakash Yadav, *Planning for People* (Kathmandu: Human Resources Development Research Centre, 1993 [1978]).

12 For a discussion in an Indian context which questions the altruism implicit in a Western understanding of philanthropic acts, such as the establishment of a hospital, in the nineteenth and twentieth centuries, see Douglas E. Haynes, "From Tribute to Philanthropy: The Politics of Gift Giving in a Western Indian City", *Journal of Asian Studies* 46, no. 2, 1987, 339–60. Haynes (p. 339) distinguishes between gift giving, which he sees as common to all societies and embedded in a particular society's values, and philanthropy, which originated particularly in Western cultures and was motivated by a desire to promote human welfare. Haynes believed local businessmen continuously adjusted their gift giving to conform to the ideology of British rule and so obtain influence and honours.

13 Marc Sidel, "Recent Research on Philanthropy and the Nonprofit Sector in India and South Asia", *Voluntas* 12, no. 2, 2001, 171–80. For the first published volume on the history and practice of philanthropy in Nepal, see Rupa Joshi, Kedar Sharma and Basanta Thapa, eds., *Twice Blessed: The Art of Giving* (Lalitpur: Tewa, 2000).

14 Mahesh C. Regmi, *Landownership in Nepal* (Berkeley: University of California Press, 1976), 17 and 19.

15 Regmi, *Landownership in Nepal*, 50 and 57.

elite. Sherpas, like the vast majority of Nepalese people, were usually poor, but the monastic revival in Khumbu in the early twentieth century was financed through Sherpa philanthropy. Most of this came from a small number of wealthy individuals but it was supported by smaller gifts from those less well-off.[16] Sherpas believed that good acts, including charitable giving, increased one's personal store of merit upon which their future rebirth depended. It was traditional to give to religious causes and Sherpas believed that they gained the most religious merit by giving to religious causes.[17] Supporting a hospital did not give them the same merit. Christoph von Fürer-Haimendorf summed up the position when he wrote in 1964 that "Generosity in the service of religion outshines in Sherpa eyes most other virtues, and covers a multitude of sins."[18]

In the early 1960s, therefore, neither the government nor local philanthropy were potential sources for a hospital at Khunde. The area was also too poor at this stage to attract a hospital as a business proposition with either internal Nepalese or external foreign funding. External interest in Nepal was nonetheless increasing. The number of visitors to the country was still small, but from the very small beginnings of a US$2000 grant by the United States of America to the Rana government in January 1951, foreign aid to Nepal grew.[19] It expanded rapidly, particularly in the late 1950s during the latter stages of the implementation of the country's First Five Year Plan (1956–1961).[20] Although the percentage fluctuated, in 1960–61 foreign aid provided 60.31 per cent of Nepal's budget.[21]

The principal donors to Nepal in the 1950s were the USA and India, with China and the United Nations emerging as significant

16 Ortner, *High Religion.*

17 They still do.

18 Von Fürer-Haimendorf, *The Sherpas of Nepal,* 282.

19 Sharma, "Half a Century of Foreign Aid", xxv. For a history of the USA's aid to Nepal, see Christa A. Skerry, Kerry Moran and Kay M. Calavan, *Four Decades of Development: The History of U.S. Assistance to Nepal, 1951–1991* (Kathmandu: United States Agency for International Development [USAID]), 1991.

20 Stiller, *Planning for People,* 164.

21 Sharma, "Half a Century of Foreign Aid", liii.

donors in the 1960s.[22] Other countries, including New Zealand, made small contributions. During this early period the USA initially emphasised agriculture and rural development, adding health and education in the 1960s. India initially concentrated on administrative reforms, transport and communication, expanding into the provision of irrigation, drinking water and education in the 1960s. Most foreign aid at this time was concentrated on the Kathmandu Valley.[23] Elsewhere, the rugged terrain was the biggest constraint against development, but most people lived in these rural and often remote areas.

Eugene Mihaly, in the first book on foreign aid in Nepal (published in 1965), found that most countries and agencies failed to meet their expected goals.[24] Plans had conceptual flaws and people seriously underestimated the problems of working in Nepal. A key issue was the sheer inability of the Nepalese government to cope either with its own plans or with the increasing demands being made by the donors of foreign aid who wanted to contribute to Nepal's development but, in what was considered good development practice, wanted the Nepalese to participate. Ludwig Stiller and Ram Yadav, in the country's first major "indigenous" study of aid, examined Nepal's planning experience between 1951 and 1976. They described how the new government had to carve out ministries from the old Rana administrative organisation and extend ministerial authority down to the district and village level.[25] The objectives of the Rana state machinery were to collect revenue and maintain law and order, but its structures and resources were ill equipped for the challenges of national development set out in King Tribhuvan's Social Manifesto. In 1952 Suvarna Shamsher, the finance minister, presented the country's first budget and an estimate of the government's income and expenditure for 1951, but the accounting

22 For a case study of this early period, see particularly Mihaly, *Foreign Aid and Politics in Nepal.*

23 Hillary had also noted this. Hillary, *Schoolhouse in the Clouds,* 6–7.

24 Mihaly, *Foreign Aid and Politics in Nepal,* 204–7.

25 Stiller and Yadav, *Planning for People*, chapter one.

procedures then in use made it impossible to produce any accurate financial information.[26]

With promises of new liberties, the Nepalese people's expectations were high. From the beginning, however, it was apparent that the pursuit of modernisation required outside help. Stiller and Yadav concluded at the end of chapter one:

> This was never really questioned. What was questioned was the *kind* of outside help that would be sought or accepted and the uses to which that help would be put. There were painful lessons in store for the administration and for the Nepalese in general. Only as they began to face the problem of development would the Nepalese learn the extent of the legacy the Rana regime had bequeathed to them in administration, education, and isolation from the world outside Nepal. The road ahead would be much harder because the Nepalese as a nation were so poorly prepared to understand, evaluate, and harness the aid that would be extended to them as soon as they asked for it.[27]

By appreciating the enormity of the task facing the Nepalese, it becomes possible to comprehend some of the difficulties and frustrations felt by both the donors and the receivers over many aspects of the aid and development processes. The limited availability of personnel for aid projects provides an example. Ideas about aid in this early period focused on technical assistance to a country, but Nepal only had a small number of appropriately educated people. In 1951, it had only three hundred graduates and 1251 high school students.[28] It would take time to increase this significantly, but while the numbers who could be trained were insufficient, people in the villages became disillusioned with the government when it had, for example, no one to staff the health clinics.[29]

The increasing number of countries that had begun to provide aid to Nepal continued to do so, despite encountering difficulties in implementing their aid programmes during the 1950s and

[26] Ibid., 114.

[27] Ibid., 27.

[28] Ibid., 22.

[29] For a historically grounded discussion of development activity and the experiences of Nepalese villagers, see Pigg, "Unintended Consequences".

early 1960s. In New Zealand's case, official aid, which was provided through the New Zealand government, became entwined with the private aid of Hillary's programme in Solukhumbu. Whether private or official, Hillary became the face of New Zealand aid to Nepal.[30]

New Zealand's involvement in Nepal began in 1955 as part of its contribution to the Colombo Plan, the Commonwealth's regional assistance programme.[31] By 1965 New Zealand had expended £104,751 in aid to Nepal.[32] Despite being a small country, New Zealand believed that if it wanted to be consulted by its allies, have a voice in important decisions and receive military assistance and protection when in need, then it had to be willing and able to assist its allies. In what was described as the "growing moral outlook" of international affairs after the end of the Second World War as well as being a response to the spread of "aggressive communism" in the region, New Zealand took an active role in the Colombo Plan for Economic Development in South and South-East Asia which was conceived during a meeting of Commonwealth foreign ministers in Colombo in 1950.[33] Asia was New Zealand's main focus for external aid and the Colombo Plan its principal programme, which was mainly implemented through bilateral arrangements with the respective countries.[34] The key components of the Colombo Plan

[30] Graeme Thompson's contemporary discussion of New Zealand's international aid performance concluded that while the people of New Zealand "probably" led the world in terms of private foreign assistance, official government assistance placed New Zealand "low" on the list of donor countries. Graeme J. Thompson, *New Zealand's International Aid* (Wellington: The New Zealand Institute of International Affairs, 1967), 113.

[31] The evolution of New Zealand foreign policy from the 1930s through to the 1980s is discussed in W. David McIntyre, "From Dual Dependency to Nuclear Free", in *The Oxford History of New Zealand*, ed. Geoffrey W. Rice, 2nd ed. (Auckland: Oxford University Press, 1992), 520–38.

[32] Thompson, *New Zealand's International Aid,* 120.

[33] R. H. Wade, "New Zealand's External Aid Programmes", in *New Zealand's External Relations,* ed. T. C. Larkin (Wellington: New Zealand Institute of Public Administration and London: Oxford University Press, 1962), 79–109.

[34] New Zealand's focus is now the Pacific region.

aid were technical assistance and capital aid, and projects selected for New Zealand support were to be of high priority in the development programme of the concerned country.[35] The scheme was not confined to Commonwealth countries and in 1952 Nepal became a member. New Zealand aid to Nepal concentrated on dairying, high country pasture development and technical education which were areas thought to be of benefit to Nepal and where New Zealand felt it had expertise to offer.

The implementation of one country's official aid to another is closely linked to diplomatic and state structures. New Zealand's external aid was administered through the Department of External Affairs. Initially, New Zealand had no diplomatic presence in Nepal, but in 1958 the government opened a High Commission in New Delhi. In the early 1960s, New Zealand's High Commissioner to India became accredited as its Ambassador to Nepal.[36] After two hundred years of keeping the West (principally the British in India) at arm's length, Nepal was only just "opening up" to people from such countries. Although individual Nepalese could be very supportive, the official attitude to foreigners was at times hostile. Hillary sought the help of New Zealand authorities to assist him in achieving his various aims, whether he was seeking permission to visit an area, climb a mountain or build a hospital. As an eminent New Zealander he was also able to take advantage of his position.[37] He had access to people at the top. Nevertheless, in the insecure international climate in the Himalayan region in the 1950s and 1960s, following the intensification of Chinese activities in Tibet and tensions and conflict between India and China, permission was neither easy to obtain nor could applicants assume a positive outcome.

[35] Wade, "New Zealand's External Aid Programmes", 93.

[36] The files of the High Commission are a valuable source of information about Hillary's activities in the 1960s and contain additional documents, such as correspondence with the British Embassy in Kathmandu, that are not found in the files from the Department in Wellington.

[37] Even so, Hillary experienced considerable difficulties and frustrations, and at times these would have required him to draw on the determination in his character that saw him succeed on Everest.

By the early 1960s Hillary was gaining experience in dealing with the Nepalese authorities, but he had also recently been in trouble with them. In this phase of Hillary's involvement with Nepal his expeditions combined adventure, science and aid. Problems over one part of his activities had ramifications for the others. Following the unauthorised ascent in 1961 of Mt Ama Dablam by members of his Himalayan Scientific and Mountaineering Expedition while Hillary was out of the country, the Nepalese government wanted to make an example of Hillary as a warning to other groups not to disregard its rules.[38] It cancelled permission to climb Mt Makalu which was intended to be the culmination of both the research and the expedition. Permission was later reinstated, but Hillary's reputation for apparently disregarding rules lingered. In 1964, while the New Zealand High Commission was assisting Hillary with his application to the Nepalese government to build an airstrip as an aid project, that importantly for Hillary would help transport materials for his building programme throughout the area, the High Commissioner confidentially informed the Secretary for the Department of External Affairs in Wellington that "We have been rather pointedly reminded that Hillary has in past given offence by departing from agreed and approved programme or route."[39]

Hillary's position was not helped by the fact that his assistance targeted Sherpas. To Hillary and other climbers, these were the people who were contributing so much to their success, yet were seen to live impoverished lives in a tough environment and deserved some help in return. The high profile given to Sherpas outside Nepal was out of step with the situation within Nepal. The government actively pursued a policy of discouraging ethnic difference and pro-

[38] For an account of the incident, including the text of the two letters from the Nepalese government, see Hillary and Doig, *High in the Thin Cold Air,* 205–8.

[39] Telegram from the High Commissioner to the Secretary of External Affairs, 15 July 1964, Himalayan Climbing Expeditions & Schoolhouse Project, ABHS 6949 W4628 NDI 64/14/2 Part 2 [ANZ].

moted a unified Nepal.[40] The new constitution in 1962 declared Nepal to be a Hindu state.

When Hillary built the first school in Khumjung in 1961, he had not envisaged it as the start of a continuing and expanding aid commitment to the people of the area, although he certainly had ideas at the time about other ways to help. The small school and other early projects were primarily funded through the support of his early expedition sponsors, but Hillary's aim was that the Nepalese government would take them over in approximately five years.[41] Building and supporting a hospital, however small, was a different proposition, particularly in terms of the finance that would be involved. The question of funding brought Hillary's private aid world into contact with the official aid world of governments. Despite a common goal of providing assistance to those deemed in need, the encounter revealed differences.

During this period (the early 1960s) Hillary discussed the possibility of funding his efforts through the Colombo Plan.[42] He commented in a letter to Sir Guy Powles, the New Zealand High Commissioner to India and Ambassador to Nepal, that the diplomatic scene was complicated when the personnel came from one country and the finance from another.[43] At this point Hillary's

[40] See David N. Gellner, Joanna Pfaff-Czarnecka and John Whelpton, eds., *Nationalism and Ethnicity in a Hindu Kingdom: The Politics of Culture in Contemporary Nepal* (Amsterdam: Harwood Academic Publishers, 1997). For an overview of the period's turbulent politics, see Whelpton, *A History of Nepal.*

[41] "Sir Edmund Hillary's Activities in Nepal", 19 August 1964, Himalayan Climbing Expeditions & Schoolhouse Project, ABHS 6949 W4628 NDI 64/14/2 Part 2 [ANZ]. This restricted brief from the Department of External Affairs for the High Commissioner's visit to Nepal in September broadly discussed Hillary's aid work and the New Zealand government's position.

[42] See Economic and Technical Assistance to individual countries—Nepal. Sir Edmund Hillary's Himalayan Projects, EA W2824 118/13/13/14 Part 1, and Himalayan Climbing Expeditions & Schoolhouse Project, ABHS 6949 W4628 NDI 64/14/2 Part 2 [ANZ]. This referred not only to Khunde Hospital.

[43] Hillary to Sir Guy Powles, 12 February 1962, Himalayan Climbing Expeditions & Schoolhouse Project, ABHS 6949 W4628 NDI 64/14/2 Part 2 [ANZ].

intended involvement was short-term and official New Zealand support through the Colombo Plan would secure valuable finance that would otherwise need raising elsewhere, would give official endorsement that would help with dealing with the Nepalese government and importantly for Hillary would make it a New Zealand contribution.

The response from the government in Wellington to Hillary's work in Nepal at this time appeared more ambivalent. As the Department of External Affairs noted in its brief to the High Commissioner before his visit to Nepal in 1964: "He may well have a chip on his shoulder over the [New Zealand] Government's apparent lack of wholehearted support of his efforts." [44] It was one thing to lend support to Hillary in his dealings with Nepalese bureaucracy and generally talk positively about his projects, but quite another officially to endorse or finance the work. A letter in October 1964 from the Department of External Affairs in Wellington to the High Commissioner in New Delhi spelt out the reasons for the New Zealand government's rejection in 1963 of Hillary's plans for a hospital: "The reason for rejection was mainly that such a project, not being directly related to the economic development of the area, was not a suitable vehicle for our aid." [45] The letter continued that: "the relatively high capital cost (£10,000) was also a factor, coupled with the fact that the Nepalese Government would have insisted that the hospital be maintained by us for 5 years, a stipulation which would have involved a further £21,000 approximately in recurrent expenses." The High Commissioner was instructed that "no encouragement should be given that we would be prepared to use Colombo

[44] "Sir Edmund Hillary's activities in Nepal", 19 August 1964, Himalayan Climbing Expeditions & Schoolhouse Project, ABHS 6949 W4628 NDI 64/14/2 Part 2 [ANZ].

[45] T. P. Davin for the Secretary of External Affairs to the High Commissioner, 16 October 1964, Himalayan Climbing Expeditions & Schoolhouse Project, ABHS 6949 W4628 NDI 64/14/2 Part 2 [ANZ] The Department's file also emphasised the issue that the Nepalese government had not requested the project and so the Department was unclear as to the project's priority. Some health work was funded at this time. A New Zealand Colombo Plan Surgical Team worked in South Vietnam. *New Zealand Foreign Affairs Review* 22, no. 1, January 1972.

Plan funds even for staffing and maintenance, the more so in view of the high level of our aid to Nepal in other fields, notably dairy equipment."

Hillary's rejected request for financial help steered Khunde Hospital along a different aid trajectory. In 1965 Hillary submitted to the Nepalese government his proposal for a hospital at Khunde which, following approval, he built towards the end of 1966. While he received some official New Zealand support such as through the deployment of VSA volunteers, Khunde Hospital was privately funded and privately administered. Yet within a few years the New Zealand government entered into a bilateral agreement with the Nepalese government to build, in partnership with Hillary, a second hospital that was bigger than Khunde and which it would support for five years. The press statement issued from the Prime Minister's office in September 1974 announced that "Here we have a good example of a voluntary agency working with the Government and with the local people".[46] Following the election of a Labour Government in 1972, New Zealand's international aid contribution increased.[47] This was also the peak period of official New Zealand aid to Nepal. While Hillary continued to administer Khunde Hospital, this second hospital was taken over by the Nepalese government after five years, and at the beginning of 1980 became the district hospital for Solukhumbu.

46 24 September 1974, Nepal: Solu Hospital, ABHS 950 W4627 118/13/13/18 Part 1 [ANZ].

47 For changing ideas and increasing New Zealand government support for international aid in the early 1970s see, for example, a report from the Ministry of Foreign Affairs, Wellington, "The Flow of Resources from New Zealand to Developing Countries 1972/73", February 1974 and Sam Buckle, "A Conscience Issue? Attitudes of New Zealand Governments to International Aid, 1967–1975" (B.A. Hons. diss., University of Otago, 1996). The aid contribution of 0.55 per cent of Gross National Product in 1975 was the most generous of any New Zealand government. Buckle, "A Conscience Issue?" 51. Ideas about the types of projects were also changing. In 1975 the New Zealand government also became involved in Khumbu through a bilateral aid agreement with the Nepalese government for the setting up of the Mount Everest (later Sagarmatha) National Park.

This change of direction on the part of the New Zealand government leads directly into the next part of the chapter which considers the question of why Khunde Hospital continued to be an aid project, because part of the answer was to be found in the more important role that health had come to occupy in the world of governments and international aid projects. It also related to the type of health aid, with a less top-down approach and an emphasis on partnership with the intended recipients. Ideas about aid and development, and the role of health in the process had, therefore, changed. As a result the goalposts in the quest for funding had shifted.

Why is Khunde Hospital Still an Overseas Aid Project?

In 1998, thirty-two years after it opened, Khunde Hospital remained an overseas aid project, mainly staffed (except for the doctors) and run from within Nepal but financed from overseas. The reasons were threefold: unlike Hillary's other hospital no other funding or medical staffing option was offered from within Nepal; donors remained both willing and able to support the hospital; and rural primary care services, such as those provided by Khunde Hospital and its village clinics, became the focus of a prominent international medical aid programme. Over this period ideas about the theory and practice of aid and development changed, although there was never one single and homogenous discourse. In this section I use the example of the Hospital Advisory Committee to discuss how one of the key concepts, "community participation", both shifted in its understanding but still failed to materialise at Khunde when, despite encouragement, local Sherpas did not become involved in the running of the hospital.

During the 1960s Hillary regularly visited Nepal to build, support or maintain a growing number of projects in the Solukhumbu district. Each time he applied to the Nepalese government for permission to carry out the planned work, bring in supplies or obtain visas for personnel, and used diplomatic support when necessary from the New Zealand High Commission staff in New Delhi or the British Embassy in Kathmandu to assist with the often lengthy process.[48] The lack of a permanent New Zealand diplomatic presence in Nepal made Hillary's task more difficult. This problem was expressed both by Hillary and diplomatic staff in New Delhi who felt out of touch with the many changes and events occurring in Nepal.

The Nepalese government preferred to deal at a government-to-government level rather than with individual people. It struggled to cope with the burgeoning number of people, organisations and governments that wanted to provide aid to Nepal but which also imposed demands that the government found difficult or impossible to meet. Mihaly's study criticised the aggregate impact of smaller aid programmes from countries such as New Zealand or Britain, because, however commendable or successful individual projects were, they created serious problems for Nepal. The number of organisations and the variety of methods by which these operated "vastly complicated" the Nepalese government's task of trying to direct the country's development efforts.[49] As a result little coordination occurred.[50] During the 1960s the Nepalese government and its staff had many other pressing and important issues. The introduction by King Mahendra of panchayat democracy, which was enshrined in the 1962 constitution, allowed limited popular representation "while the king ruled unhindered by the pressures of parliamentary democracy".[51] At a national level governments changed, but this translated into job insecurity for individuals and an unwillingness to make decisions that could jeopardise a person's own position.[52]

[48] See chapter one concerning the involvement of the British Embassy.

[49] Mihaly, *Foreign Aid and Politics in Nepal,* 202–3.

[50] Stiller and Yadav in *Planning for People* discuss this problem in detail in connection with planning, but problems relating to coordination and regulation have continued to the present.

[51] Whelpton, *A History of Nepal*, 101. Documents in the High Commission files similarly refer to the king's absolute power within the country. King Tribhuvan had died in 1955.

[52] Also see Alan Macfarlane, "Fatalism and Development", in *Nepal in the Nineties,* ed. Michael Hutt (New Delhi: Oxford University Press, 1993). A central feature of what Dor Bahadur Bista sees as part of the "fatalism"

The king had requested foreign assistance to help with Nepal's problems, but increasing acceptance of aid brought mounting exposure to the aims and agendas of the donors. There were no easy solutions to the enormous task facing the government, but in accepting aid the question arose as to who was in control of the process? The Nepalese government's underlying concern was to continue as before to promote the Nepalese position in order to keep the country's needs at the forefront of aid. Donors sought to exert more authority over, or at least influence, Nepal's affairs. While earlier the British mostly had respected the Nepalese position, Stiller and Yadav in *Planning for People* describe an unstable Nepalese political situation and the aid programme getting out of hand in the late 1950s. Opinions vary as to the degree that a country's foreign policy influenced its aid strategy, but the Nepalese government was well aware of the international interest in the wider region's politics and deliberately pursued its own policy of friendly relations with India, China and the USA.[53] Countries, such as New Zealand, offering smaller aid packages had less influence. Hillary's difficulties during the 1960s, whether concerned with climbing mountains or aid to Sherpas, need to be understood within this wider context of the Nepalese government wishing but struggling to remain in control of what was happening in their own country. Hillary was also aware of the international political dimensions and hoped the Nepalese government would expand its presence in the border area to try and counter the spread of communist influence from China.[54] He saw his practical aid projects further contributing to the effort.

Throughout the 1960s, Hillary was relying on the goodwill and services of other people to assist his increasing work in Nepal. While Hillary was personally reluctant, pressure was mounting

---

in Nepalese ruling groups is the fear of decision-making and the taking of responsibility (p. 119).

53 For a study that views foreign aid in Nepal as an extension of foreign policy, see Narayan Khadka, *Foreign Aid and Foreign Policy: Major Powers and Nepal* (New Delhi: Vikas, 1997).

54 Hillary, *Schoolhouse in the Clouds,* 7. Also see documents in Himalayan Climbing Expeditions & Schoolhouse Project, ABHS 6949 W4628 NDI 64/14/2 Part 2 [ANZ].

from different quarters to formalise his working relationship with the Nepalese government. By the end of the decade it was becoming harder to gain permission for voluntary efforts such as those of Hillary. Ralph Naylor, from the New Zealand Forest Service, joined Hillary in Nepal in 1970 on a Colombo Plan assignment for the Department of External Affairs. His brief was to examine forestry and related land use in Solukhumbu and to comment on "Hillary aid". After listing Hillary's considerable achievements in the region, Naylor wrote that "Many aid leaders acknowledge that these attainments are greater than theirs and that they have been attained with far less administrative effort."[55]

He believed that Hillary aid would "snowball", but of concern to the Nepalese officials in the area was the issue that:

> Through no planned seeking of power on his part, but by virtue of the money and resources at his disposal, Sir Edmund is perhaps the most powerful person in Solu-Khumbu where changes are occurring. He alone can order an aluminium roof for a monastery or a Darjeeling teacher for a school.

Officials in Kathmandu expressed concern about the lack of an agreement that would have sorted out a number of procedural and practical issues prior to commencement of aid.[56] Problems such as those that occurred in 1966 over the levy of heavy customs duties for Khunde Hospital supplies would have been avoided. Leaders of aid missions acknowledged the "outstanding aptness and effectiveness of Hillary aid" and envied his independence within Nepal, but

55 R. Naylor, "Afforestation in the Khumbu: A Colombo Plan Assignment", New Zealand Forest Service, 1970, in "Forestry in Sagarmatha National Park—Nepal: A Collection of Unpublished Reports, 1970–1995", prepared by G. C. Baker, New Zealand Forest Research Institute, PO Box 465 Rangiora, New Zealand, August 1995. This collection was held at the Sagarmatha National Park headquarters at Namche Bazar. I am grateful to the park warden Nima Wangchu Sherpa for allowing me to consult this and various other publications. At ANZ, Naylor's forestry report (but not these comments on Hillary) is in Nepal: Solu Hospital, ABHS 950 W4627 118/13/13/14 Part 2 [ANZ].

56 As already noted, the lack of a permanent New Zealand diplomatic presence in Nepal compounded the problem.

believed that "within a couple of years, H.M.G. would completely curtail all aid not formally negotiated at diplomatic levels".

The official opening of Khunde Hospital in December 1966 encapsulated the uncertainty regarding official Nepalese support for Hillary's work at this time. While Louise Hillary conveyed the happy completion of a successful aid project, documents in the High Commission files reveal considerable concern.[57] The New Zealand High Commissioner, John Farrell, wrote confidentially to Wellington about the "delightful occasion" and that "the completion of this attractive hospital in record time is an outstanding achievement. It is just a pity that aid projects generally could not be carried out so expeditiously."[58] Yet only the Assistant Minister for Education, Gyarendra Bahadur Karki, had attended the event representing the Nepalese government. He gave a long, mainly political speech in Nepali that ended with three cheers. Farrell wrote that "we thought they were for Sir Edmund and his team" but from the press release he learned that they were for the King. He believed that a combination of factors, some of which were due to the expedition and the voluntary nature of the aid but others had nothing to do with Hillary, had irritated the Nepalese and as a result they showed their displeasure not in words but through "non-cooperation" (Farrell's words). While the question of customs duties was under consideration by the Nepalese government, in February 1967 Farrell wrote that "it is recommended that this should be noted officially as an embarrassing situation" and that it "could occur if subscriptions were collected for a similar project in this country".[59]

Staff at the New Zealand High Commission in New Delhi were caught in the middle; they wanted to help Hillary but had few means

[57] Louise Hillary, *A Yak for Christmas,* 88–99.

[58] J. E. Farrell, High Commissioner, to Secretary External Affairs, "Hillary Hospital Expedition", 23 December 1966, Himalayan Climbing Expeditions & Schoolhouse Projects, ABHS 6949 W4628 NDI 64/14/2 Part 3 [ANZ].

[59] Farrell to Secretary of External Affairs, 7 February 1967, Himalayan Climbing Expeditions & Schoolhouse Projects, ABHS 6949 W4628 NDI 64/14/2 Part 3 [ANZ].

of doing so.[60] Hillary was aware of the difficulties surrounding the implementation of his projects, but was reluctant to lose some of the independence that he personally enjoyed and which had enabled him to carry out a lot of work. Writing in August 1970 to Brian Lendrum, the High Commissioner, he agreed with the need to formalise his working relationship, as Lendrum was suggesting, but "I can see problems in adopting the procedures you suggest".[61]

Nevertheless negotiations began in late 1970 with the text for an agreement submitted by Lendrum to the Nepalese government.[62] On 20 January 1972 Hillary, as Chairman of the Himalayan Trust, signed a three-year agreement with Bharat Raj Bhandary, the Foreign Secretary for His Majesty's Government of Nepal.[63] The Agreement outlined the terms and conditions under which the government (referred to as HMGN) and Hillary (referred to as the Trust) would work together "desiring to co-operate in promoting the economic and social welfare and the development of educational and health services" in Eastern Nepal.[64] Appendix A listed the various schools built by Hillary that were to be included and also noted that it was agreed:

[60] See correspondence between Pearl, Hillary and Lendrum in 1970, Himalayan Climbing Expeditions & Schoolhouse Projects, ABHS 6949 W4628 NDI 64/14/2 Part 4 [ANZ].

[61] Hillary to Lendrum, 15 August 1970, Himalayan Climbing Expeditions & Schoolhouse Projects, ABHS 6949 W4628 NDI 64/14/2 Part 4 [ANZ]. Other Sherpa Trust members were also reluctant.

[62] See Himalayan Climbing Expeditions & Schoolhouse Projects, ABHS 6949 W4628 NDI 64/14/2 Part 4 [ANZ]. The proceedings in Kathmandu were mostly handled by New Zealander John Claydon, who had been a pilot with Hillary in Antarctica and was in Nepal as Airport Management Adviser with the Asian Development Bank's Air Transport Development Project.

[63] Louise Hillary described the occasion in Louise Hillary, *High Time* (London: Hodder and Stoughton, 1973), 180–84. The Hillary's tent in Kathmandu contrasted with the formal surroundings of the former palace of Singha Durbar which housed government offices.

[64] Agreement between His Majesty's Government of Nepal and the Himalayan Trust regarding Educational and Health Services Projects, Trust Agreements [HTK].

> that the Kunde Hospital built by Sir Edmund Hillary and helpers with the co-operation of local village committee and the approval of HMGN be recognised and incorporated in this Agreement, and that its maintenance, provision of medical supplies, equipment and the provision of medical staff, be the responsibility of the Trust for the duration of this Agreement.

The Foreign Ministry released a press-note which reported that the agreement "regularizes" existing projects and allowed for additional projects in the future.[65]

This agreement, with subsequent renewals, became the basis of Hillary's operations within Nepal. From 1976, the agreement for Khunde Hospital and the new hospital at Phaphlu was with the Ministry of Health and included a clause that reserved the right for the Nepalese government "to nationalise the hospital whenever it so decides".[66] In January 1980 the government took over the management of the hospital at Phaphlu with continued assistance from the Trust, but has not availed itself of this opportunity in relation to Khunde Hospital.[67] The hospital at Phaphlu was close to the Solukhumbu district headquarters of Salleri and in the increasing decentralisation of the 1980s and 1990s became the centre for health activities in the district.

Similarly, the wider Sherpa community has not been particularly keen in either wanting to participate in running the hospital or taking it over, although Sherpa staff became involved with the management of the hospital. Yet "community participation" in development, as Linda Stone comments, is "an established, even revered" strategy in development programmes around the world.[68]

65 "Nepal Press Digest" 16, no. 3, 24 January 1972, 25. The "Digest" was first produced by the Regmi Research Project, Kathmandu, in 1956.

66 Dr N. D. Joshi, Director General, Directorate of Health Services, Ministry of Health, His Majesty's Government, to Sir Edmund Hillary, Chairman, Himalayan Trust, 28 April 1976, Trust Agreements [HTK].

67 L. Poudayl, Director General, Department of Health Services to Hillary, 21 March 1980. This letter was in reply to Hillary's letter of 31 October 1979. Trust Agreements [HTK].

68 Linda Stone, "Cultural Crossroads of Community Participation in Development: A Case from Nepal", *Human Organization* 48, 3, 1989, 206–13.

It was the guiding principle of the primary health care programme in Nepal.[69] Encouraging participation by the beneficiaries of these programmes was necessary if development was to be "relevant, sustainable and empowering".[70] In the past ten years participation has become a highly contested subject as programmes often failed to achieve the desired social change for society's poor and marginalised groups, mainly, it is argued, because they did not engage with underlying issues of power and politics.[71]

It is beyond the scope of this book to analyse participation in terms of development theory, but some of these issues are relevant to discussing the role of community participation at Khunde Hospital. First of all, Stone raised concerns about the cultural appropriateness of international development efforts since "the style or approach of development, the rhetoric and the fads all bear the cultural imprint of the West."[72] Furthermore, however meritorious the programmes, the focus, for example on nutrition and "Women in Development", arose when these issues became prominent in the West. Participation was a means to implement these already defined health programmes.[73] Stone's research was undertaken in Nepal where she found that the ideas about participation of the villagers differed from those of project staff.[74] Both understood participation, but foreign project staff expressed Western notions of self-reliance, equality and individualism while villagers thought in terms of obeying a panchayat order to contribute land, money or labour for some development project. Stone found that over 80 per cent of the sample households had contributed in this way, although not always willingly.[75] While Stone carried out her research among different

[69] Stone, "Primary Health Care for Whom?"

[70] Sam Hickey and Giles Mohan, "Relocating Participation within a Radical Politics of Development", *Development and Change* 36, no. 2, 2005, 237–62.

[71] Hickey and Mohan, "Relocating Participation", 237.

[72] Stone, "Cultural Crossroads", 206.

[73] Stone, "Primary Health Care For Whom?" 301.

[74] For a discussion about the conceptualisation of the Nepalese village in relation to development, see Pigg, "Inventing Social Categories Through Place".

[75] Stone, "Cultural Crossroads", 211.

ethnic groups in the middle hill region of Nepal, there were parallels with the situation at Khunde Hospital.

Case study: Khunde Hospital and "community participation"

The initiative for a Hospital Advisory Committee came from Hillary in New Zealand. In May 1971 he wrote to the Langs at Khunde Hospital to inform them that the Himalayan Trust Board had decided to establish a Hospital Advisory Committee with the main aim "to encourage the Sherpas to become familiar with the running of the hospital and of the costs and other problems involved".[76] In this letter Hillary suggested that the committee could consist of the doctor and his wife, Mingma Tsering who was Hillary's "Sherpa manager", two representatives appointed by the Khumjung panchayat and one from Thame or Namche, and possibly the headmaster of Khumjung school. He thought the committee should meet monthly and discuss issues such as monthly finance, firewood, visits by children and adults to the hospital for public health lectures, village water supplies, hospital staff and "greater financial participation" by Sherpas in the hospital. Hillary saw the committee as advisory and educational, both about health and management, but final decisions were to be left to the "Kunde Doctor".

Hillary believed that community participation was important for the overall success of the project. The inaugural meeting was held on 20 June 1971.[77] In November, at a meeting also attended by Hillary, it was agreed that the committee should have some financial responsibility.[78] Initially meetings were held monthly along the

[76] Hillary to S. and A. Lang, 1 May 1971, Hospital Advisory Committee Book (hereafter HACB). A separate file, Minutes HAC (hereafter MHAC), contains minutes for 1995 and 1996 plus some other material. Documents are mostly in English, with some in Nepali when addressed to Nepalese government officials.

[77] Shyam Pradhan Krishna, who became supervisor of the Hillary schools, provided a Nepali translation of the minutes of the meeting.

[78] The meeting was held at Mingma Tsering's house in Khunde, 19 November 1971. The meeting appointed a treasurer and the committee was to have an account which was to be used for transporting "poor patients" to Kathmandu for treatment. This account was separate from the two kept by the

lines Hillary had earlier suggested, but gradually their frequency declined. Only two meetings were held in 1973 and two in 1974, after which the committee ceased to operate, although there was no formal decision taken to do so.[79]

The question of community participation in the running of the hospital was raised again in 1976 following the renewal of the Trust's agreement with the Nepalese government, but no meetings were held.[80] Towards the end of 1981 another attempt was made to establish a committee.[81] The Canadian doctors at the hospital, Dawson and Uhrig, discussed the situation with Mingma Tsering and Kami Temba, the senior of the two medical assistants at the hospital. They tried to identify people who would participate. Representatives were chosen from the various villages and were approached individually and accepted.[82] The first meeting was held two days

Khunde doctor. Money could only be spent from this account if approved by the committee. The treasurer was Tsering Doma, one of the Khumjung representatives. Both Khumjung panchayat representatives were women. The other was Ang Dooli, Mingma Tsering's wife, from Khunde.

79 Meetings were held in June, July and August 1972 but then there was a gap until July 1973, when the minutes noted that this was the first meeting of 1973 as previously many of the committee members had been away on expeditions or business.

80 In his annual report for 1978 Dr Jim Jerram mentioned that he had corresponded with the Chief District Officer at Salleri "who would like to see the formation of a Hospital Committee with himself as chairman", but subsequently had not heard from him for "some months". Kunde Hospital Annual Report for the Year Ending 30th November 1978.

81 McKinnon to Drs Penny Dawson and Jamie Uhrig, 3 December 1981, Trust Letters, 1981–82 [KH]. The HACB, 7 February 1982, refers to a letter from McKinnon to Dawson and Uhrig that they establish a hospital advisory group. The HMG agreement with the Trust refers to a board for the running and maintenance of the hospital. McKinnon, who had assumed the chairmanship of the Trust's medical sub-committee following Pearl's death in 1980, wrote to Dawson and Uhrig that the Trust did not really want them to reconstitute the Hospital Board unless there was "pressure" from the Nepalese government to do so. He said that it had been an unworkable organisation in the past, and the Trust would prefer an informal, advisory group.

82 7 February 1982, HACB. Mingma Tsering was one of the Khunde representatives and Kami Temba represented Thame.

later. This committee was no more successful. The following year it ceased to function. The next attempt to revive the committee was in 1988, with sporadic meetings being held since then. [83] An important step was taken at the meeting held in December 1992, making Kami Temba chairman instead of the Khunde doctor, but this did not revitalise the committee. By the mid-1990s it appeared that the staff of the hospital, the Trust and the local community did not see this structure as an essential part of the management of the hospital.

Complicating the situation in the 1990s was the pressure placed on the hospital and the Trust, particularly from the Canadian International Development Agency (CIDA) through the Sir Edmund Hillary Foundation (SEHF), to implement better community participation. This brings into focus another key aspect relating to the development discourse regarding community participation. It changed over the period being discussed. In 1993 independent consultants in Canada, Community Based Initiatives in Health Inc., carried out an institutional evaluation of the SEHF on behalf of the Foundation and the Ontario International Development Program (OIDP). In its main findings the report stated that:

> At its inception in the mid 70's, the SEHF leadership were visionaries in their time. This was a time when development organizations had not fully incorporated community participation in their activities. Sir Edmund and the SEHF responded to the needs as expressed by the communities through creating projects such as the Kunde Hospital and health clinics. [84]

Hillary's insistence from the early 1960s on the importance of involving the local community emerged before it became a mainstream idea in development activities, and illustrated his independ-

[83] 10 June and 13 July 1988, 22 March 1990, 23 December 1992, 11 August 1993, 30 March 1994, 26 July 1995 and 22 May 1996 [HACB].

[84] Report by Community Based Initiatives in Health Inc., conducted on behalf of the Sir Edmund Hillary Foundation and the Ontario International Development Program, "Sir Edmund Hillary Foundation: An Institutional Evaluation", 31 March 1993, iii [SEHF]. In December 1990 the SEHF's project files and management responsibilities were transferred from CIDA/NGO Division to OIDP. OIDP funds continued to originate from CIDA.

ent approach and distance from the development discourse that underpinned the international aid programme.

By the 1990s international development policy ideas had overtaken Hillary's interpretation of participation. The report believed there was "less evidence" of community participation in the Foundation's projects.[85] Praise had now become criticism. On the ground, the hospital had not changed the way it worked in Khumbu, but at an international level a shift had occurred in ideas about the nature of a community's participation. Although the idea of people's involvement had been around since the 1950s as part of the process of community development, it now became transformed into the idea of "empowering" the local community. This would enable the necessary social change to occur which the top-down approach of international aid and development had failed to achieve.[86] The report on the SEHF recommended that the Foundation, Hillary and Khunde Hospital similarly move on in its ideas and ways of working. One of its recommendations was that the SEHF should "broaden the expertise on the Board to include more professional(s) who are active within the NGO community and knowledgeable about international health and development."[87] The same could have been said about the Himalayan Trust in New Zealand which was the Foundation's sole "implementing partner and grantee" in Nepal.

Returning to the issue of the Hospital Advisory Committee, the question of the divergence over many years between the desire for community involvement in the running of the hospital, and the failure to achieve it in practice, needs further exploration as it raises a number of points that suggest a greater complexity to the issue than is first apparent. Part of the reason for the committee's failure lay in

85 Ibid.

86 See, for example, Alice F. Purdey, Gyan Bahadur Adhikari, Sheila A. Robinson and Philip W. Cox, "Participatory Health Development in Rural Nepal: Clarifying the Process of Community Empowerment", *Health Education Quarterly* 21, no. 3, Fall 1994, 329–43, and Marko Ulvila and Farhad Hossain, "Development NGOs and Political Participation of the Poor in Bangladesh and Nepal", *Voluntas* 13, no. 2, 2002, 149–63.

87 "Sir Edmund Hillary Foundation: An Institutional Evaluation", iv.

people's deference to the Khunde doctors, the different views and approaches of the various Khunde couples that have run the hospital locally since the beginning, and also a lack of direction from the Trust overseas that might have ensured a more consistent policy.[88] The revised Hospital Handbook in the mid-1980s mentioned that the volunteers could hold a meeting if they wanted, but that they were rarely called. In contrast, one of the volunteers was expected to represent the Trust and play an informed role on the Khumjung school committee.[89]

Another issue is related to who or what was the "community" for the hospital staff. In the 1950s, von Fürer-Haimendorf described a society that was remote from the main centres and rarely visited by government officials, so that there was a minimum of outside interference in practice if not in theory. The village was the key unit and von Fürer-Haimendorf saw a high level of community responsibility for the preservation of natural resources, the maintenance of public peace and harmony and the ritual activities of the whole village. "The foremost principle underlying Sherpa village organization is the allocation of civic tasks by rotation".[90] Village officials were elected by villagers and spoke for the village as a whole, although real authority in the village generally lay with a number of men who combined wealth and social prestige. Although von Fürer-Haimendorf's view of Khumbu Sherpa society is considered "rosy" by other researchers, Sherry Ortner after thirty years of research that began among Solu Sherpas agreed that Khumbu Sherpas appeared "more cooperative and community oriented".[91]

Khunde Hospital provided services not for one village but for several, including small settlements that were separate from the

[88] We did not hold any meetings between 1996 and 1998. As I went through hospital files I realised they had been held in the past, but thought they appeared ineffectual. In the end we became too busy with the hospital's clinical load, particularly after Kami Temba left to train as a doctor in Fiji, and we did not come up with any alternative way to involve community participation. Local people also did not raise the issue.

[89] Kunde Hospital Handbook, 1985, 1: no page numbers.

[90] Von Fürer-Haimendorf, *Sherpas of Nepal,* 100 and 114.

[91] Ortner, *High Religion,* 6.

permanent villages to which most Sherpas belonged. The principal monastery of the area at Tengboche showed that a wider sense of belonging also existed as people from throughout the area assisted with its construction from 1916–19.[92] Both Khunde Hospital and the celibate institution of the monastery of Tengboche were new organisations for Khumbu.[93] A wider community uniting for a single event such as a building project was, however, different from the ongoing commitment subsequently required to run such institutions. Tengboche monastery is presided over by the senior religious figure, the rinpoche, who is given great respect and is immensely influential within the area.[94]

Khunde Hospital represented change as part of a general modernising process that was occurring within Nepal. In their book, published in 1970, Leo Rose and Margaret Fisher provide an account that was contemporary to the setting up of Khunde Hospital's Hospital Advisory Committee. They describe a country in transition and wrote with a vein of optimism that would be missing today. The vigour and speed of change in Nepal in the early 1960s surprised them.[95] Hillary's two key personnel in Nepal illustrated the changes taking place. Mingma Tsering, who began working for Hillary in the early 1960s, operated well in the village environment of Solukhumbu, but felt out of place in the offices of urban Kathmandu. The well-educated Ang Rita, who began working in the Trust office in the mid-1980s, lives and works in Kathmandu. Ang Rita was the top School Leaving Certificate student in the country in 1969, but Rose has highlighted recently the continuing involvement of Nepalese elite groups both at a national and regional

[92] Ibid., 135–36. The monastery has been rebuilt twice after being destroyed first by earthquake in 1933 and then by fire in 1989.

[93] Sherpas were familiar with such monasteries in Tibet, but in Khumbu the monastery at Thame was not a celibate institution.

[94] Although he does not have authority in secular affairs, he was involved, for example in the establishing in 1993 of the Sagarmatha Pollution Control Committee.

[95] Leo E. Rose and Margaret W. Fisher, *The Politics of Nepal: Persistence and Change in an Asian Monarchy* (Ithaca: Cornell University Press, 1970), 82. Also see Stiller and Yadav, *Planning for People*.

level in government.[96] Ang Rita and other Sherpas remained on the outside.[97]

Lastly, another aspect of community participation and running a hospital related to the actual and perceived complexity of knowledge about hospital issues. This particularly referred to technical knowledge. Researchers, such as Ortner and Draper, wrote that in reply to many of their questions people would refer them to a "lama" as he was considered the person who would have the necessary knowledge to answer their questions.[98] Draper developed his thesis around Foucault's idea that the control of knowledge is a fundamental aspect regarding issues of power and domination and their asymmetrical relationship within a society. Tsering Doma, who was chairwoman of the Khumjung Village Development Committee (VDC), found in the mid-1990s that her lack of knowledge was hindering her ability to run VDC affairs.[99] Doctors at Khunde Hospital, like the religious leaders Draper examined, also had control of knowledge.[100]

Nevertheless, not all management issues required modern technical knowledge. For local representatives on the Khunde Hospital Advisory Committee in the early 1970s the question of the community supplying firewood or potatoes to the hospital did not present a "knowledge" problem. Indeed community representatives would have had a much better level of knowledge than the overseas volunteers in regard to such matters. Similarly, one of the biggest medical issues for the volunteers at this time was tuberculosis and they tried to involve the Hospital Advisory Committee to help with the problem of people not taking their medicine.[101] Again this was not a technical problem, but one where a community understanding was important. Again they were unsuccessful.

★ ★ ★

96 Rose, "The National Political Culture and Institutions in Nepal", 136.

97 Weiner, "Source Force", 669.

98 See, for example, Ortner, *High Religion,* 7–8, and Draper, "Lama Knows".

99 Conversation with Tsering Doma, Khumjung, 1998. The VDC replaced the panchayat as the local unit of government after 1990.

100 Draper, "Beyond Medicine".

101 19 August 1971, HACB.

Community participation to help run a hospital was one level of local involvement. Could the community go a step further and take over the project so that it was no longer an aid project? This raises the issue of the finance required to sustain the hospital. The development of tourism in the Everest area has brought about increasing wealth in the region. Much of people's earnings from tourism was used for better housing, clothing, food and education, but Sherpa religion also benefited in terms of people being able to afford to hold more ritual ceremonies or even sponsor new ones such as were introduced in the mid-1980s.[102] When Tengboche monastery burned down in 1989, US$50,000 was raised from the local community towards the rebuilding.[103] Sherpas paid for traditional forms of treatment when sick, and the income from fees introduced at the hospital now provides part of the costs of running the hospital, but the hospital has rarely received financial donations from the community. In other areas senior religious figures are now telling people that causes such as hospitals are also worthy.[104]

Hillary was well aware of the situation. At a meeting of the newly established Himalayan Trust Sherpa Committee in Lukla in 1992 he challenged those present:

> And what have the local people done? Some hard work certainly, some carrying of loads, a little raising of money (except for Tengboche Monastery where they were very generous). But often just asking, asking—more money, more pay, more buildings, more clinics, more high schools, more monastery roofs, more bridges.[105]

Hillary continued that he was not about to stop his work; he said it was why he was there in Nepal, but his increasing age (he was then 73 years old) and that of others involved, both in New Zealand and overseas, had prompted discussion about the future. Hillary's com-

[102] Adams, *Tigers of the Snow and Other Virtual Sherpas,* 212.

[103] Johnston, *Sir Edmund Hillary,* 205.

[104] Conversation with Dr Lhakpa Norbu and Helen Sherpa, Dunedin, January 2005.

[105] "Lukla Meeting. Introductory remarks by the Chairman, Sir Edmund Hillary. 27 March 1992." I would like to thank Dr Lynley Cook who was present at the meeting for a copy of this document.

ment also highlighted his vision of aid. Hillary's approach to his aid work was that he would continue as long as he was wanted. Sherpas present at the meeting were his senior Sherpas and they were the people he looked towards to take over. When they did, Hillary would withdraw. He had worked hard for the Sherpa, but he derived a lot of personal satisfaction. [106] He was not looking to finish one project and then find another, as were many of those working in the aid sector. His activities in Nepal had become a way of life for Hillary, but he was never part of Kathmandu's large and thriving international aid community. [107]

When Hillary first began helping the Sherpa, his was the only aid for the region which was of low priority for the Nepalese government. In 1970 Naylor commented in his review of Hillary's work that "to some extent, the offer of specific aid in quite large measures to the single defined Himalayan area of Solu-Khumbu is an anathema in Khatmandu because of their low priority for the area." [108] The state's presence nevertheless slowly grew in the area. With the development of tourism, the establishment of a national park in 1976 and the increasing affluence of the Everest region in the 1980s and 1990s, it could be thought that outside aid would become less necessary. Yet many individuals, organisations and also other countries became involved in aid in the region. Vincanne Adams discusses the idea of people being needy but also worthy of receiving help. [109] Involvement with tourism can be construed as Sherpas helping themselves to develop. This is seen as something positive, but Sherpas continue to be seen as "in need" to people who come from wealthy countries who then want to continue to give and so help them further. Hillary's comments to Sherpas at the meeting in 1992 could be viewed as Sherpas being greedy and no longer worthy of helping. Yet Hillary continued with his work. His projects and the Sherpa remain attractive for a lot of prospective donors. Some

[106] Conversations, Hillary, 2002–5.

[107] See Justice, *Policies, Plans, & People,* 38–39. In 1979 over seven hundred foreigners worked with donor aid programmes and the diplomatic corps in Kathmandu.

[108] Naylor, "Afforestation in the Khumbu", 4–5.

[109] Adams, *Tigers of the Snow and Other Virtual Sherpas,* 90–92.

individual Sherpas are wealthy, but most are not. The area also lacks many basic amenities. Some, such as the need for safe water supply and sanitation, are important for good health.

As part of the outside world's encounter with the Everest area, Khunde Hospital has received aid from various sources. One type of aid that has been essential to the running of the project has been the volunteer medical aid of the doctors. Not only did they provide the medical services for which the hospital was established, but the continuing need for their presence was another reason for the hospital remaining an aid project. Hillary had to rely on overseas doctors because initially there were no Sherpa doctors and the area was unappealing to Nepalese doctors from other parts of the country.[110] Ang Rita was the first Sherpa to begin medical training overseas, but a revolution in Burma ended his studies in 1975. While a few Sherpas from various parts of the Solukhumbu district have trained in medicine, it was not until 1996 that a Sherpa doctor, Nawang Karsang from Namche Bazar, worked at Khunde Hospital for nearly a year after training in Beijing.[111]

The aid given by the volunteers was a particular form of aid. It was both practical and financial, and was sustained over a lengthy period of time. The volunteers had various reasons for wanting to go and work at Khunde Hospital, but, whatever the reason, each was prepared to accept the low pay and basic living conditions entailed in being a volunteer in a Third World country.[112] This contrasted to the often highly paid consultants who were employed to carry out much of the international aid programme. Hillary believed that volunteers living in close contact with the community in which they worked were more likely to create the kind of goodwill he was seeking to achieve with his aid projects. The presence of the volunteers considerably influenced the way the hospital worked, the nature of its relationship with the local community and its wider dealings

[110] In 1990, 70 of Nepal's 75 districts had a district hospital with three positions for doctors, but "rarely are all three posts filled". Ali, *Status of Health in Nepal,* 55.

[111] Nepalese doctors at Khunde Hospital are not volunteers.

[112] See chapter one. Some volunteers are less well off than individual members of the local community.

with the Nepalese administration. They were at the heart of the relationship that Hillary sought and recognised as important in the quote at the beginning of this chapter.

As well as the unofficial support from individual people or organisations, the hospital has also received assistance from official sources in New Zealand. Nepal was not a priority area for official New Zealand aid, but Hillary was a New Zealander and became widely recognised internationally for his work to help the Sherpa and Nepal. New Zealand's image gained from the association. As discussed earlier, one official link between the hospital and New Zealand aid was through Volunteer Service Abroad (VSA), which was the employer of the volunteers between 1966 and 1979.

Most New Zealand government aid to the Himalayan Trust, however, was provided in the form of a varying and relatively small annual grant that could then be directed where needed. Hillary was able to operate fairly independently and Khunde Hospital was part of this overall programme. Although the government in 1963 declined to fund the building or operation of Khunde Hospital, in 1969 it approved a grant of $1,000 for equipment and supplies. [113] After gaining permission, Hillary later used this to pay for the repair of the X-ray machine. [114] Hillary did not use or request money that he did not need, but while he had sufficient donated medicines, the repair bill was a substantial item. Hillary, via the Trust, was accountable to the Department of External Affairs for the money the Trust received and submitted an annual statement of the Trust's accounts, but this was generally all that was required for most of Hillary's programme. [115] The larger sums of money and the formal bilateral agreement between New Zealand and Nepal regarding the build-

[113] Secretary of External Affairs to the High Commission, 14 October 1969, Himalayan Climbing Expeditions & Schoolhouse Projects, ABHS 6949 W4628 NDI 64/14/2, Part 4 [ANZ]. The telex noted that Hillary did not consider he needed government assistance for the schools.

[114] Correspondence between Pearl and the Department in November and December 1973, Nepal: Solu Hospital, ABHS 959 W4627 118/13/13/18 Part 1 [ANZ].

[115] Interview, Joplin, 2002.

ing of the hospital at Phaphlu and its operation during the first five years, however, did require a greater relationship.

Khunde Hospital was part of Hillary's broad-based aid programme that covered education, health, forestry and other community projects; foundations were set up over the years by enthusiastic supporters in Canada, the USA, Britain and Germany to help fund his work. These organisations were private and voluntary, but in Canada the Sir Edmund Hillary Foundation received considerable long-term funding from CIDA, the federal organisation for most official Canadian government aid which was established in 1968.[116] The SEHF project with which CIDA was most involved was Khunde Hospital; and it is in the hospital's relationship with CIDA that the effects of changing development discourse were most apparent.

The Canadian connection with Khunde Hospital may be explained by Hillary's employment with Sears and the private North American financial support of Hillary's expeditions and early aid projects. William "Zeke" O'Connor, former Toronto Argonauts football player and the national Marketing Manager for Sporting Goods for Sears, which was Canada's largest retail company, first met Hillary on a camping trip in Canada in 1971.[117] Two years later he made his first visit with Hillary to Khumbu where he was impressed with the schools and Khunde Hospital. He also met Pearl who ran the Trust's medical committee. At this time Hillary and the Trust were involved with the New Zealand government in plans to

116 The Canadian aid programme in Nepal began in 1958 with support for the aviation sector. In 1965 Canada established diplomatic relations with Nepal. A Canadian Co-operation Office in Kathmandu oversees Canadian aid projects which include some health projects, but Khunde Hospital is not part of this. As already discussed, the hospital comes under Hillary's Agreement with the Nepalese government. CIDA's support to Khunde Hospital goes via the SEHF in Canada. For an analysis of Canadian aid to Nepal, see Byas Jee Poudel, *Canadian Development Assistance to Nepal* (Kathmandu: Sharad Shashi Poudel, 1991 [1989]).

117 Interview with William "Zeke" O'Connor, Toronto, December 2004. Also see Gelaine Camelon, *Rising to New Heights: The Sir Edmund Hillary Foundation of Canada* (Toronto: Sir Edmund Hillary Foundation of Canada [1999]).

build the hospital at Phaphlu. The small New Zealand organisation's resources, both human and financial, were being stretched as its Nepal programme expanded. In 1974, Pearl was in Canada and approached O'Connor about the possibility of helping; O'Connor agreed. He set up the Sir Edmund Hillary Foundation, which was incorporated in the province of Ontario in 1976 and had its office in the Sears building in Toronto.

Although the Canadian organisation would fund Khunde Hospital, Pearl made it clear that the Trust in New Zealand would administer the project and direct the use of funds.[118] The relationship between the two organisations and countries has generally worked well, because in practice Hillary identified what he wanted to do and O'Connor, the SEHF's long-serving president, agreed to find the money.[119] The structure reflected O'Connor's personal commitment to supporting Hillary's work.[120]

The division of responsibility was significant, not just because it determined the relationship between the SEHF, the Trust and Khunde Hospital, but also because almost from the beginning of Canadian involvement CIDA allocated funds for the SEHF to assist the hospital and health services in the area. Byas Jee Poudel commented that, based on the funds allocated during the 1970s to the mid-1980s, the SEHF was one of the most active of about thirty Canadian NGOs operating in Nepal.[121] Both the SEHF and the Trust had its own aims, constraints and method of working that have influenced Khunde Hospital. Using the case histories of two "well-established" NGOs in western India, Alnoor Ebrahim has

118 Interview, O'Connor, 2004. O'Connor has a letter from Pearl (which unfortunately he was unable to find) in which Pearl was quick to point out that the SEHF did not "run" Khunde Hospital. Pearl's papers were destroyed after his death, and so the only letters to survive are those still held by the recipients.

119 Ibid.

120 Also see Brian H. Smith, *More Than Altruism: The Politics of Private Foreign Aid* (New Jersey: Princeton University Press, 1990). Smith finds that Canadian and European non-governmental organisations focus more on political change as part of development efforts than do those of the USA. Hillary, however, preferred to keep out of politics.

121 Poudel, *Canadian Development Assistance to Nepal,* 54.

discussed recently how shifts in "development discourse" influenced the behaviour of these NGOs.[122] While he emphasised "the embeddedness of NGO behaviour" in the discourses prevailing at the time of an organisation's founding, he believed that subsequent shifts also have an important influence on a project. Discourses have constantly changed and have been transmitted through to an NGO by mechanisms such as the use of consultants, conditions attached to funding and reporting requirements.[123]

These ideas provide a useful framework for considering the involvement of the SEHF and CIDA with Khunde Hospital. Although the SEHF and CIDA became involved with an ongoing project rather than one in an establishment phase, Ebrahim's view of the importance of the prevailing discourse is pertinent. In order to attract assistance, the project had to appeal. O'Connor liked what he saw when he visited Nepal and set about raising money to support Hillary's work. CIDA's agreement to co-fund arose because Khunde Hospital and Hillary's work fitted into CIDA's views at the time about aid.

By the mid-1970s international ideas about aid had changed from the time when the hospital was built. Although the phases overlapped, the emphasis had shifted from the provision of curative services to prevention. The focus, particularly after the Declaration of Alma Ata in 1978, became primary health care as the way to bring health to people living in rural areas. Donor agencies in Nepal acknowledged that their previous hospital-based approach typically brought services to urban areas where few people lived.[124] The ongoing support of an official aid agency such as CIDA provides an example of how the services provided from Khunde Hospital engaged

[122] Alnoor Ebrahim, "NGO Behaviour and Development Discourse: Cases From Western India", *Voluntas* 12, no. 2, 2001, 79–101. Ebrahim refers to development discourse as not only how development is described or talked about, but also how it is thought about and practised. His ideas have been expanded in Ebrahim, *NGOs and Organizational Change*.

[123] Nevertheless, the relationship also had a two-way dimension in that the NGOs were able at times to challenge and adapt some of the discourses to better suit their own needs.

[124] Justice, *Policies, Plans, & People,* 51.

with these evolving ideas and objectives of international medical aid. On the one hand Khunde Hospital was working at a grassroots level in a rural area, but primary care in itself did not require hospitals and a medical model of health care services. Also, earlier ideas of basic services shifted in emphasis towards community services. For areas, such as those served by Khunde Hospital, there was an additional cautionary note in a 1979 World Bank country economic study of Nepal. The final point in its chapter on the development of human resources stated:

> In planning such programs, basic needs considerations should not be allowed to obscure the fact that the provision of social infrastucture to many unusually remote and sparsely populated areas can never be automatically viable. In these cases, it would be unwise to squander Nepal's meager resources for programs that would delay, but not put off, the migration which will inevitably occur. [125]

The SEHF first applied to CIDA for a grant in 1976. The language and content of the different proposals, as well as the SEHF meeting increasingly demanding reporting and auditing requirements, show how the SEHF responded to CIDA's changing ideas and requirements, while at the same time continuing to emphasise the ongoing nature of the project which was to provide medical services to the people of the Everest area. [126] Early proposals focused on the provision, maintenance and expansion of services. The training of village health workers and the building of village clinics allowed the project by the latter part of the 1980s to change emphasis from Khunde Hospital to "Khunde Hospital and its Medical Clinics". In the 1990s proposals had to specify how interventions promoted the health of women and children, the project's environmental impact, linkages with other organisations, governance and sustainability. O'Connor

[125] Yukon Huang, *Nepal: Development Performance and Prospects* (Washington: South Asia Regional Office, World Bank, 1979), 50.

[126] See files at SEHF office in Toronto: FIC (CIDA) Projects TSEHF; CIDA Project Submissions, 1993–1995; CIDA—miscellaneous, 1995; CIDA Project Submissions, 1996–1998, and Khunde Hospital Proposal, 1995–1998.

followed CIDA's recommendation and hired consultants to write these later proposals.[127]

The Sir Edmund Hillary Foundation was the link between the hospital and the Trust and CIDA, presenting interim and final project reports, audited accounts and addressing issues raised by CIDA. In practice the SEHF was also a buffer that enabled the Trust to continue to administer the hospital as it had been doing. The 1993 evaluation of the SEHF showed that the SEHF continued to operate as much as it could within the philosophy of support for Hillary, which had been O'Connor's intention from the beginning. While some changes did occur after the report, such as new bank accounts for the hospital which better suited Canadian auditing arrangements, life and work for those at Khunde Hospital continued much as before.

How Have staff at Khunde Hospital Negotiated the Aid Framework?

While the previous section discussed issues that have been important in defining the wider framework in which Khunde Hospital functioned as an aid project, staff at Khunde Hospital directly engaged with some of these, but not others. Here I examine how Khunde Hospital operated in this aid environment. The first part considers the different types and levels of relationship that occurred and the mechanisms of control employed by the different parties outside the hospital. The second examines the role played by visitors who have had a considerable impact on the hospital's daily functioning. Finally, the section discusses the hospital's engagement with health programmes provided through the Nepalese government. The three main ones affecting Khunde Hospital were vaccination, family planning and tuberculosis control.

Although supported by the Trust and the SEHF to carry out their work, the overseas volunteers at Khunde Hospital operated for most of the time on their own. Khunde Hospital was an isolated aid project. Limited and slow means of communication combined

[127] Interview, O'Connor, 2004.

with the rugged topography, cold climate and remoteness created the need for independent activity. This applied both to relationships with people and places in Nepal as well as overseas. Although the physical distance from Khunde to New Zealand was very much greater than from Khunde to Kathmandu or the Solukhumbu district centre of Salleri, at times this did not matter. The most isolated period of the year at Khunde was the monsoon when poor weather prevented flights operating in the mountains for days and sometimes weeks at a time. This isolation resulted in staff having to make decisions about what to do or not to do, both for medical and non-medical issues. One of the criteria VSA used for their selection of volunteers was an ability to take the initiative and function on one's own in difficult circumstances. [128] Hillary wrote how aid-work "demands a pioneering spirit, an ability to adapt and improvise". [129] Most of the time the volunteers at Khunde Hospital relished their independence.

While Khunde Hospital became the main provider of Western medical services in Khumbu, it operated on the margins of Nepal's system of health care and had only limited contact with government officials or government health services. A hospital at Khunde was not part of the government's planned nationwide development of health services. [130] In October 1967 McKinnon sent a review of the hospital's first nine months work to the Director of Health, Dr Joshi, at the Department of Health Services in Kathmandu. [131] McKinnon's successor, Evans, also sent reports to Kathmandu, but by the time the first hospital handbook was compiled in 1976 these reports had been replaced by the submission of monthly statistical

128 Clark, *The Two-Way Street,* 62.

129 Hillary, *Schoolhouse in the Clouds*, 5

130 See Dixit, *The Quest for Health,* and Padma Mathema, *Primary Health Care in Nepal* (Kathmandu: Vijaya Ram Mathema, 1987), for an overview of health service development during the different Plan periods. While health services expanded considerably throughout the period, achievements and targets were a long way apart. Mathema discusses weaknesses (pp. 101–8) such as government policy that promoted uniformity in a country where diversity prevailed.

131 McKinnon, "Health Problems of Khumbu", 6 October 1967.

returns. As the role of district administration developed in the 1980s and decentralisation increased, these returns were submitted also to the district health office in Salleri. [132] Although this was a way for the government to monitor health activities at Khunde Hospital, in practice, except for the obtaining of relevant supplies, the reports and returns were a one-way transmission of information from the hospital to the government, whether at the central or district level of administration. What mattered was that the hospital sent in the required information as and when it was specified. Without such statistics government staff were unable to write the reports required by their superiors or donor organisations.

Staff at the hospital also played no part in the negotiations for the 1972 Agreement between the Trust and the Nepalese government that provided the basis for the operation of Hillary's aid programme. The 1976 renewal stipulated the formation of a hospital board for the running and maintenance of the hospital under the chairmanship of Solukhumbu's chief district officer or his appointee. The Khunde Hospital doctor was the vice-chairman and responsible to the board for "all medical, administrative and disciplinary matters". [133] The only two occasions that a meeting took place under these circumstances were on 19 April and 10 September 1982. In April, the senior government official in Namche Bazar represented the chief district officer and Hillary was also present. The context of the meeting was also significant, because those present agreed to introduce a one rupee charge for each course of medication and the money collected would be used to buy more drugs. [134] Consultations would remain free. In August, the doctors at Khunde received an urgent letter from the branch officer at Salleri in which it acknowledged that their office had chaired the meeting at which

[132] Kunde Hospital Handbook, 1985, 2: 28.

[133] Note from Dr N. D. Joshi, Director General, Directorate of Health Services, HMG Ministry of Health to Hillary, April 1976, Trust Agreements [HTK].

[134] This was permitted under the terms of the Agreement between the Trust and the Nepalese government. Phaphlu Hospital had such a charge from the beginning. Much of the wording of the Agreements for each hospital is identical.

it was agreed to impose the charge, but that they had received complaints both about the charge and that also "we have heard that your charging system is unregular [*sic*]". The letter continued with the instruction "So please stop it at once and let us know the total accounts of the sum of money that you have raised up to the date of Today."[135] The doctors replied that a further meeting of the board would be needed if the decision was to be reversed and that they would supply a full account of the funds collected.[136] The meeting was held on 10 September. The charge was retained, but the Khunde doctor was instructed to ensure that the hospital and its village clinics kept proper records of the funds collected and that these would be presented to each board meeting. The board also approved that these funds would be used to buy more drugs and that the Khunde doctors were to send yearly reports to the Department of Health.[137]

This August 1982 letter from the district office to the hospital is one of few to be found in the hospital's records and illustrates the limited contact between the two organisations. Such direct monitoring of hospital affairs was unusual, as was the confrontation. Indirect methods were more usual, so that the volunteers were always aware of their insecure guest status in Nepal. The Khunde Hospital Handbook impressed upon the volunteers the need for caution when presenting information to the media and to not write anything "that might be construed as criticism of the Nepalese Government".[138] Throughout his involvement in Nepal, one of Hillary's "golden rules" for working in the country was to refrain from interfering in Nepalese politics.[139]

135 24 August 1982, HACB.

136 3 September 1982, HACB.

137 10 September 1982, HACB. Apart from a letter in the file dated 25 February 1983 referring to the Board decision, this appeared to be the end of the matter as far as the hospital was concerned. I have not found any yearly reports.

138 Kunde Hospital Handbook, 1985, 1, no page numbers.

139 Interview, Hillary, June 2002. The other was religion, but Hillary respected that Buddhism was extremely important to Sherpas and throughout has assisted Sherpas with religious projects. CIDA, however, did not support

This 1982 debate was also significant in another way. It was an official acknowledgement of some local unhappiness over a hospital policy. Those at the meeting expected that there would be some resistance.[140] Yet the imposition of the charge was an attempt to engage with the wider health environment in Nepal, and not unreasonable given that the Nepalese government recently had taken over Phaphlu Hospital and from the beginning this hospital had charged such a fee. The previous doctor at Khunde had written in the hospital's annual report for 1981 of the importance of planning for the future because funds would be insufficient to maintain services if the government was to take over the hospital. To guard against a possible deterioration in services he supported the idea of a fee in "an effort to educate the local population into accepting a user pays service".[141] He believed the area could now economically support such a move, which had been tried elsewhere.[142] He added that local people went to Kathmandu where they paid for medical services as well as being prepared in Khumbu to pay "considerable sums" for consulting spirit mediums.[143]

Being an aid project outside the government system also had practical implications for the hospital in that Hillary could set up the hospital as he thought appropriate. Independence thus gave flexibility. The basic structure that he implemented in 1966, consisting of a doctor supported by local staff, has continued until the present, as has the type of worker and their terms and conditions of employment. Just as Hillary could determine and arrange that the hospital would have a doctor, so the doctors at Khunde were

---

funds being used for religious projects and so O'Connor sought alternative funding for such projects. Interview, O'Connor, 2004.

140 Also see Adams, *Tigers of the Snow and Other Virtual Sherpas,* 118.

141 Kunde Hospital Annual Report from 1 September 1980 to 31 August 1981. For a discussion that illustrates the changing preoccupations of international health economists, see Anne Mills, "Leopard or Chameleon? The Changing Character of International Health Economics", *Tropical Medicine and International Health* 2, no. 10, October 1997, 963–77.

142 For example, the drug scheme run by the Britain-Nepal Medical Trust.

143 Kunde Hospital Annual Report from 1 September 1980 to 31 August 1981.

responsible for hiring and organising the local staff and were able to adapt structures and wages to the Khumbu situation where the cost of living was high and trained staff often non-existent.[144] The Khunde doctor was subject to the authority of the hospital's board, but, as has already been discussed, this board rarely met. Similar flexibility occurred regarding the working hours of both the hospital and individual staff. While government institutions operated fixed government hours and days per week, staff at Khunde Hospital arranged their own schedule.

In the same way that staff at Khunde Hospital took no part in the highest level of negotiations between the Trust and the Nepalese government, so they had no direct input into Trust and Foundation meetings in New Zealand and Canada and the relations between these overseas partners who supported Khunde Hospital. CIDA was even more distant. As the Trust administered the hospital, most communication occurred with New Zealand. In medical matters the volunteers turned to Pearl, but they also dealt directly with Hillary in financial matters and areas where the volunteers also acted as Trust representatives for Hillary's other work. The first Canadian volunteers arrived in September 1981. They were more familiar with the Canadian organisations, but also continued to deal with the Trust in New Zealand. By this time, however, Trust personnel in Kathmandu were playing a much greater role in the support of the hospital.

Tensions periodically surfaced relating to the New Zealand and Canadian volunteers. One of the most difficult times for any of the volunteers at Khunde was the hand-over period at the end of what generally had been around two years of very intense involvement with the hospital, the people and the area. Usually the hand-over lasted a few days.[145] At times frustrations between the two sets of volunteers resulted in letters being sent that complained of the vol-

144 For example, the Agreement between HMG/N and the Trust from 1 January 1980 to 31 December 1982 specified that the board could pay "special allowances".

145 The two sets of volunteers had already had contact with each other through letters. At the end of the period the hospital had a telephone, fax and email.

unteers in terms of them being Canadians or New Zealanders. The tension, however, needs to be understood in relation to the stresses of being a volunteer at Khunde, the emotional time of the departure or the excitement of arrival, and the individual characteristics of the different volunteers as people. Difficulties, in any case, also occurred when the two couples were both from New Zealand.[146] All this went on at the same time as the normal work of running the hospital and treating patients.

Despite the distance and relatively infrequent contact, the volunteers were influenced initially by the Trust in New Zealand and then by both the New Zealand and Canadian organisations in the running of the hospital. Staff sent details of the accounts and annual reports to both, as well as writing letters and responding to other requests for information. Justice comments on the considerable administrative demands placed on aid advisors in Kathmandu by the donor agencies and that these were geared towards these organisations' procedures and needs.[147] Initially the overseas volunteers undertook all such work, but particularly from the early 1990s local staff took on more of the administrative tasks and responsibilities. Communication between the staff at the hospital and the various overseas organisations differed because of the particular interests and concerns of each. Communication to and from the Trust in New Zealand was primarily about the operation and finances of the different Trust projects, while that with the SEHF in Canada also reflected the SEHF's role as fundraisers for Hillary's work and specific auditing and reporting requirements within Canada, both to Ontario province and CIDA.[148]

Hospital staff became used to what was required and the way things worked. Most of the time communication from the Trust and the SEHF was supportive, but at times criticism of the volunteers occurred. As discussed in chapter one, often it was about non-medical matters such as the accounts or the non-medical responsi-

146 McKinnon to the new volunteers, 26 July 1989 [KH].

147 Justice, *Policies, Plans, & People,* 42.

148 The SEHF in Canada faced more onerous demands than the Trust in New Zealand.

bilities of the volunteers.[149] Misunderstandings occurred. With the physical isolation of Khunde and the slow turnaround of letters, the volunteers became frustrated, angry and demoralised before being buoyed once more when an issue was resolved.

As chapter one also noted, the means of communication improved greatly in the mid-1990s, particularly after the arrival of a telephone and fax machine in 1995 and email in 1997. These methods were much quicker and allowed issues to be discussed with the Trust office in Kathmandu or people overseas. The telephone was particularly useful in 1997 in sorting out arrangements regarding Kami Temba's admission and departure for medical training at the Fiji School of Medicine.[150] The introduction of new methods of communication coincided with increasing demands by CIDA on the SEHF, who then communicated directly with Khunde to provide the relevant information to help write a report or proposal. Although communication with CIDA continued to be via the SEHF, the staff at Khunde became much more aware of CIDA's priorities.[151] The hospital's annual reports of 1996 and 1997, for example, reflected this knowledge and emphasised the role of the village clinics and public health work carried out in the area.[152]

Although most communication between the concerned overseas donor organisations and the staff at the project occurred on paper and from a distance, some of the donors also visited the hospital. Once the volunteers arrived in Nepal they rarely left, except for a mid-term break, until their time at the hospital had finished. Visitors came to the hospital where they would familiarise themselves with what was happening at the hospital and in the area, meet the staff and undertake specific tasks. Visits enabled those at Khunde

[149] Each set of volunteers has its own episode or episodes. Together these illustrate another aspect of the continuity in the volunteers' experiences at Khunde throughout the period.

[150] Personal participation.

[151] Ibid.

[152] Similarly, in an example that reflected the changing international discourse regarding the importance of women in development, the Nepalese government required the hospital's statistics to specify what percentage of people using the services were women and children.

to meet or maintain links with the people with whom they were dealing.

The most important visits were those of Hillary. While Pearl was responsible for medical matters, the visit of Hillary reinforced his philosophy and the low-key, practical approach to his aid. In the early years the hospital depended on supplies and services from New Zealand and Hillary was actively involved with various other building projects. He would communicate via the hospital with Mingma Tsering, who came from Khunde village. Hillary came to Khumbu one or more times each year for visits that could last for several weeks. During that time the lives of the volunteers at the hospital revolved around the visit. Dr Selwyn Lang described in the *NZ Listener* Hillary's three-week visit in November–December 1970. Lang met Hillary in Lukla, accompanied him on various visits to villages in the area as Hillary inspected schools and then climbed over the high pass into the Rolwaling valley, where Hillary promised a school for the village of Beding while Lang treated sick villagers. He then walked out to Jiri and Kathmandu before flying back to Khunde.[153]

When Hillary went to Nepal, family and other visitors accompanied him. Staff at the hospital had to deal with each of these and take into account their particular relationship to the hospital. O'Connor, for example, was a regular visitor. Having formed the SEHF in 1976, he took on responsibility for funding the hospital and visited annually. These visits were cited in his proposals and reports to CIDA as part of his mechanism for monitoring the progress of the project.[154]

As Hillary grew older and was less able to tolerate the high altitude, his personal and practical involvement with his projects lessened. Other Trust members visited and reported back to Hillary. Sometimes these visits were more social, as people enjoyed travelling in Nepal, while others, for example, were work parties to undertake specific projects such as maintenance or new building.

153 Lang, "The Highest Schools in the World", 10–11.

154 Dr Joan Ford, who became the Foundation's medical adviser, built up her knowledge of the hospital from doing several locums there from the early 1980s.

Visitors provided company and were also welcome for bringing in items for the hospital or for the volunteers' personal use that could not be bought locally.

Until his death in 1980, Pearl was the principal medical contact with the Trust. After 1980 other Trust doctors went to the hospital. These medical visits were partly to keep in touch, but they were also to report on how the volunteers were coping and how they were regarded in the area. [155] Whoever the visitor was, whatever the reason for the visit and whether they were connected with the New Zealand or Canadian organisation, staff at the hospital were also aware that the visitor was part of the hospital's ongoing monitoring by the donor organisation. [156] As the volunteers were rarely able or invited to attend medical meetings or conferences in Nepal, medical isolation was significant. Doctors from the Trust, therefore, were also an important avenue for discussing the medical work of the hospital, either in general terms or relating to specific issues. [157] After McKinnon left Khunde in 1968 he specialised in ophthalmology. Staff at the hospital continued to seek his advice about eye conditions and surgical expertise for operations such as cataract removal.

Looking after visitors took time and inevitably impinged upon the hospital's medical work. Khunde Hospital enjoyed a high (international) profile as an example of Hillary's aid. As a result, it attracted a large number of other visitors each year due to the rise in tourism in the Everest area. Image and publicity are important features of the aid world, encouraging assistance, educating others about the project and the work being done or promoting the role of the donor. The hospital acted as a flagship for Hillary's work,

[155] Linda Gill, *Living High: A Family Trek in the Himalayas* (Auckland: Hodder and Stoughton, 1983). Linda Gill relates their family holiday, but Mike's specific role (p. 19) was to visit the two Trust hospitals and the clinics. "The Trust has found that the hospitals run more smoothly if a doctor goes over every other year to experience first hand what is happening, to 'get the feel' of the place, its medical priorities and the qualities needed by those wanting to work there."

[156] As the Trust's activities were also supported by foundations in Britain, Germany and the USA, members of these also visited.

[157] The doctors at the hospital also sought specific medical advice and assistance at times from other doctors visiting the area.

but this general role was of considerably less interest to the SEHF and CIDA as their main concern was with the hospital that they were funding and not Hillary's other projects.[158] The SEHF hoped that Canadian visitors would return to Canada and donate to their organisation. CIDA was keen to see that its support was publicised, both in Canada as well as at the project.

> We ask all recipients of CIDA funds to acknowledge this fact in their annual reports, financial statements and other publications. We do so not to seek gratitude but as a form of development education—to inform the public, parliamentarians, media and others how CIDA funds are used. Such acknowledgements also help organizations which receive CIDA funds because they demonstrate the confidence that CIDA places in them.[159]

Hillary's approach was different. Although visitors went to Khunde Hospital and his other projects to see what he had done, Hillary did not advertise his own role. He did not put up plaques. He saw the projects as belonging to the people and did not want to overemphasise his contribution.[160]

The annual number of visitors to the hospital is not known, but throughout the period the issue of tourists and the work they created was discussed regularly in reports and letters. The number of visitors peaked during the spring and autumn trekking seasons and was least during the monsoon when few planes were able to fly. Usually, people just turned up at the hospital. Visitors were often a welcome change at the beginning when the medical work was less, but as the hospital became busier with patients and tourism increased, the (limited) staff were under pressure, particularly the volunteers who mostly dealt with visitors. Even if the hospital's staff

158 The SEHF was also the principal funder of the Trust's reforestation project in the Sagarmatha National Park.

159 Letter of agreement to Zeke O'Connor, President, Sir Edmund Hillary Foundation, from Kendel Rust, Director, Anglophone NGO Section (Asia), Non-Governmental Organization Division, CIDA, 20 November 1990, FIC (CIDA) projects [SEHF].

160 Conversation, Hillary, February 2005. Nevertheless, he also probably did not need to because more people knew of his work in the area than that of other organisations.

accepted that creating goodwill was important, there was no direct correlation between time spent and donation given, if any, either at Khunde or overseas.[161] A small number of tourists were patients, but most just came to visit; some were both.

Many people gave financial donations of varying amounts either at the hospital or subsequently from overseas. Others brought medicines or equipment that supplemented the basic range stocked at the hospital. Some brought items specifically requested by the overseas volunteer doctors. Usually visitors gave one-off donations with no strings attached, but a significant number of people visited the hospital regularly and provided ongoing support. They were keen to help the hospital's work, but also needed to see that the hospital continued to merit their assistance.

While these visitors' principal interest was helping the hospital, others went to Khunde who worked for aid organisations or were associated with the international health agencies or with the diplomatic missions. In the 1990s networking was an important consideration for CIDA which applicants for project funding had to adequately address. Kathmandu is the point of entry into Nepal for international air travel and aid projects in the vicinity of the capital were visited regularly because of their ease of access. Kathmandu is also the centre of Nepal's aid industry. Nevertheless, despite Khumbu's physical location, it became relatively easy to visit Khunde Hospital compared to many parts of Nepal.[162]

161 Personal participation.

162 Most visitors took the one-hour flight by small plane or helicopter to Lukla and then embarked on a three-day walk, staying overnight either in tents or lodges that from the late 1970s were built along the route. The visit to the hospital was usually part of a general trek to see the magnificent scenery of the Everest area and the home of the Sherpa. Despite the high altitude of 3,840 metres some official visitors, such as the American, British and New Zealand ambassadors who came to the opening of the hospital in December 1966, chose to directly fly to Khunde landing in a field by the hospital. Not only was it a more efficient use of their time, but also these visitors returned to low altitude within a few hours and so avoided the health hazards associated with the hypoxia and being exposed further to the freezing temperatures of winter in Khumbu.

At a general level visits provided contacts and helped develop networks that could be tapped when specific issues arose. For example, in spring 1997 representatives from the Kathmandu office of the United Nations High Commissioner for Refugees (UNHCR) visited the hospital and discussed their role in Nepal.[163] When in December a group of Tibetans arrived in Khunde and spent several weeks at the hospital suffering from frostbite, staff contacted the UNHCR who were able to assist both with the costs of looking after them and their onward travel.[164] Trekkers visiting the hospital were happy to donate warm clothing. Further publicity occurred when the story of a young Tibetan girl and a nun, who were helped by other trekkers to reach Khunde Hospital, was the cover story of a subsequent issue of *Reader's Digest.*[165]

This use of the visit as a tool to help networking with other organisations also applied locally. Both the staff at the hospital and the Trust more generally within Nepal, have throughout focused on their own work rather than engaging with what was happening around them, although the amount of contact with other aid or overseas personnel varied among the different volunteers and local staff and the issues at a particular time. In the 1960s there was little interest, apart from that of Hillary, in aid to such a remote area and so the volunteers at Khunde Hospital as the only foreigners in the area on a long-term basis had the place to themselves.[166]

During the 1970s there was increasing interest in the region from outside organisations keen to provide aid, both in terms of conserving the environment with the establishment of a national park in 1976 and in developing the area with a World Bank study on tourism. As part of the international rise in prominence of NGO involvement in international aid and development, a number of

163 Personal participation.

164 Ibid.

165 David Moller, "Challenge on the Roof of the World", *Reader's Digest* (UK edition, May 1999), 92–104. No such outside help was forthcoming for a Nepalese porter who came to the hospital a few months later with frostbitten feet. The hospital paid for an operation in Kathmandu to enable him to walk and so continue to earn a living.

166 The International Red Cross left as the Tibetans moved on to other areas.

other small aid projects started in the area and some, such as the small electricity scheme for Namche Bazar established in the early 1980s, had foreign staff for varying periods of time.[167] In 1988 the Nepalese and Austrian governments signed an agreement to build a hydropower plant in the Bhote Kosi valley. In 1993 an Austrian INGO Eco Himal took over responsibility for the final phase of its construction, training of a Sherpa team of technicians and implementation of the scheme and also became involved increasingly in the area with a variety of other projects. Both Eco Himal and Khunde Hospital had expertise that could assist the other. The hospital benefited from the electricity and technical help when there were problems, while the hospital provided medical support for Eco Himal through health services and first aid training.[168] A further link was developed in 1997 when hospital staff provided medical training for Eco Himal's mountaineering course.

Further layers of relationships arose through the hospital's local staff and their involvement with aid projects. For example, in the mid-1990s Kami Temba was treasurer to the Sagarmatha Pollution Control Committee (SPCC) and a director of Khumbu Bijuli Company. With a small population and a limited pool of educated and people willing to participate in the running of the many organisations that developed in the area, an overlap occurred in organisational affiliations.

Lastly, a third and increasingly important area in which staff at Khunde Hospital engaged with the world of international aid was in the interaction between some of the health programmes offered by staff at the hospital and those offered by the Nepalese government's health department. Nepal was one of the poorest countries in the world and its health status "uniformly poor", both in absolute terms and in comparison with neighbouring countries.[169] The government focused on preventive health and basic needs to achieve the maximum gain on a population level for the minimum

[167] Official support for NGOs was closely allied to the disillusionment with the results of official development assistance.

[168] Dieter Rachbauer, ed., *Energy from the Top of the World: Small Hydropower Plant Thame-Namche Bazar, Nepal* (Kathmandu: Eco Himal, 2001).

[169] Ali, *Status of Health in Nepal,* 18.

amount of resources, but also sought to incorporate Nepal's specific needs with those of international policies. While Khunde Hospital offered a wide range of outpatient and inpatient, curative and preventive services, the health department had very limited financial and human resources to establish, expand and maintain its activities. Khumbu was also at the far end of the district and difficult to support from Salleri.

Much of the government's preventive health programme work was funded through foreign aid support of specific projects that were then implemented in Nepal through the Ministry of Health. The United States Agency for International Development (USAID) was the largest bilateral donor of health aid to developing countries, including Nepal.[170] Its policy was to assist and advise, but not take control of projects. Such a process of working through a country's government structures or local organisations to achieve the donors' aims also had an additional desired effect as it lessened the visibility of foreigners.[171]

When Khunde Hospital opened in 1966 the government's preventive health programmes had made little inroads into either the densely populated hill areas or the more remote and sparsely settled mountains. Virtually no health service delivery system existed outside the Kathmandu valley. The government health programmes in the 1960s were separate and centrally organised on a vertical basis, each with its own particular structures and way of working.[172] Apart from the small clinic at Namche Bazar, visits to the area from other government health workers were infrequent. It was also difficult to retain staff in the clinic at Namche due partly to Khumbu's "harsh conditions".[173] Most of the time staff at Khunde Hospital provided preventive health services independently, but when government health workers did occasionally come into Khumbu to offer a serv-

170 Justice, *Policies, Plans, & People,* 26–29.

171 Ibid., 28.

172 Mathema, *Primary Health Care in Nepal,* chapter two.

173 Mingmar Gyelzen Sherpa, "Himalayan Trust, and Health in Solu Khumbu", in *Triumph on Everest,* ed. Ang Rita Sherpa and Susan Höivik, 122. Dr Mingmar Gyelzen (in chapters two and three his name is spelt Mingma Gyelgen) was the district's chief medical officer.

ice then Khunde Hospital staff sought to complement but not compete. For example, in 1969 government smallpox vaccinators came into the area and gave smallpox vaccinations in Namche Bazar, but none in any of the other villages.[174] Later in the year, during his annual vaccination programme, Dr Richard Evans went round most of the other villages in the area on a house-by-house basis and gave 807 doses.[175] The smallpox vaccine was supplied free-of-charge by the WHO in Kathmandu.

Other regions in Nepal were not so fortunate, and few had any alternative but to wait for the gradual expansion of government services. Large areas of the country remained without modern health services. The terrain, which made it even more difficult for people to get to a health post or a health worker out to the people, compounded the situation.

As well as smallpox vaccinations, Evans offered BCG vaccination against tuberculosis. In 1965, the government established a national Tuberculosis Control Project, but initially activities were confined to the Kathmandu Valley. The aim of the WHO, which provided the vaccine, was to cover the whole population. In 1968 the Britain-Nepal Medical Trust began to work in Eastern Nepal to combat tuberculosis.[176] Staff at Khunde Hospital also provided tuberculosis treatment. The annual report for 1976/77 recorded that 13 of the 94 inpatient admissions were for tuberculosis, that the hospital had 30 patients currently undergoing treatment and that they were managed in cooperation with the government's Tuberculosis Control Project.[177] Most of the new cases came from outside Khumbu.[178] By 1986 the Tuberculosis Control Project operated in 31 of Nepal's 75 districts.[179] Data from 1992 showed that further expansion had occurred and that 60 of the 75 districts were covered by the na-

174 R. Evans to Dr C. G. I. Gordon, WHO Representative in Nepal, 14 May 1969, assorted papers [KH].

175 Hillary Sherpa Hospital Report 23 August 1968 to 27 February 1969.

176 Dixit, *The Quest for Health,* 103.

177 Kunde Hospital Annual Report for the Year Ending 30 June 1977.

178 Kunde Hospital Annual Report from 1 September 1980 to 31 August 1981.

179 Mathema, *Primary Health Care in Nepal,* 48.

tional tuberculosis programme with a variety of INGOs and NGOs having the responsibility in 24 of the districts.[180] Despite the seriousness of the country's tuberculosis burden and the amount of aid, the fact that not all of the country could access treatment even by the early 1990s illustrated the ongoing problems for providing health care in Nepal.

Family planning was another service that Khunde Hospital was able to offer people in the area. USAID was actively involved with Nepal's family planning programme, but national programmes were only able to advance slowly as they were implemented gradually in an increasing number of districts. In Khumbu, however, staff at the hospital initially obtained their supplies from the central agencies independently and provided services. Gradually, as government services expanded, the hospital was drawn into the government programme. The provision of long-acting progestin implants (Norplant) from 1991 was offered wholly within the government programme. Staff undertook an approved training course, and the service operated within the official protocol.[181] The hospital reported to the district health office from where it also obtained its supplies. By the late 1990s, if the district had problems ensuring sufficient supplies to provide the service for the district, then so did Khunde Hospital.[182] If the policy guidelines changed, then Khunde Hospital was expected to comply.

While expansion of services through vertical projects such as tuberculosis control or family planning was one aspect of the developing government role in health, the other was the provision of personnel and facilities in a growing number of places throughout the country. The building of a health post in a rural area became a base from which health services could spread out into the surrounding villages. By 1970 the total throughout Nepal was 113.[183] At the end

[180] In 1993 the WHO declared tuberculosis to be a global emergency. It was also reappearing as a problem in developed countries.

[181] J. A. Litch, R. A. Bishop, M. T. Sherpa, G. N. Sherpa and K. T. Sherpa, "Hormonal Contraceptive Use in a Rural District of Nepal", *Journal of Nepal Medical Association* 39, 2000, 199–202.

[182] Personal participation.

[183] Dixit, *The Quest for Health,* 47.

of the Fourth Five-Year Plan in 1975 the number had climbed to 351. The main problem, however, was "the poor state and lack of proper functioning of the health posts". [184] For example, many did not have their own premises. An expansion of facilities required the training of an increasing number of health workers of various grades to staff these health posts, but staff retention in remote rural areas was a problem. Despite such difficulties, the move to district level administration in the 1980s following the 1982 Decentralisation Act continued these activities towards the stated, if by the 1990s increasingly unrealistic, goal of achieving basic minimum health services for all Nepalese by the year 2000.

The implication of this expansion for Khunde Hospital was considerable. Reviewed broadly, what happened was that staff at Khunde Hospital continued to offer services as they had done from 1966 onwards, but the distance between services provided by the hospital and places where services were offered through the government's programmes gradually decreased. The 1991 National Health Policy proposed that each VDC would have one sub-health post. [185] Khunde Hospital covered an area with three VDCs. Curative services occupied a lower priority in the government's plan, and so this aspect of the hospital's operation was less affected. The number of outpatients attending Khunde Hospital continued to increase from 6,066 in 1990 to 7,294 in 1997. In preventive health work, however, Khunde Hospital slowly adjusted its activities so that it operated its programmes within the government framework for the area and from the 1980s dealt primarily with the District Health Office in Salleri.

Khunde Hospital's experience with government vaccination programmes illustrated the shifting ground in this relationship. During the early 1970s Khunde Hospital staff continued to provide both smallpox and BCG vaccinations to people throughout Khumbu and further afield as Hillary's school building activities led to widening involvement in the Solukhumbu district. With the opening of Phaphlu Hospital at the beginning of 1976, Khunde Hospital staff

[184] Ibid., 52.

[185] Ibid., 223.

were able to concentrate on Khumbu and the adjacent area of Pharak. In 1978 the Department of Health Services planned to give BCG vaccinations to all of the Solukhumbu district and it asked Khunde Hospital to vaccinate all the under-16s in Khumbu and Pharak.[186]

During the 1980s Khunde Hospital's role in vaccination changed. With the Nepalese government taking over Phaphlu Hospital in 1980 and with decentralisation and the establishment of district health services, Phaphlu and the nearby government centre in Salleri became the focal point from which preventive services radiated and from where supplies increasingly came. By the late 1980s the government health service was providing the Expanded Programme on Immunisation (EPI) for the district, including Khumbu, although Khunde Hospital's annual report for 1988/89 comments that visits were sporadic and often poorly organised with local communities not knowing when the vaccinators were coming.[187] Whether due to lack of supplies or manpower, problems continued to occur and by the early 1990s the Khunde doctors believed coverage must be low.[188] When a year passed by with no visit, the doctors at Khunde Hospital thought they would have to resume the service. In this instance and with the immediate concern of an outbreak of measles, a letter to the Salleri office brought a team into the area seven days later.[189]

Paradoxically this lack of involvement with vaccination put the hospital in a weaker position vis-à-vis CIDA with its emphasis on prevention and strategies to promote women and children's health. Vaccination had been one of the most important roles of the hospital. Following requests from the local people, however, it became a designated vaccinator again in 1994 and restarted giving immunisations.[190] Vaccine was delivered each month from Phaplu and offered regularly on the 21st of each Nepalese month. In 1995

[186] Kunde Hospital Annual Report for the Year Ending 30 November 1978.

[187] The Kunde Hospital Annual Report, August 1988 to June 1989.

[188] Kunde Hospital Annual Report, 1 June 1991 to 31 May 1992.

[189] Dr Lynley Cook to Director, Immunisation Services, Salleri, 27 August 1992, Vaccinations [KH].

[190] Khunde Hospital Annual Report, February 1994–January 1995.

Khunde Hospital was donated a fridge which helped with some of the supply problems and also led to the hospital acting as a depot for government vaccinators. During the winter of 1996/97 Nepal participated in the international campaign to eradicate polio, holding national immunisation days in December and January. Khunde Hospital coordinated activities in the three VDC areas of Chaurikharka, Namche and Khumjung with its staff and village health workers working with government staff and volunteers to run 11 centres throughout the region.[191]

While Khunde Hospital operated independently, particularly in respect of the curative services it provided, its preventive programmes by the mid-1990s were, therefore, much more aligned with the work of the government's health services.[192] In 2003 Dr Mingmar Gyelzen Sherpa, chief medical officer for Solukhumbu, wrote of Khunde and Phaphlu hospitals that "the District Health Office Solu Khumbu has received much support from Himalayan Trust. The health of the local people has been significantly improved through programmes for tuberculosis and leprosy control, immunisation (TB, measles, tetanus, polio, and diphtheria), family planning, and nutrition."[193]

Another aspect of this increasing alignment with the government's programmes can be seen in the issue of health worker training, although here progress was much slower. While the Agreement between the Trust and the Nepalese government allowed the Trust to bring in an overseas doctor, other staff working at the hospital and in the villages were drawn from the local community and were trained at the hospital. When there were few alternatives such independent action was acceptable, but this became less satisfactory as government training programmes developed. In the mid-1970s, the

[191] Kunde Hospital and Village Clinics Annual Report 1996.

[192] In its curative services Khunde Hospital policy emphasised basic provision at a health clinic level with some secondary services such as inpatient provision for obstetrics. The level of services also depended on the particular skills of the different volunteers.

[193] Mingmar Gyelzen Sherpa, "Himalayan Trust, and Health in Solu Khumbu", in Sherpa and Höivik, *Sherpas on Everest*, 122. Khumbu only had a few cases of leprosy.

government introduced a programme for integrated health services and community health volunteers and so the Khunde doctor, Jim Jerram, sent four of the village health workers on a six-week government course "to come in line".[194]

The issue of health worker training was complicated by a problem that illustrated the enormous gap that could exist between the promotion of a policy and its implementation in the field.[195] For example, the government sought to raise health service standards and so it raised the entry requirements for admission to government health worker courses. In the mid-1990s the Trust, the SEHF and CIDA all supported the concept of well-educated trained female village health workers and the District Health Office emphasised that these health workers should undertake government approved courses. Apart from the issue that employment in the tourism industry often appeared more attractive, there was a lack, particularly in the outlying villages, of local Sherpa girls with sufficient education to be accepted on to the government courses. Hillary responded by offering increased financial sponsorship to encourage more girls to stay at school.[196] In the short-term the hospital retained its staff and thus at least provided a basic level of services, but the situation was unsatisfactory. Even when a suitable person was found and went for training outside the area, there was no guarantee he or she would complete training, return or stay.[197] In trying to negotiate the world

194 Kunde Hospital Annual Report for the Year Ending 30 November 1978. Some confusion also occurred when government village health workers were sent into areas where the Trust had workers. After correspondence between the District Health Office and the Chief District Officer these were recalled.

USAID was the primary donor for the Integrated Community Health Programme.

195 See Justice, *Policies, Plans, & People,* although the example used is different.

196 Minutes of the Annual General Meeting of the Himalayan Trust, 25 October 1997.

197 For example, a girl from Khumjung topped in the entrance examination for a nurse/midwifery course at Jiri Technical School and began studies in early 1992 with the promise of a job at Khunde Hospital when she finished. Finding the course boring, she withdrew and returned to Khumbu and

of international aid, therefore, the volunteers at Khunde Hospital were also encountering the Sherpa world of Khumbu.

Conclusion

The gradual and increasing alignment of Khunde Hospital's preventive health programmes with those provided by government services, which provided most Western medical health care in Nepal, provides a fitting point to end this discussion of Khunde Hospital as an aid project. Situated in a poor isolated area that had a limited government presence and limited Western medicine services, the hospital was built in 1966 as a private aid project but had also remained one. No other funding or medical staffing option was offered from within Nepal in the ensuing period (more than thirty years), a change in orientation had occurred among international medical aid programmes towards rural primary care initiatives and donors remained both willing and able to support the hospital. Nevertheless, for much of its history, and in much of its work, Khunde Hospital functioned independently in Nepal, operating since 1972 through Hillary's Agreement with the Nepalese government. From the late 1970s, however, most funding came from Canada through the Sir Edmund Hillary Foundation and the Canadian International Development Agency, although the hospital continued to be administered by the Himalayan Trust from New Zealand. The relationship worked in practice because of the way O'Connor supported Hillary's work.

That Hillary and the Trust worked in a rural rather an urban area, and worked with a community rather than adopting the more common top-down approach, made the hospital acceptable to CIDA in the 1970s. By this time the focus for international aid had shifted to the development of Nepal's rural areas, where most of the population lived, and to preventive health rather than curative services. Proposals by the SEHF to CIDA subsequently reflected a continually evolving discourse surrounding medical aid. The implementation of aid programmes in Nepal, however, was fraught with diffi-

Class 10 at Khumjung School. Kunde Hospital Annual Report, 1 June 1991 to 31 May 1992.

culties and was hampered by Nepal's lack of modernisation, trained personnel and infrastructure. Other factors also need to be considered. A case study of the failed Hospital Advisory Committee analysed the difficulties of achieving a key aid concept of community participation, ideas about which also changed over the period. The failure or abandonment of the Committee by the late 1990s emphasised that this specific problem, as with the overall provision of health services from the hospital, was grounded in the specific local conditions of Khumbu and the general issues of aid and the provision of health services in Nepal.

While many accounts about the implementation of aid over-generalise and often assume that outsiders are able to impose their priorities on unquestioning and supposedly undifferentiated recipient countries and communities, they also ignore the bonds of expectation and obligation that come with the gift of aid. Khunde Hospital had multiple donors with different types of aid and different degrees of involvement with the project. While Justice's study on foreign aid and health development in Nepal showed the complexities and layers between formulating a policy at an international aid agency level and implementation in the field, this chapter has reversed the focus and looked upwards and outwards from a project as it responded to the many expectations and obligations placed upon it. Furthermore, this occurred within a shifting framework throughout the period in the ideas and delivery of aid at an international level. Staff at the hospital had to continually locate themselves within a matrix of multiple official and unofficial aid relationships that operated at varying levels and in varying ways, defining how the hospital existed and operated. Each donor had specific ideas, interests and expectations. Reporting from and visits to the project were monitoring tools that took up a considerable amount of staff time and ensured that the staff at the hospital were always aware of the bonds that were an integral part of the gift of aid.

Despite its remote physical location and overseas financial and organisational support, the hospital was not isolated from developments within the local area in which it was situated and more widely within Nepal. Each was very different in the late-1990s and the hospital had become firmly embedded within both. By then,

Khunde Hospital's earlier isolation had gradually lessened as international aid supported the expansion of government health services throughout the country and with the establishment of district level mechanisms from the 1980s. Nevertheless, by the end of the period, although the hospital was now much more closely integrated into Nepal's health programmes, Khunde Hospital remained on the outside in a situation that continued to allow the hospital flexibility in what kind of health care it provided for the local population and how it did so. It was also one that the local community appeared not to be in a hurry to change.

Conclusion

In the Introduction I argued that a book about the history of a small hospital in the mountains of Nepal, in itself a small country sandwiched between the regional giants of India and China, had a wider relevance. I suggested that despite all the literature we know remarkably little about the practical implementation of the international aid that has been a key feature, whether overtly or more invisibly, of international health programmes and state health services throughout much of the world since the 1950s.

Khunde Hospital, International Health and Aid: Multiple Worlds of Place, People and Relationships

Foreign aid has had its critics and supporters, but a large and expanding industry grew around the world involving individuals and institutions, national and international agencies and organisations of varying size working in the field or involved with funding, training and research. Many policies and projects were formulated and carried out as ideas and practices developed or changed throughout the period. Some were "successful"; but many failed or did not achieve the expected results, took much longer than anticipated or even collapsed after a period of apparent success. Success and failure, of course, are open to different interpretations and many reasons and theories were put forward to explain both. These in turn led to the ongoing formulation of new policies and projects that sought, and continue to seek, to address particular concerns, whether at an international, national or local level.

Far from being a narrative about the implementation and resulting diffusion of ideas, policies and practices, this history of Khunde Hospital has explored encounters and interaction between various global, national and local forces. In assessing what happened when

Western medicine and international aid came into contact with Sherpas in Khumbu through the institution of this small hospital, it has emphasised the fractured, pragmatic and selected nature in which international health policies and practices were received and that the dialogue was ongoing. As Nancy Hunt has written about childbirth practices in the former Belgian Congo, the encounter was not "one epic-like meeting between two, and too homogeneous, groups".[1] Western medicine was not in itself changed or weakened in the process[2], but it was not, however, taken up in the way that it was supposed to, and it also occurred much more slowly than expected. Practising medicine at Khunde Hospital was both a proactive and a reactive process as the doctors responded not only to health issues but also to how people did and did not use the hospital's services. The diverse and complex issues and multiple layers of different kinds of relationships resulting from ongoing encounters and interaction were all a part of the hospital's history as was the agency of those involved at every stage of the process.

This study concludes, therefore, that if a small project like Khunde Hospital shows such complexity and diversity, then it is unlikely that there are simple answers, or "one-stop" or "quick-fix" solutions to the current and ongoing health needs of the mainly poor populations of Third World countries. If at times the medical practice at Khunde Hospital appeared submerged within many other concerns, it is because it really was, and continues to be so. That Khunde Hospital has survived the challenges of its location and its prosperity has to be seen as a considerable achievement; however, it did not just happen because, for example, it met a need or was a well-designed project, and so on. The introduction and spread of Western medicine and the implementation of this aid project need to be seen as an ongoing and adaptive process with its ups and

[1] Nancy Rose Hunt, *A Colonial Lexicon: Of Birth Ritual, Medicalization, and Mobility in the Congo* (Durham: Duke University Press, 1999), 160. Sherpas also homogenised outsiders.

[2] Andrew Cunningham and Bridie Andrews, "Introduction: Western Medicine as Contested Knowledge", in Cunningham and Andrews, *Western Medicine as Contested Knowledge,* 1–23.

downs, successes and failures, that required continued and continuing input from all concerned.

By focusing on this one small project of Khunde Hospital and by using a conceptual device of what I called "worlds" with the hospital as the site for analysis, I have argued that the practice of medicine needs to be placed and understood within multiple contexts and that all these mattered. (The worlds of Sir Edmund Hillary, the Sherpa of Khumbu, Western medicine and international aid were those that I identified as being important for the questions I was looking at.) Khunde Hospital was an integral part of these multiple worlds, each with their different aims and agendas and their many layers of relationships that bound people and place, and that separately and together influenced events and practices at the hospital. The device of worlds also allowed me to move away from a binary explanation of opposing medical systems or a monolithic sense of tradition versus modernity—which, nevertheless, at times it was. Whether by Sherpas, other Nepalese or outsiders, tradition was associated with backwardness and the village, and development with modernity and urbanisation. The hospital was a symbol of that modernity even if located in a remote village.

Each chapter in the book closes with the conclusions drawn. Here, I bring together the different parts of the study and consider a number of points that have been significant for Khunde Hospital, but also have a wider relevance for those today concerned with the design, implementation, ongoing management, monitoring and evaluation of health programmes. Finally, I will revisit the hospital as an area of research.

"Multiple"

For more than thirty years (between 1966 and 1998) the provision of health services at Khunde Hospital revolved around the intersections of Western medicine, different kinds of foreign aid, Sherpa beliefs and practices and Sherpa desires for modernisation in their mountain home. It involved multiple people, organisations and places in Nepal and overseas.

Although the spread of Western medicine and foreign aid were (and remain) linked because of Western medicine's role as the main paradigm of international medical aid projects and programmes, they were also separate globalising forces. Khunde Hospital was an institution that operated within a medical system that has its particular ideas and practices, institutions and practitioners and an institution that functioned within an aid process, also with its own ideas and practices, institutions and practitioners. At Khunde Hospital the worlds of Western medicine and aid met. In the 1960s many Sherpas had heard of "modern medicine" and some had even used it, but Hillary's successful efforts to build and provide ongoing assistance to a hospital in the remote Everest region introduced this type of medicine on a long-term basis and more widely within the area. Nevertheless, the hospital's subsequent experience demonstrated that even when services existed staff could not assume they would be used as anticipated or even used at all. This suggests that some rethinking is needed about widely held Western assumptions by those providing or promoting such medical services, whether or not in an aid context, that once people see the superiority of Western medical services they will use them and use them exclusively, and that imparting such knowledge through health education programmes will then inevitably lead people to adopt these ideas and practices. That such assumptions about health education remain problematic in "the West" also seems to be overlooked.

In many respects the opening of Khunde Hospital still presented a "first contact" situation for most Sherpas, although unlike much of South Asia the process in Nepal was not associated with colonialism. As elsewhere, Western medicine did not enter a vacuum. In Khumbu, the spirit-based beliefs and practices of Sherpas remained important and dynamic and continued to inform people's responses to the hospital in the 1990s as they had done in the 1960s. The coexistence of multiple healing systems is widely documented in Nepal and in the wider Himalayan region Western medical services, if available, continue to be regarded as an option.[3] In Khumbu, Sher-

[3] Nevertheless, even where a state today formally recognises and supports other healing systems, Western medicine occupies a dominant position in almost all nationally supported health systems in Asia (less so in Bhutan). In Khumbu, government medical services are biomedical, not Ayurvedic. For the situation in Bhutan, see McKay, *Their Footprints Remain*.

pas incorporated Western medicine and the hospital in a way that was neither antagonistic nor did it displace other avenues for dealing with sickness. Its being seen as "modern" did not translate into it being inherently "superior". People used the hospital pragmatically and selectively based on their perceptions of appropriateness and efficacy, with local staff playing a key role mediating between hospital and community. Patient numbers at the hospital increased, but attendance was, for the most part, on Sherpa terms with people using the services of Khunde Hospital as part of a plural strategy for dealing with ill health.

As part of Hillary's world, the hospital was the visible expression of a particular form of aid. From the 1950s an expanding number of international donors entered Nepal for various strategic and humanitarian reasons and the popular perception that Khunde Hospital was doing a good job in a difficult environment benefited Hillary's overall programme. Khunde Hospital, however, has always had multiple donors and each organisation or individual had their own expectations of the project. Despite a common goal of providing assistance to those deemed in need, differences also occurred. While Hillary thought in terms of providing overall services as a way to improve people's health, CIDA's expectations over time changed and became more targeted towards different groups of the area's inhabitants as thinking evolved about international health at a global level.

For staff at the hospital, multiple donors meant multiple sets of relationships that varied with each donor's degree of involvement. These ranged from a visitor leaving a donation at the hospital, to CIDA's indirect involvement through the Sir Edmund Hillary Foundation, to the overall responsibility of Hillary and the Trust in New Zealand for administering the hospital. A degree of donor competition and questions of "Whose project is Khunde Hospital?" arose. Both New Zealand and Canada acknowledged the important role of the other, but each saw Khunde Hospital as their project.[4] Further, those at the hospital most involved with the overseas

[4] Khunde Hospital became one of Hillary's flagship projects and other organisations associated with assisting Hillary's programme also liked to mention that they supported Khunde Hospital in some way.

donors (the volunteers) were themselves overseas donors. While the overseas staff who went to Khunde were people who liked an adventurous environment, unlike many aid workers in Nepal and other parts of the world those at Khunde Hospital were volunteers and received only small financial allowances. Like other donors, however, they had expectations about the project. The volunteers needed to believe in Hillary's work, especially that Khunde Hospital was a worthwhile project. Once they reached Khunde, they then expected to have the infrastructure support to provide health services, whether this was done through Hillary, the Himalayan Trust or the Sir Edmund Hillary Foundation. It was up to Hillary, therefore, to negotiate an agreement with the Nepalese government that allowed the hospital to be located there and it was Hillary's responsibility to provide the necessary funds for staff, medicines and other supplies.

Lastly, one of the key factors influencing the day-to-day provision of health services from Khunde Hospital has been the many and varied aspects to living and working at Khunde. Over the years, hospital staff, whether overseas or local, have had to cope with a multiplicity of both expected and unexpected issues relating not only to medicine and aid, but also to being part of the Sherpa world of Khumbu. Khunde Hospital was a small project with correspondingly few staff and while people could focus on some tasks all of the time, in practice it was not possible to devote the same amount of energy to each issue all of the time.

Similarly, staff could not both be in the hospital and out in the community, although the medical workload could be divided when both volunteers were doctors. Nevertheless, however important public or preventive health issues were, treating a patient with an acute serious condition came first and could occupy the attention of all the staff for many hours. Preventive health promotion was built upon this foundation of ongoing successful curative services. Ultimately, neglecting the sick person who had sought hospital treatment would have damaged the hospital's standing within the community and so weakened its objective of implementing the preventive health programmes and education that would improve the overall health status of the community.

Place

While mountain peoples around the world share many common features in their lives, "each association of a people, place, and their shared history", as geographer Barbara Brower wrote in her study of the pastoral system of the Sherpa of Khumbu in the Sagarmatha National Park, "makes for a singular situation, a unique interaction of man and landscape."[5] Khunde Hospital is firmly grounded, literally and metaphorically, in the spectacular and rugged, mainly Sherpa region close to the world's highest mountain. The love of climbing and the lure of Mt Everest first drew Hillary to the area. Together with the Sherpa, Mt Everest remains the principal draw card for the tourism industry that developed subsequently and both contribute to the ongoing high international profile that the area enjoys. They also explain why Hillary built a hospital at Khunde as an aid project in the first place and why it has been able to remain one. Despite the poverty and needs of people living in adjacent valleys, it is to the Everest area that visitors are drawn and aid is given.

Despite the area's fame, the challenges of providing health services in the region remain considerable. Although situated at high altitude with its associated problems of cold and hypoxia, much of the hospital's work was related to the low socio-economic status of most of the population, not with altitude. In common with many other areas around the world, and mountain areas in particular, the region's soil is deficient in iodine. Since iodised salt only became a viable option in recent years, the prevention and control of iodine deficiency disorders through the use of iodised oil injections was an important activity. General features such as the hospital's rural, isolated and mountainous location have influenced the size of the hospital, its building and maintenance issues. Khunde Hospital needed Hillary's commitment to exist and survive. The transportation of supplies remains expensive and until recently methods of communication slow. The rugged terrain and lack of roads make access an issue for patients and staff. Both have to walk, while seriously ill

[5] Brower, *Sherpa of Khumbu,* 8.

patients are carried. Air evacuation of patients is too expensive to be used other than sparingly in emergencies.[6]

The hospital became an integral part of the wider development of the region. Staff were involved with Hillary's other work and so the hospital was not only a place to go when sick. If the events post-1950 changed the face of Khumbu forever, they were still part of Fisher's tradition of change.[7] The hospital was both part of the change by bringing in a different medical system, a new institution and outside personnel, but was itself also affected by the transformation occurring around it. Rising prices, increasing education, changing population dynamics, employment issues and tourism have all had an impact on the hospital. Modernisation has occurred in Khumbu and Sherpas have fostered this process to encourage the economic development of the area, to improve their standard of living and to increase their links not only with other parts of Nepal, and Kathmandu in particular, but especially with other parts of the world where individually and collectively Sherpas often enjoy a high and favourable profile. How much these changes have influenced the internal world of Sherpas is more difficult to ascertain. Beliefs about life and death are core concepts in any society and the hospital's experiences with these events reveal a considerable continuity throughout the period.

Khumbu remains a Sherpa world. Sherpas continue to predominate, despite the presence today in the area of the Nepalese army, use of the national Nepali language and non-Sherpa officials in the district and national park's administration, police, bank, post office, schools and government health post. The mainly Sherpa population mostly speak Sherpa amongst themselves, intermarry, own the land and control the tourist industry. The visual impression of Khumbu is of a Sherpa cultural landscape with its lay and religious architecture, way of life and dress. Tourism has encouraged an intensification of Sherpa culture and Sherpas are "massively reinforced" for

[6] Tourists are advised to carry travel insurance that allows for this.

[7] Fisher, *Sherpas,* 64.

being Sherpa.[8] Khunde Hospital today provides health services in a confident Sherpa society.

Khunde Hospital and Sherpas, however, were also caught up in wider happenings occurring in Nepal. The area became a much more integrated part of the state. Of particular concern in the late 1990s was the political uncertainty. A Maoist uprising tempered nascent hopes of increasing democracy following the success of the "People's Movement" in 1990–91. In 1998 Maoist violence was still contained mostly within western Nepal and Khumbu continued to be largely untroubled. Tourists still visited and people carried on with their lives. Nevertheless, Khumbu was no longer the same *beyul,* the hidden valley that brought Sherpas to this sanctuary from troubles in their home in Tibet nearly five centuries earlier.

People and Relationships

This study has analysed the broader political, social, economic and cultural contexts in which Khunde Hospital operated and discussed the population-based health programmes that are aimed at improving the overall health status of a community. Throughout it has underlined the importance of people and relationships in all of these.

Underpinning Hillary's aid programme was his relationship with Sherpas which determined what he did, and even more significantly, how he conducted it. It strikingly emphasises the influence of the aid donor, although Hillary was a very unusual aid donor. The friendship and respect that existed between Hillary and Sherpas is the key to understanding Hillary's work in Nepal and the extraordinary bond that developed between this donor and the recipients of his assistance.[9]

[8] Fisher, *Sherpas,* 137. Fisher also refers to "Sherpaization" occurring where some non-Sherpa groups say they are Sherpa. This counters the widespread process in South Asia of "Sanskritisation" where people adopt high-caste Hindu behaviour. For a discussion in a Nepalese context, see Rex L. Jones, "Sanskritization in Eastern Nepal", *Ethnology* 15, no. 1, January 1976, 63–75.

[9] New Zealanders also identify with his modesty and down-to-earth, practical approach.

In the 1960s most aid was conceived and administered in a top-down approach, but Hillary was far ahead of most development thinking at this time and worked at a grassroots level with the people he was assisting to achieve their wants. He responded to their requests rather than assuming that he knew best, was involved practically with his building projects and was the principal fund-raiser. His ability to organise, gain sufficient funding (not always easily) and his celebrity status from climbing Everest gave him a degree of independence to pursue his small-scale private aid programme. Although the volunteer overseas staffing for Khunde Hospital was an affordable system for Hillary, more importantly it fitted with his view of aid and the relationship between the givers and the receivers. Hillary's language in the 1960s may well have resembled what Ortner and Lionel Caplan called "paternalism", but Hillary never saw Sherpas as weak or inferior.[10] The partnership on the mountains was translated into one in their home in Khumbu. Unlike many visitors to the area, Hillary did not idealise Sherpas. He respected them and their way of life and those who worked with him understood the importance of that relationship. He may at times have appeared saddened by some of the changes he saw, but he did not deny Sherpas their right to determine what they should or should not do.

Even if Hillary was restless and wanted to get on with things in his own life,[11] these characteristics were not carried over into his dealings with Sherpas. He was prepared to wait. In many respects, Sherpas in the late 1990s appeared in no hurry to change the way they had worked with Hillary since the early 1960s. After all, he had provided so much and had started at a time when little other support was available for Sherpas who were isolated socially, politically and geographically within Nepal. Having someone in a sponsorship role, such as Hillary or other visitors from around the world who have provided assistance, fitted Sherpa ideas and traditional patterns

[10] For example, see Ortner, *Life and Death on Mt. Everest,* 46, and Lionel Caplan, *Warrior Gentlemen* and "'Bravest of the Brave': Representations of 'The Gurkha' in British Military Writings", *Modern Asian Studies* 25, no. 3, July 1991, 590.

[11] See Hillary, *Nothing Venture, Nothing Win* and *View from the Summit.*

of behaviour. In this, Hillary gained merit for his work and those he helped did not have to reciprocate. Local people quickly adjusted to petitioning Hillary on his visits, while Hillary and those with him were very aware of the ritual being performed and what was expected. Hillary provided the most long-term and wide-ranging support for the Sherpa and to some extent in recent years had to propel those seeking his help along a more independent course hoping that his continuing presence would assist the transition. [12]

Hillary expected the volunteers at the hospital to show similar respect to their Sherpa patients. Over the years, hospital and community became used to each other in a relationship that was in practice a coexistence of difference. Medical historians examining the introduction of Western medicine have argued in terms of diffusion, resistance and more recently encounter. Transformation occurs in the process. In this study, however, I suggest that hospital and community could each acknowledge and incorporate aspects of the other's beliefs and practices when dealing with a person's sickness, but that they remained separate. Use and non-use of the hospital or Western medicine by Sherpas, or an accommodation with indigenous beliefs and practices on the part of the hospital staff, did not result in a fundamental weakening of either. Use of Western medicine was also not part of a debate about nationalism or identity; being Sherpa was not threatened by Western medicine.

Discussions about the introduction and spread of this medical system and its practice have often focused on the different conceptual basis of each medical system or on religion. They acknowledge but place less emphasis on issues affecting individual patients and their experience of sickness such as accessibility of services, staff or the physical aspects of the treatment. [13] Yet such concerns are cen-

[12] This view is based on discussion with Sir Edmund Hillary since 2002. He also had to convince members of the Himalayan Trust of the appropriateness and timing of this step. Sherpas seeking continuing assistance from outside supporters was not a sign of weakness as they also used such aid for other agendas such as improving their position within Nepal.

[13] In contrast to this trend, Bhattacharya, Harrison and Worboys' recent account of control measures against smallpox in colonial India examines economic, scientific and political issues and emphasises the unpleasantness

tral to what people do in sickness. Sick people and family members travelled hours and sometimes days to reach Khunde Hospital, but in so doing expected to find it open and with staff and medicines to treat their problem. This often contrasted with the situation in other areas of rural Nepal.[14] Patient registers show, not unexpectedly, that most patients came from the villages closest to the hospital. Yet, people's response to sickness was and remains an individual and family affair. Khunde Hospital in 1998 had provided a continuous service for more than thirty years, but the overseas and local staff at the hospital knew that even in Khunde village some people for a variety of reasons had never used the hospital.

Time

Considerations of time are implied within historical research. In this study, however, a number of aspects also need highlighting in their own right because of the influence they have had for the hospital and the importance time has in the structuring of aid.

When Hillary built the school at Khumjung in 1961, or even the hospital at Khunde in 1966, he had not envisaged the long-term involvement that developed in his aid to Sherpas. He also did not have the short-term project or programme focus of much international aid work. Hillary set out to remedy the lack of something, whether bridge, school or hospital and when the Nepalese government took over the schools, or the second hospital at Phaphlu, he continued to support them. He planned to provide help for as long as he was asked and was in a position to do so. If the Himalayan Trust's agreement with the Nepalese government, which provided the framework under which Hillary operated in Nepal from 1972, was renewable every three to five years, the Trust did not conceive of its administration of the hospital or the schools in these cycles. In contrast, while CIDA provided funds for Khunde Hospital that

---

of vaccination itself. Bhattacharya, Harrison and Worboys, *Fractured States*. Bhattacharya continues this approach in the second volume. Bhattacharya, *Expunging Variola*.

14 If no Western medical facility existed, then a discussion about the conceptual basis of the different medical systems is far less relevant.

in practice turned out to be on a long-term basis, each donation of money was based on a specific proposal for a limited period although Zeke O'Connor emphasised the ongoing aspect of the hospital's work throughout his dealings with CIDA.

Time has also been a factor helping to provide stability and continuity within the different organisations through the long-term involvement of many people. On a personal level, they grew older together. In 1998 Hillary was seventy-nine years old. Many people, both New Zealanders and Sherpas, were present from the early days and each over time became used to the ways of the other, whether they were similar or different. In some cases the association was intergenerational. These long-term and personal relationships were also often more influential than formal bureaucratic structures. The Canada–New Zealand connection worked through O'Connor's support of Hillary, but each had different ideas about how to conceptualise this relationship in terms of formal lines of responsibility between the different organisations. Such relationships may have fostered the development of a level of conservatism within the different organisations, but (and probably more importantly) they allowed the accumulation of knowledge and experience of working in Nepal. Long-term associations were also evident in the Trust's medical sub-committee and this continuity could counter the inherently stop-go situation implicit in the two-yearly cycle of volunteers.

Some of the time Hillary's ideas fitted closely with the shifting discourse of the wider world of international aid, but on other occasions they did not. Differences, tensions and fractures are revealed. In the early 1960s, the New Zealand government did not consider a hospital at Khunde an appropriate project for their aid. A decade later, they supported Hillary in the construction of a hospital at Phaphlu. Similarly, in the 1970s, Hillary's project at Khunde providing health services in a remote rural area and his method of working closely with the people he was helping, appealed to CIDA's aid programme. In the 1990s CIDA, while still supporting the project, criticised the hospital for its apparent lack of community participation.

Time is also an important and often inadequately acknowledged factor in the introduction and spread of both curative and preventive health services. Changes in people's use of Khunde Hospital's services have occurred, but more slowly and in more piecemeal a fashion than anticipated. Over the period considered, patient numbers rose and more people used the hospital for more conditions, but staff remained aware that people used the hospital pragmatically and selectively. The use of iodised oil injections and more recently the increasing use of iodised salt within the community has reduced the level of IDD significantly, although it continues to need monitoring. Yet this was a problem where a technical solution was available and eradication possible. A case study of the hospital's response to this major issue illustrates the complexities of medical practice and also the ebbs and flows of a policy over the years with changing personnel, new knowledge and different organisations involved.

It also took time (often a long time) for people to see any relevance in using some of the hospital's services. For example, although antenatal care was offered from the hospital's opening, only in the 1990s was attendance more widespread and even then the multiple visits that remain the norm in the volunteers' own countries were uncommon.

Of course, thirty years is not long and so the question remains that, if use of Western medical services continues to increase, will such coexistence still occur in another thirty years? There seems to be no reason to suggest that dialogue will not continue, but equally there seems to be no reason to suggest that this dialogue will not follow—as it has been doing—its own course as global and local forces negotiate their relationship among Sherpas in Khumbu.

Infrastructure

Randall Packard has noted how in the 1950s a number of post–Second World War international health programmes—especially the Malaria Eradication Programme—were unworkable because of inadequate rural health infrastructures.[15] While the initial attack phase was successful and malaria morbidity and mortality fell, the programme encountered problems in the consolidation or follow-

[15] Packard, "Visions of Health and Development", 102–3.

up phase. Smallpox remains the only eradication success and it did not require the existence of a local health infrastructure, but the belief remained that such success could be replicated easily for other diseases and "that health for all could be provided without health services for all".[16]

In Nepal, many of the reasons for lack of infrastructure in the 1950s continue to count despite continued attempts to improve the situation and develop rural health services. Issues of finance, staffing, supplies, terrain and poor communications are ongoing and compound the pressures placed by a rapidly increasing population; maintaining the status quo is difficult enough, let alone improve services. In the relatively stable demographic situation of the Everest area, however, Khunde Hospital provided a local infrastructure that was also used by others at times—by Hillary for his wider aid programme in the area, the local community for communication and more recently Government health personnel for storing vaccine in the hospital's fridge. International health policies may emphasise the role of basic village health services and community programmes, but Khunde Hospital has provided a pivotal role on which these other programmes relied—in the same way that Khunde Hospital itself has needed support to function as intended. The strategy in Khumbu to implement the current global polio eradication policy relies on community participation and cooperation between government and Khunde Hospital services, but the hospital provides the infrastructure support to coordinate the programme and ensures the vaccine remains cold in its fridge and organises its distribution.

Despite the close association between the hospital and the rise of scientific medicine in Europe and North America and an extensive literature, remarkably little is known about "the hospital" in non-Western societies and countries such as Nepal. A decade ago Roy Porter wrote that "Today, surgery and hospitals go hand in glove. . . . Without surgery, or at least without a battery of invasive treatments, the hospital would lose its unique place in the medi-

[16] Ibid., 103.

cal system."[17] Yet at Khunde the first doctor noted how Sherpas refused such surgery. The hospital did not offer a battery of invasive treatments. Its laboratory occupied a corner in the clinic and offered only a few basic tests, with blood samples rarely taken because Sherpa beliefs opposed this. We should not, therefore, make assumptions about hospitals that are based on an understanding of mostly Western institutions. Historical research in non-Western societies has followed other lines of enquiry. Hospitals are included in discussions about medicine as a "tool of empire" or about patient "resistance", but the hospital itself is not a central focus. When a general discussion includes a section about hospitals in the "Third" or "developing" world, it tends to be short and with a small number of references. Yet the point that Joel Howell emphasises is that hospitals in the twentieth century in other parts of the world present a very different and varying picture to that of Europe and North America. "A hospital always reflects the larger world."[18]

Undoubtedly there are similarities as well as differences between hospitals that reflect their location; and it is important to understand both and their influences. Many issues discussed in relation to Khunde Hospital, such as appropriate facilities and services for the small scattered population of the area, questions of distance and accessibility, or recruitment, training and retention of staff are pertinent to considering hospitals and services in any rural area, whether in the "First" or "Third World", or indeed anywhere in the world. On the other hand a hospital doctor in the "First World", except perhaps in treating some immigrant communities, is unlikely to have to worry about hospital ghosts. Hillary built Khunde Hospital to provide Western style health services and the overseas volunteers set out to implement them, but quickly found that the hospital had a mixed response from people who used the hospital for some conditions and not others or might decline to be admitted or travel at night. Throughout its history, Khunde Hospital patients as well as doctors have shaped and re-shaped patterns of health care delivery.

17 Roy Porter, ed., *The Cambridge Illustrated History of Medicine* (Cambridge: Cambridge University Press, 1996), 202.

18 Joel D. Howell, "Hospitals", in Cooter and Pickstone, *Medicine in the Twentieth Century*, 513.

From the outside it may be easy to dismiss spirit beliefs as "superstition", but from the perspective of being at Khunde and trying to practise medicine it quickly became apparent that people's beliefs underpinned their responses to sickness. Fear of a malevolent ghost is a very real concern for someone who believes in its power.

If we do revisit the hospital as an area of research, then it is also important to avoid "framing" the hospital or other health care facilities or services in non-Western societies as being a less "developed" version of what is to be found in the "First World". Throughout the time I spent living and working at Khunde Hospital and during subsequent research I observed, participated and gathered multiple pieces of evidence that cumulatively testified not only to the multiplicity of factors concerning health care delivery at Khunde Hospital that were not only a consequence of the place, but also of the relationships that were established and their influence on the hospital. What this study of Khunde Hospital makes clear is that there is no simple one-way diffusion between policy and practice. This history provides evidence to reveal the complex interactions that occur in Khunde Hospital's relationship with the local community and it also elucidates similarly complex interactions occurring between public (government) and private health care provisions of all types, between official and private aid and between national and international health agencies. The hospital in a non-Western society may be different, but to see it in terms of being less "developed" continues an oppositional approach to health issues that is as simplistic and unhelpful as it is arrogant and patronising.

Epilogue

We left Khunde in early October 1998. The monsoon had passed and the temperature was beginning to fall. In and around the village the grass had been cut, gathered and stored in the houses and in the fields people were digging up the year's potato crop. Another trekking season was underway and at the hospital a new volunteer couple settled in. Like volunteer couples before us, the handover period was not always an easy time; we sought to pass on knowledge and understanding and discuss ongoing projects, while the new couple, both doctors, brought in their own fresh outlook and particular interests that they wanted to develop during their time at Khunde. After final farewell cups of sweet milk tea and with khatas draped around our necks, we departed. As we walked up to the small pass and looked back on our home of the past two and a quarter years, we wondered if and when we would be back. Like Sherpas leaving to visit other parts of Nepal or overseas, we hung our khatas at the pass that would help ensure our safe return to Khunde. Then we walked on and down to Namche Bazar where we drank more cups of tea and said further farewells before descending steeply to the bridge over the Dudh Kosi. We had left Khumbu, were now in Pharak and on our way out.

This sequence of events and the powerful emotions contained within were all elements in the themes of continuity and change that have been an integral part of these narratives and analysis of Khunde Hospital. Embedded within the continuities was the constant presence of change. If the inhabitants of the area were used to the volunteers changing every couple or so years, then they as well as the supporting organisations in New Zealand and Canada also had had to get used to the particularities of each set of incumbents at the hospital. Three years later we did return to cover the hospital for six weeks while the then volunteers, Dr Carol and Ian Nicholson and their family, went away for their mid-term break. Mingma Temba and Gayse Nuru (our medical assistants) and Tsumje (our cook/cleaner) were still there but the hospital now had a qualified nurse, Nima Yangen.[1] Many of the patients remembered us from before; they and we filled in the gaps of who had done what in our respective families and resumed our relationships from where we both had left off. Nevertheless, it was winter and many of the area's residents had left for the warmer temperatures of lower altitudes, although other people still came up to the hospital from outside the area despite the seasonal cold weather. Perhaps the most unexpected example of one kind of continuity was a father who for five days had carried on his back his very sick 18-year old daughter to bring her through the mountains to Khunde. The last occasion that he had been to the hospital was when we were the volunteers from before and so he saw the same doctor. The people and the place were familiar to him.

Importantly, however, when we left Khunde in 1998 we knew that within a few years a very major change would take place at the hospital which would end its reliance on overseas medical staff. In 1997 the hospital's senior medical assistant set off from the mountains of his home in Khumbu to travel to the heat and low altitude of the Pacific where he had been accepted for medical training at the Fiji School of Medicine, joining part way through in a programme for experienced medical assistants. Despite a political coup in Fiji in 2000 that saw many of the overseas students return to the different island states of the region, the school remained open and at the end of the year Dr Kami Temba Sherpa graduated and returned to Nepal. Initially he worked at Patan Hospital in the Kathmandu area enabling him to gain a wide variety of clinical experience and fulfil the requirements for registration with the Nepal Medical Council.[2] Later, in October 2002, he flew to Lukla and began the walk

[1] Ang Lhamu, Mingma Temba's wife, shared the cooking with Tsumje.

[2] Patan Hospital began in 1954 as Shanta Bhawan Hospital, one of the initial projects of the Christian United Mission to Nepal (UMN), and is a joint venture between the UMN and the Government of Nepal.

up to Khumbu as the new doctor-in-charge of Khunde Hospital. His years away had seen him lose some of his high-altitude acclimatisation and as he walked up the steep hill into Namche Bazar he appreciated the struggles of those who normally live at low altitude. He also wondered how after years of "white medicine" the inhabitants of Khumbu would take to his "brown medicine".[3]

For Sir Edmund Hillary, members of the Himalayan Trust and the Sir Edmund Hillary Foundation it was the fulfilment of a dream.[4] Between them, they had funded Dr Kami Temba's training and supported him and his family while he was away. The small boy who began his education at the school built by Hillary in Thame was now returning to provide health services to the people of the area. After Kami Temba's departure for Fiji, Mingma Temba increasingly took over the administrative and management duties at Khunde Hospital while Gayse Nuru was introduced to the multiple tasks of being a medical assistant. For the next few years they provided, as Mingma Temba had done before with Kami Temba, the underlying continuity at Khunde. Overseas volunteer doctors continued to work at the hospital, but as time passed their role was increasingly seen, both in Nepal and overseas, to be a holding one and transitional. Decisions about future developments, such as implementing the recommendations of a CIDA review of the project carried out in 2000, were made in consultation with Dr Kami Temba or put to one side until his return to Khunde.[5] The Nicholsons were the last

3 Conversation with Dr Kami Temba, Khunde, June 2003. These terms were his.

4 The SEHF (although not CIDA) provided the finance for Kami Temba's medical training and has since funded further medical scholarships.

5 This review was prepared by an independent Kathmandu consultant, Rudra P. Devkota. Overall the report was favourable, but identified four themes for further action: the need to put more effort into preventive as opposed to curative medicine; the need for the project to become more independent of finance from the SEHF and the Trust; the need for a defined organisation chart, business plan, budget and review/upgrade of administrative skills at the hospital; and the need for more community input into fund-raising, planning and selection of medical goals. Minutes of Meeting of Himalayan Trust (NZ) Medical Advisory Group, 6 October 2001, Auckland [Heydon papers].

of the "regular" volunteers and were followed by a series of mainly Canadian volunteer doctors working for a few months at a time at the hospital. These were organised by former Khunde Hospital volunteer, Dr Robert (Bob) Zimmerman (1995–96) who had joined the Board of Directors of the SEHF and has recently become its Senior Medical Officer.

With the rising number of patients at the hospital the question of staffing levels was an important concern. For much of the 1980s and 1990s the hospital had two doctors and the Trust and the SEHF intended this to be the situation when Dr Kami Temba took control. In 2000 a New Zealand work party converted one of the hospital buildings to provide accommodation for a second doctor.[6] Issues of the area's remoteness, medical isolation and the need to ensure time-off were also important considerations. While the longest the volunteers stayed was around two years, the Trust and the SEHF saw Dr Kami Temba's appointment as a long-term arrangement.

Initially overseas volunteers filled the second (and junior) doctor position, but increasing efforts were made to appoint another doctor from Nepal. Throughout the period since 1998, Ang Rita has remained the senior member of staff for the Trust in Nepal and he and the office in Kathmandu have had, and will continue to have, a vital role in this recruitment.[7] From July 2005 the hospital has obtained its medical staff from within the country. Initially these came from other parts of Nepal, but when Dr Sonam Zangbu joined the staff in January 2007 Khunde Hospital had two Sherpa doctors. The situation, however, remains unstable because, like other rural institutions around the world, Khunde Hospital faces the challenges of not only appointing but also retaining staff for more than a few months at a time. This uncertainty places considerable burdens on the existing staff. A key area of concern at Khunde, as the 2006/07

[6] The addition of plumbing led to the introduction of a new item of modernisation for the hospital—the installation of a washing machine.

[7] Elizabeth Hawley continues to live in the upstairs flat, still collects the widely acknowledged mountaineering data from the expeditions and remains as New Zealand's Honorary Consul in Nepal.

annual report notes, has been the difficulty of planning and implementing continuing medical education for Dr Kami Temba.[8]

The 2006/07 annual report also identifies that the hospital's two main objectives continue to be to provide "prompt and quality" medical care to all patients and to continue existing public health and health promotion programmes. From a total of 8,597 outpatients at the hospital in 1998/99, numbers fell to 7,281 the following year during an unsettled period at the hospital.[9] Since then outpatient numbers have risen; in 2006/07 the total was 8,013.[10] The inpatient total of 117 has remained at much the same level as it has since the hospital opened.

The number of patients seen by the village health workers over the past decade has fluctuated, being influenced by the particular circumstances of each clinic and health worker. The most significant development has been the recent availability and introduction of trained health workers to the clinics at Phortse (2005), Thame (2006) and Monjo (2007). As discussed earlier in the book, this has been a long-term goal, but after many years is now being realised. The aim for these new staff, who are all female, is to be "more proactive rather than reactive".[11] They act as health educators in their communities and give classes on "public/environmental health" in the schools, as well as treating patients who come to see them. As has been an important theme throughout the hospital's history, Dr Kami Temba stresses the continuing need to support these workers with medical supplies, educational materials, refresher training and medical visits.

While fluctuations in patient numbers at Khunde Hospital or the village clinics may indicate problems or popularity, patient totals do not indicate the reach or effectiveness of a particular programme. Shortly after his arrival, Dr Kami Temba initiated a health census of the whole of Khumbu and Pharak that involved staff carrying out door-to-door interviews at every residence. Given the terrain

[8] Kunde Hospital and Village Health Clinics Annual Report – 2006/2007.

[9] Kunde Hospital Annual Report, August 2001.

[10] Appendix 3; Kunde Hospital and Village Health Clinics Report, 2006/2007.

[11] Kunde Hospital and Village Health Clinics Annual Report, 2006/2007.

and that it was done in the staff's "spare time", the undertaking was both a considerable achievement and commitment. [12] Gathering data for the period 1998/2002, the study showed a high contraceptive prevalence rate (the proportion of married women of reproductive age, usually 15 to 49 years, who use contraception) at 67.0 per cent compared with 38.8 per cent for the Solukhumbu district as a whole and 40.0 per cent for Nepal. Spacing methods, particularly the use of Depo Provera, were more popular than the permanent methods employed in most of Nepal. [13] The neonatal mortality (43.8 per 1,000 births) rate remains high, although lower than in other parts of Nepal (49.9 in 1996). Unfortunately, information about the cohort of under-five children is incomplete and the report's figure of 55.5 per 1,000 births compared with 118 for Nepal as a whole is very likely to be an under-representation. [14] The maternal mortality rate in the area was also lower than the national rate at 292 per 100,000 births compared with 539, but with just two maternal deaths reported in the area over the period surveyed the sample was too small to have much confidence in this rate. Complete immunisation status was achieved by 78.2 per cent of infants with a further 9.6 per cent having some coverage, but although this

[12] Assistance was given by the Canadian volunteers at the hospital at the time, Drs Katie Morgenstern and Simon Pulfrey, and further technical support was provided in New Zealand with analysis of the data. These comments are drawn from the following report "Khumbu and Pharak Demographic and Health Survey: 2003". Report by Isla Dobson, Summer Studentship, Christchurch School of Medicine and Health Sciences, University of Otago, 20 May 2006 [Heydon papers]. She was supervised by Dr Lynley Cook and Professor David Murdoch, former Khunde Hospital volunteers. That there were some technical flaws to the survey does not undermine these comments and findings and its overall value.

[13] Depo Provera is injected every three months.

[14] I am grateful to Dr Lynley Cook for her comments and for a copy of the report. The two commonest causes of death among the under-fives in countries such as Nepal are acute respiratory infection and diarrhoea. The annual report for 2006/2007 comments on the significant decline in cases of diarrhoea over the previous decade at the hospital and the village clinics and attributes this to community education programmes, a rising standard of living in the area and access to safe water supplies. An Eco Himal project installed a piped water supply in Namche Bazar in 2000.

total is relatively high it is low compared with the given rates for Nepal as a whole—a country where gathering statistics, however, remains a challenging task.

The survey is important for a number of reasons. It provides information for the hospital staff about their services, about what has been achieved and about what needs doing. For example, staff were able to follow-up infants who had not been immunised. The survey also provides data for reports to donors, although not surprisingly it also raises questions and adds to speculation generally about the collection and reliability of statistics in Nepal. At a wider level, the survey results reinforce the point that even if there is a policy, committed workers, supplies and so forth (as has been the case with Khunde Hospital) they do not necessarily translate into population compliance and complete coverage. As has been discussed in this book, other factors have also influenced the uptake of services.

Throughout the decade since 1998 Khunde Hospital has continued to function within a plural and changing medical environment. Further links developed with the government's health clinics which consisted of a new clinic at Pangboche, the longstanding one at Namche and one at Choplung in Pharak, and the Trust also agreed to the government request to provide a financial subsidy to government health workers in view of their remote location. [15] Pangboche clinic, however, has been closed since the end of 2004. Khunde Hospital continues to receive its immunisation supplies from the government and is the designated immunisation centre for Khumbu (Namche and Khumjung VDCs), while Choplung provides these services in the upper part of Pharak. A major development in the region has been the building and opening in late 2005 of a Swiss-funded hospital at Lukla. [16] Lukla is situated on the periphery of Khunde Hospital's catchment area and, as occurred earlier when Phaphlu Hospital opened in the 1970s and took over the provision of services in the Solu area, the new facility has seen Khunde Hospital revert to concentrating on upper Pharak and Khumbu. The

[15] The clinic at Pangboche was built with Trust support and was part of the government plan to have one government health clinic in each VDC area.

[16] Lukla community clinic, which was originally established by a French group and then supported by the Trust, closed.

hospital at Lukla, for example, now provides immunisation services for lower Pharak. Nevertheless, despite a reduction in population coverage, the total number of patients attending Khunde has not declined.

Increased interest in Western countries with other medical systems and a fascination with anything Tibetan has fostered a different kind of NGO health initiative in Khumbu. [17] The Sacred Land project was founded by and is under the chairmanship of the Tengboche Rinpoche and aims both to provide "traditional healthcare" for the community but also cater for the large number of visitors to the area. [18] It supports a clinic in Namche (since 2005 called the Namche Healing Centre) which is staffed by an amchi. The clinic uses medicines brought in from India, but the project has also established medical herb gardens and begun to make medicines.

Visitors to the area also remain important for Khunde Hospital, whether they come to look or as patients because they are sick. Donations of money, drugs and equipment continue to be received and major projects such as the construction of a new long stay ward and patients kitchen (2005) and patients waiting room (2006) were funded from visitor donations. The latter project was also made possible through the donation of land in front of the hospital. [19] A new health clinic at Thame is also built on locally donated land, thus enabling the previous clinic which was located on the school complex to be handed over to the school to help with space in its expansion to a middle school.

Despite their continued significant support to the hospital, the number of visitors to the area and trekker patients at the hospital fell sharply after the escalation of Maoist activities throughout the country in 2001, the declaration of a state of emergency and the

[17] In Nepal, for political and registration reasons the ancient Himalayan origins of "amchi medicine" are emphasised. Amchi Tenzin Bista and Amchi Gyatso Bista, *Himalayan Doctors and Healing Herbs: The Amchi Tradition and Medicinal Plants of Mustang* (Kathmandu: Mera Publications for Lo-Kunphen Mensikhang [2005].

[18] http://www.sacredland.net/medintro.htm (13 December 2007).

[19] Kunde Hospital Annual Report, 2004/2005.

resulting uncertain political situation.[20] Although the Everest area was less affected than other parts of the country, and indeed visitors to Nepal were encouraged to come to the region instead of going elsewhere, tourism throughout the country slumped. For the hospital, the relentless pressure from the rising number of visitors in the 1990s came to a sudden but temporary halt. Fewer visitors also had a considerable impact on the local economy and employment opportunities. The highest number of visitors to the Sagarmatha National Park was recorded in 2000 with 25,291, but in 2002 the total fell to 13,786.[21] Numbers increased in 2003 with the fiftieth anniversary Everest celebrations and rose to 19,300. Despite the continuing political uncertainties, visitors continued to come to the area with a total in 2006 of 20,036. The number of trekker patients at Khunde Hospital has also risen, but in 2006/07 at 91 (which is just over 1 per cent of the total number of outpatients) both the total and the proportion is less than the 265 or 3.7 per cent in 1996.[22]

Although Khunde Hospital's medical services were not affected by Nepal's political troubles, these did impact on the hospital in a variety of ways and serve as a reminder of how the hospital is embedded in Nepal, despite its overseas connections. The loss of its telephone and email connection, after destruction of network infrastructure in the lower hill region, badly affected communication and restored the hospital's isolation both within the country and in its relations with people and organisations outside Nepal. Both Nepalese army and Maoist personnel regularly stopped the hospital's mail runner, although he was always allowed to continue. The carriage of supplies for the hospital also became more irregular. With fewer visitors, the number of planes flying into the area decreased and the Jiri area, where the road ended and where porters left to walk to the Everest area, was very unsettled.

While the 2003 survey provided information for health services it also provided useful demographic data, particularly as it divided

[20] Nepal had already made world headlines with the killing of many members of the royal family during the evening of 1 June 2001.

[21] See Appendix 5.

[22] Kunde Hospital Annual Report, 2006/2007; Kunde Hospital and Village Clinics Annual Report 1996.

household occupants on the basis of their residency about which very few statistics are available.[23] The total population of Khumbu and Pharak was 7005. Residents (82.1 per cent) (defined as having their primary residence in Khumbu–Pharak, were registered with the VDC and whose family owned land in the area) are almost exclusively of Sherpa or Tibetan ethnicity. The ethnicity of non-residents was mixed, but the significant size of this group confirms that it has been rising throughout the period the hospital has been open, whether through coming into the area as government employees or seeking other kinds of employment as tourism developed.[24] This increase in the number of other groups in the community is reflected in the rise in the number of non-Sherpa patients at the hospital. The impact on the village clinics varies. In Khumbu, Namche Bazar has the highest proportion of non-Sherpa inhabitants.

Temporary or permanent migration is a significant factor in the overall population in Khumbu remaining stable. Of the resident population, the most common reason for both male and female residents being in the area for less than six months each year was to attend an educational establishment in Kathmandu. In view of the high costs involved, this practice occurs especially among more affluent families although others may have the cost paid by overseas sponsors.[25] The next most common reason was work either in Kathmandu or abroad. The survey, however, could not quantify the number of Sherpas who had left the region.

Another way in which demographic patterns revealed by the survey are reflected in the patient population at Khunde Hospital relate to the continuing situation of there being more male than female attendance. This was a concern raised in the 2000 CIDA review re-

[23] Dobson, "Khumbu and Pharak Demographic and Health Survey 2003", 2006.

[24] Ivan Pawson's survey had shown that this was already well under way by 1982 with a rise in other Nepalese groups from 3 per cent of the total population in 1970 to 10.9 per cent. Pawson, Stanford and Adams, "Effects of Modernization on the Khumbu Region of Nepal".

[25] Some of the children leave at a very young age. The changing nature of Sherpa migration and its impact on Sherpa society and Khumbu needs further investigation both at a macro and a micro level.

port, particularly as international aid and development policies were trying to increase the percentage of women using health services.[26] This, of course, underlines the importance of having detailed local knowledge of specific situations. Of the resident population, females outnumbered males but in the non-resident population, males outnumbered females especially among those who had been in the area less than six months (70.5 per cent). A large number of those working in the area whether as porters, or in the army or other government workers are male.

With the appointment of Dr Kami Temba Sherpa and the decline and ending of overseas medical volunteers running the hospital, the role of the overseas organisations funding and supporting the hospital has changed and a shift in emphasis has occurred further towards the Nepalese base of its operations. The Kathmandu office became increasingly important both in implementing Hillary's programme but also because of its liaison role with different Nepalese government departments and organisations. On 9 April 2002, at a meeting in Kathmandu, Hillary handed over responsibility for the running of the major part of the Himalayan Trust's work in Nepal to the Himalayan Trust Advisory Committee under the chairmanship of Ang Rita. Finance was assured for at least ten years. Although Hillary's increasing age and the inability to continue his practical involvement was a major reason for the increasing handover to the Nepalese organisation, Hillary for many years had intended to do this. While he hoped to influence the transition, his intention was not to control, and he believed that if those in Nepal subsequently decided to do things differently then so be it.[27]

While it is beyond the scope of this book to discuss in detail the wider activities and developments of the Trust, the shifting of responsibility for running Hillary's Nepal programme to Nepal and the establishment of a Council as the Trust's working group in New Zealand has thus seen a decline in New Zealand links and involve-

26 In Western countries female attendance rates are higher than those for males.

27 Discussions with Sir Edmund Hillary since 2002. Hillary made his last visit to Khumbu briefly by helicopter during his regular annual visit to Nepal at the end of April 2006.

ment with the hospital.[28] Even if agreeing with this direction, in practice the "letting-go" of something that has been an important part of many people's lives is not easy. In Canada, the Sir Edmund Hillary Foundation continues with its considerable financial support. As part of its planning for the future, the SEHF'S Board of Directors in 2007 appointed Zeke O'Connor as Founder and Executive Director and unanimously elected Karen O'Connor to succeed her father as President for a three-year term.[29] As the Trust remains the Foundation's implementing partner in Nepal, less change has occurred for the SEHF and the way it has operated in relation to Khunde Hospital. With the New Zealand organisation having handed over to the Nepal Himalayan Trust organisation, in practice the Canadian links may now become more visible.

Other changes in relationships (referred to as "linkages" in the current language of aid project proposals and reports) have also occurred for the Trust and these have varying consequences for the hospital situated as it is further down the organisational structure. In 2007 the New Zealand Government, through its official aid agency NZAID, carried out its first review of the hospital.[30] During the fanfare surrounding the fiftieth anniversary Everest celebrations in 2003, the government acknowledged publicly Hillary's work in Nepal and considerably increased its financial support to NZ$290,000 per annum, requesting that it be used to support health and education and with details to be discussed with NZAID.[31] From the

[28] The year 2006 was the fortieth anniversary of the hospital's establishment and in mid-April many former volunteers (not only from New Zealand) gathered in Kathmandu for a reunion and then visited Khumbu and the hospital.

[29] I am grateful to Zeke and Karen O'Connor for this information.

[30] The semi-autonomous NZAID was established in 2002 with its main focus on poverty reduction in the Pacific. The review of the Trust's work was described as "a low key 'stock-take'". Mike Bird, "Report on the Review of The Annual Funding Arrangement for Support of the Projects of the Himalayan Trust in SoluKhumbu, Nepal. New Zealand NGO Strategic Relationships Programme", October 2007 [Heydon papers].

[31] Letter from Helen Clark, Prime Minister to Hillary, Chairman, Himalayan Trust, undated but in reply to Hillary's letter of 19 June thanking her for the news of the Government's pledge [Heydon papers].

first meeting of NZAID with the Himalayan Trust Council at Hillary's home on 29 September 2003, it was also clear that a greater degree of monitoring would be part of the process. [32] The review included Khunde Hospital. Similarly, the Social Welfare Council, with whom the Trust now has its Agreement in Nepal, carried out an "Observation Report" in 2007 visiting for the first time Khunde Hospital, Khumjung High School and the tree nurseries in the Sagarmatha National Park. [33] The New Zealand and Nepalese reports are both favourable but also contain ideas or proposals for consideration or adoption. [34] Both see Khunde Hospital as continuing to be an integral part of the Trust's ongoing work and both anticipate continuing involvement.

Despite its very strong links with overseas people and organisations, Khunde Hospital is located in Nepal and has had to (and will continue to have to) operate in its Nepalese environment. It is appropriate, therefore, to conclude by quoting comments on the hospital and the conclusion from the Social Welfare Council's "Observation Report" about the Trust's work that provides a worthy, and perhaps surprising, tribute to this small hospital in the mountains of Nepal:

> Situated at an elevation of 13500 ft, Khunde hospital is the only hospital of Nepal, completely operated by an international donor agency providing modern facilities to people of high altitude. This hospital was established in very remote Khunde village when one had never imagined

32 Notes from Himalayan Trust Council meeting, 29 September 2003 [Heydon papers].

33 "Observation Report of Khumjung High School, in Khumjung V.D.C., Khunde Hospital in Khunde V.D.C. and Nurseries Operated by Himalayan Trust in Solukhumbu District 2064", presented by: Mrs Subhadra Dahal, Mr Kiran Bhakta Shrestha and Mr Shiva Kumar Basnet, Social Welfare Council [Heydon papers]. In the Nepali calendar the year 2007 is 2064. The Social Welfare Council monitors and coordinates the activities of local and international NGOs in Nepal.

34 A verbal report only was presented to the Himalayan Trust Council meeting on 2 November 2007. Personal communication Dr John Heydon, member, Himalayan Trust Council. For an article featuring the Himalayan Trust and its work, see NZAID, "The Heights of Development", *Currents* 6, 2007, 8–13.

> a hospital in any area of the entire Solukhumbu district. It has won heart of local residents by providing service to place neglected by Nepal government and least imagined by any one. . . . All sectors admire the operation of free services and drugs provided by Himalayan Trust through its hospital and all health posts, despite the prevalent system of selling expensive drugs in urban areas and government and non-government institutions charging high fees for their services.
>
> The decades of work done in the remote area like Solukhumbu in the field of health and education is highly commendable. The dedication and hard work of all staff members of the organization to achieve this level is a matter of pride for all. Although we have very recently entered into agreement with this organization, looking at the past, present and it's future strategies, we should encourage such organization, while regularly observing and evaluating as per the provision of the agreement. Social workers living and enjoying the facilities of cities like Kathmandu can also learn and implement the lessons learnt in the Solukhumbu region.

★ ★ ★

Since writing this Epilogue a new chapter has begun for Khunde Hospital. On 11 January 2008 Sir Edmund Hillary died in hospital in Auckland. News flashed around the world and tributes poured in to honour the passing of one of the great international figures of his time. Hailing the first ascent of the world's highest mountain and more particularly what Hillary had done with his fame and how, eulogies once again made the partnership between Hillary and Sherpas headline news. Even if in later years his involvement had been less, he had continued to watch over the work carried out under his name and he had entrusted both the running and the decision-making to Sherpas and the organisation in Nepal.

In the Introduction I wrote how in 2003 those involved with Khunde Hospital were an integral part of the fiftieth anniversary celebrations in Kathmandu for the first ascent of Mt Everest. At Hillary's state funeral in Auckland on 22 January 2008 the scene was reenacted.[35] Among the five Sherpas offering and placing khatas on

[35] A state funeral is a rare occasion in New Zealand and was a public acknowledgement of Hillary's stature within the country.

the coffin was Dr Kami Temba.[36] In the preceding days of extensive press, internet and television coverage, his name, rather than reference to the generic "Sherpas", and that of Khunde Hospital were heard or read about in homes around New Zealand as one of the flagships for Hillary's work.

In the days following Hillary's death, many references were made to continuing his work in Nepal. Part of his greatness, however, is not just what he did. It is also about how he did it. In this book I have highlighted the contrast between Hillary's approach as an aid donor and the ongoing paternalism, even imperialism, within much of the international aid process. Tributes to Hillary acknowledge how he listened to Sherpas and worked with them—a partnership that operated in practice as well as theory. With his accustomed modesty, he did not assume that he knew best and he did not presume to tell people what he thought they needed. Will those who pledge to continue his legacy also honour his legacy and, as Hillary did, respect the wishes of those they are helping? That will be the greatest tribute that could be paid to Hillary; but it would also be a challenge because it requires a fundamental change in attitude throughout the world of international aid and development.

[36] With him were Ang Rita, Chief Administrative of the Himalayan Trust in Nepal, who spoke at the funeral; Ang Rita, son of Hillary's sirdar and great friend Mingma Tsering; Ang Thukten, a businessman but better known in the Hillary story as Philip—the baby born as his mother walked to Kathmandu in 1961 to meet the Queen of England; and Phurba, widow of Mingma Norbu.

Appendix 1

Overseas Volunteers at Khunde Hospital

McKinnon, John* 1966–68
McKinnon, Diane

Evans, Richard* 1968–69
Evans, Lesley

Lang, Selwyn* 1969–71
Lang, Ann*

Strang, Lindsay* 1971–73
Strang, Genevieve

Silvester, Paul* 1973–75
Silvester, Glen

Riley, Rob* 1975–77
Riley, Leigh

Jerram, Jim* 1977–79
Jerram, Hilary

Reekie, John* 1979–81
Reekie, Sue

Dawson, Penny*† 1981–83
Uhrig, Jamie*†

Gilchrist, Wendy*† 1985–87
Kokernot, Bruce*†

Maclaurin, Simon* 1987–89
Wood, Marianne*

Hagen, Catherine*† 1989–91
Schokking, Ian*†

Cook, Lynley* 1991–93
Murdoch, David*

Bush, Diane 1993–95
Harding, Elizabeth*

Macdonald, Sally*† 1995–96
Zimmerman, Robert*†

Heydon, John* 1996–98
Heydon, Susan

Litch, Jim*† 1998–2000
Bishop, Rachel*†

Buswell, Keith* 1983–85
Kroef, Elly*

Nicholson, Ian	2000–02
Nicholson, Carol*	

* Doctor

† Appointed by the Sir Edmund Hillary Foundation

Note: This list does not include volunteers who worked at the hospital for a few weeks or months to cover various gaps or holidays or those who assisted during the transition to the hospital being staffed from within Nepal.

Appendix 2

Nepalese Staff at Khunde Hospital

Nima Yangen	1966–68	Dawa Phuti	1978–79
Ang Pemma	1966–69	Yangen	1979–80
Purba Gyalgen	1967	Mingma Temba	1979–
Mingma Norbu	1969–70	Tsumje	1991–
Kanchi	1969–?71	Pemba Doma	1992
Pemba	1969–70	Lhakpa Doma	1996–97
Ang Pasang	1970–79	Dr Nawang Karsang	1996–97
Nima Yangin	1971–72	Gayse Nuru	1997–
Da Yangi	1972–73	Ang Lhamu	1998–
Pemba Tenzing	1973–75	Nima Yangen	1999–2003
Nima, Mokhu	1975	Dr Jaggart Chettri	2000
Meyer and Urkien		Kanti	2001–02
Nima Wangchu	1975–76	Nima Yangi	2004–
Doma Leh	1976–79; 1980–91	Dr Sonam Zangbu	2007
Kami Temba	1977–78; 1979–97; and	Dr Kami Temba	2002–

Source: Compiled from annual reports and files held at Khunde Hospital, with further assistance from Mingma Temba. (Precise dates are not available. Although the year is given, some staff stayed for much shorter periods of time.)

Appendix 3

Outpatients at Khunde Hospital

A. 1967–97

1967	1,924	1983	2,868
1968	1,536	1984	3,828
1969	1,314	1985	4,234
1970	incomplete	1986	4,137
1971	1,681	1987	5,172
1972	2,125	1988	4,688
1973	incomplete,	1989	5,375
1974	due to	1990	6,066
1975	missing register	1991	5,795
1976	4,263	1992	5,572
1977	4,374	1993	5,702
1978	3,144	1994	6,176
1979	3,093	1995	7,592
1980	2,722	1996	7,224
1981	3,108	1997	7,294
1982	3,015		

Source: Khunde Hospital outpatient registers. (These totals refer to the year January to December.)

B. 1998/99–2006/07

1998/99	8,597
1999/2000	7,281
2000/01	7,737
2001/02	7,993

2002/03	8,180
2003/04	8,990
2004/05	8,703*
2005/06	8,588*
2006/07	8,013

Source: Khunde Hospital annual reports. (These totals are for split years – from 2000/01 referring to the fiscal year from 1 July to 30 June. *These figures are taken from the 'patient distribution' totals minus inpatients.)

Appendix 4

Population of Khumbu

1970	2,761	(Lang and Lang, "The Kunde Hospital and a Demographic Survey", 2)
1971	2,578	(CBS, Population Census 1971)
1982	3,108	(Pawson, Standford and Adams, "Effects of Modernization on the Khumbu Region of Nepal", 75)
1991	3,456	(Digital Himalaya, Census of Nepal 2001, http://www.digitalhimalaya.com/collections/nepalcensus/)
2001	3,335	(Digital Himalaya, Census of Nepal 2001, http://www.digitalhimalaya.com/collections/nepalcensus/)

Appendix 5

Visitors to Khumbu/Sagarmatha National Park

1964	20	1990/91	10,343
★★★★★		1991/92	10,110
1971/72	1,406	1992/93	12,124
★★★★★		1993/94	12,824
1973/74	3,503	1994/95	14,151
1974/75	4,254	1995/96	15,971
★★★★★		1996/97	17,412
1979/80	4,348	1997/98	18,511
1980/81	5,310	★★★★★	
1981/82	4,117	1998	20,014
1982/83	5,667	1999	24,561
1983/84	5,103	2000	25,291
1984/85	5,840	2001	21,570
1985/86	6,906	2002	13,786
1986/87	9,117	2003	19,300
1987/88	8,430	2004	21,396
1988/89	7,963	2005	19,063
1989/90	7,954	2006	20,036

Sources: Stevens, *Claiming the High Ground*, 362 (to 1980/81); SNP, Jorsalle (1981/82 to 1996/97) in SPCC Annual Progress Report for the fiscal year 1997–98; SNP, Jorsalle (1997/98). (Split years are from 1 July to 30 June.) Visitor totals for 1998–2000 (January to December) are from SNP, Jorsalle and 2001–06 (January to December) are from "Visitor surveys and monitoring of visitor flows in Sagarmatha National Park: Feasibility study and preliminary design", draft 22 May 2007, www.hkkhpartnership.org

Glossary

acclimatisation	physiological process by which the body adjusts to a new environment; in this study, high altitude and a reduced level of oxygen
amchi	practitioner of Tibetan medicine
beyul	sacred, hidden valley
Bhot	Nepali term for Tibet. Other terms are *Bhote* and *Bhotia* or *Bhotiya*
chamba	mild cold/cough/headache type of illness
chang	locally brewed beer, usually now made in Khumbu from rice
chorten	Buddhist monument often containing sacred relics
cretinism	a spectrum of defects caused by congenital iodine deficiency
Dumje	important community Buddhist festival
endemic	a disease present in a geographical area or population at a relatively high rate compared with other areas or populations
episiotomy	surgical incision to prevent traumatic tearing of the perineum during childbirth
goitre	enlargement of the thyroid gland in the neck, usually due to iodine deficiency
gompa	temple or monastery
guthi	form of tax-free land tenure used for endowment of a religious institution or hospital
Helicobacter pylori	bacterium implicated in the cause of duodenal and gastric ulcers
hrindi	ghosts
hypoxia	reduced oxygen

hypothyroidism	deficiency of thyroid activity
jhindak	sponsor or patron/protector
khata	felicitation scarf
lama	"high" monk; religious teacher
lha	god
lhawa	shaman, spirit medium
lhungtar	luck; spiritual protection
Losar	Tibetan/Sherpa new year
lu	serpent spirit
mani	prayer; sacred stones
Mani Rimdu	important Buddhist festival
menkhang	"medicine house", hospital
mindung	"junior" lhawa
mortality rate	number of deaths in a particular population at a given time
	under-five (child): deaths within the first five years after birth per 1,000 live births
	infant: deaths under one year per 1,000 live births
	maternal: maternal deaths related to child-bearing per 1,000 live births
	neonatal: deaths during the first 28 completed days of life per 1,000 live births
	perinatal: stillbirths plus deaths in the first week per 1,000 total births
nerpa	malignant spirit of deceased person
panchayat	council of five, one of the elected bodies set up at different levels under the 1962 constitution; also refers to the political system in Nepal between 1962 and 1990
pang	a type of depression that mainly affects women, particularly after childbirth
phangni	summer festival
pem	"witch" spirit; unconscious projection of negativity

prevalence	number of cases of a disease present in a particular population at a given time. (Note: "incidence" refers to the number of new cases) contraceptive prevalence rate: the proportion of married women of reproductive age (usually 15 to 49 years) in a given population who use contraception
puja	worship
Rana	family who ruled Nepal from 1846 to 1951
rilbu	long-life pills
rinpoche	"precious"; term of address and reference for a reincarnate lama
Sagarmatha	Nepali name for Mt Everest
sahib	boss or master
Sharwa	Sherpa, meaning "easterner" and derived from *sha*—east and *wa* or *pa*—people
sirdar	foreman of an expedition
tawa	monk
thip	spiritual pollution
torma	offering cake
yul	earth, soil, place. *Khumbu yul lha*—the god of Khumbu

Bibliography

PRIMARY SOURCES

1. Archives in Nepal, New Zealand, Canada, India and England

Nepal

Archives held at Khunde Hospital [KH]:

Annual Reports, 1967–1983
Annual Reports, 1983–
Boxes of assorted files and loose papers
Dear Successor
Forestry
Health Workers
Hospital Advisory Committee Book
Kunde Hospital Handbook
Kunde Hospital Handbook, 2 vols, revised February 1985
Kunde Hospital Village Health Worker Manual, 1980
Inpatient Registers
Minutes HAC
Outpatient Registers
Various files of correspondence (incomplete)
Teas, Jane. "Some Epidemiological Considerations of Children Under Fifteen Treated by the Staff of the Kunde Hospital, Nepal, 1966–1972". Department of Local Development/UNICEF, Research-cum-Action Project, Paper no. 1, Kathmandu, Nepal, 1973.
Wood, Dr Marianne. "1989 Survey of Khumbu Region of Nepal".

Archives held at the Himalayan Trust, Dilli Bazar, Kathmandu [HTK]:

Trust Agreements with HMG

New Zealand

Archives held at New Zealand/Te Rua Mahara o te Kawanatanga, Head Office, Wellington [ANZ]:

a. Department of External Affairs [EA]
W2824 Economic and Technical Assistance to individual countries: Nepal—Sir Edmund Hillary's Himalayan Projects, 118/13/13/14 Part 1

b. Ministry of Foreign Affairs and Trade [ABHS]
Series 950:
Nepal General 118/13/13/1, Parts 2 and 3
Nepal: Mount Everest National Park, 118/13/13/14 Part 2
Nepal Solu Hospital: 118/13/13/18 Part 1
(Volunteer Service Abroad) General 118/80/1 Part 5
(Volunteer Service Abroad) Volunteer Workers NZ: Conference Papers, 118/80/2 Part 1
Series 6949 (New Zealand High Commission, New Delhi, to 1982):
(Nepal) General NDI 64/14/1 Parts 1, 2 and 3
(Nepal) Himalaya Expeditions, NDI 64/14/2 Part 1
(Nepal) Himalayan Climbing Expeditions & Schoolhouse Project, NDI 64/14/2 Part 2
(Nepal) Himalayan Climbing Expeditions & Schoolhouse Projects, NDI 64/14/2 Parts 3 and 4
(Nepal) Himalayan Climbing Expeditions & Schoolhouse Projects: Khumjung Hospital, NDI 64/14/2 Part 5
(Aid to Nepal) Khumbu National Park: Agreements etc. NDI 72/19/6A Part 1
(Aid to Nepal) Himalayan Trust, NDI 72/19/10 Part 1

Canada

Archives held by the Sir Edmund Hillary Foundation, Toronto [SEHF]:

CIDA Project Submission, 1993–1995
CIDA – Miscellaneous, 1995
CIDA Project Submissions, 1996–1998
FIC (CIDA) Projects TSEHF
Khunde Hospital Proposal, 1995–1998
Khunde Hospital 1984–1989, Doctors' reports, correspondence, etc. Book. 1, 1990 –
President's Newsletter
Self Assessment Profile, 1995 SEHF
Community Based Initiatives in Health Inc. "Sir Edmund Hillary Foundation: An Institutional Evaluation". Conducted on behalf of the Sir Edmund Hillary Foundation and the Ontario International Development Program, 31 March 1993.

India

Archives held at the New Zealand High Commission, New Delhi, which was reopened in late 1984:

51/2/1. Vols. III and IV. Overseas Development Assistance: NZODA to South Asia: General
54/1/1. Vol. II. Aid to Nepal: General
54/2/1. Vols. VI and VII. Aid to Nepal: Training
54/3/1. Vol. 1 and 2. Aid to Nepal: Projects: Miscellaneous HOMF (Head of Mission Fund) requests
54/3/2. Vol. 1. Aid to Nepal: Projects: Himalayan Trust
54/4/1. Vol. II. NZ aid to Nepal: General: Volunteer Service Abroad (VSA)
NPL/NZ/8/1. Vol. 1. Nepal: Bilateral – Development Assistance: General
NPL/NZ/8/3. Vol. 1. Nepal: Bilateral: HOMF Projects
NPL/NZ/8/4. Nepal: Bilateral: Himalayan Trust

England

Oriental and India Office Collection and Records held at the British Library in London [OIOC]:

L/P&S/11 Political and Secret Annual Files
L/P&S/12 Political and Secret (External) Files

These contain a few assorted files related to the British Residency/Legation in Kathmandu and Annual Reports for 1911–12, 1912–13, 1914–15, 1919–20, 1920–21.

2. Private Papers

Documents from the personal papers of:
Murray Ellis, Dunedin, New Zealand
Dr Richard and Lesley Evans, Christchurch, New Zealand
Professor James Fisher (sent from USA)
Drs John and Susan Heydon, Dunedin, New Zealand
Sir Edmund Hillary, Auckland, New Zealand
Professor H. Kaye Ibbertson, Auckland, New Zealand
Mrs Betty Joplin, Auckland, New Zealand
Drs Selwyn and Ann Lang, Auckland, New Zealand
Jack Tait, Christchurch, New Zealand
Dr Jim Wilson (sent from Christchurch, New Zealand)

3. Publications and unpublished work by Sir Edmund Hillary, family and members of the Himalayan Trust (excluding Khunde Hospital volunteers)

Gill, Linda. *Living High: A Family Trek in the Himalayas.* Auckland: Hodder and Stoughton, 1983.

Gill, Michael. *Mountaineering Midsummer: Climbing in Four Continents.* London: Hodder and Stoughton, 1969.

——. "The Sherpas: A Survey of an Isolated Mountain Community". Department of Preventive and Social Medicine diss., University of Otago, 1961.

Hardie, Norman. *On My Own Two Feet: The Life of a Mountaineer.* Christchurch: Canterbury University Press, 2006.

——. *In Highest Nepal: Our Life Among the Sherpas.* London: George Allen & Unwin, 1957.

Hillary, Edmund (Sir Edmund). *View from the Summit.* London: Doubleday, 1999.

——. *From the Ocean to the Sky.* New York: Viking Press, 1979.

——. *Nothing Venture, Nothing Win.* London: Hodder and Stoughton, 1975.

——. *Schoolhouse in the Clouds.* London: Hodder and Stoughton, 1964.

——. *No Latitude for Error.* London: Hodder and Stoughton, 1961.

——. *High Adventure.* London: Readers Book Club, 1957 [1955].

Hillary, Edmund, and Desmond Doig. *High in the Thin Cold Air.* London: Hodder and Stoughton, 1963 [1962].

Hillary, Edmund and Peter. *Two Generations.* London: Hodder and Stoughton, 1984.

Hillary, Louise. *High Time.* London: Hodder and Stoughton, 1973.

——. *A Yak for Christmas.* New York: Doubleday, 1969.

——. *Keep Calm if You Can: Round the World with the Hillary Family.* London: Hodder and Stoughton, 1964.

Hillary, Peter, and John E. Elder. *In the Ghost Country: A Lifetime Spent on the Edge.* Auckland: Random House, 2004.

Lowe, George. *Because it Is There.* London: Cassell, 1959.

Mulgrew, Peter. *No Place for Men.* Auckland: Fontana Silver Fern, 1975 [1964].

Pearl, Max. "Kiwi in the Khumbu". *New Zealand Medical Journal* 64, 1965, 584–88.

4. Publications by Sherpas

Ang Rita Sherpa and Susan Höivik, eds. *Sherpas on Everest: A Tribute from the Sherpas of Nepal.* Kathmandu: Mandala Book Point, 2003.

Ang Tharkay (recueillis par Basil P. Norton). *Memoires d'un Sherpa*. Trans. into French, Henri Delgove. Paris: Amiot Dumont, 1954.

Mingma Norbu Sherpa. *Sherpa Culture: Way of Life, Festivals and Religion of Sherpa People.* Kathmandu: Mingma Norbu Sherpa, 1982.

Tenzing, Judi and Tashi. *Tenzing and the Sherpas of Everest.* Sydney: HarperCollins, 2001.

Tenzing Norgay Sherpa (as told to Malcolm Barnes). *After Everest: An Autobiography.* London: George Allen & Unwin, 1977.

——. (as told to James Ramsey Ullman). *Man of Everest: The Autobiography of Tenzing.* London: The Reprint Society, 1956 [1955]. The book was also published as *Tiger of the Snows: The Autobiography of Tenzing of Everest.* New York: G.P. Putnam's Sons, 1955.

Zangbu, Ngawang Tenzin (as told by). *Stories and Customs of the Sherpas.* Frances Klatzel, ed. Kathmandu: Mera Publications, 2000. The earliest version is a small leaflet "Information on Khumbu Sherpa Customs, on Sherpa Religion, on Tengboche Monastery, and on Mani Rimdu". Compiled by Tengboche Reincarnate Lama and translated by Sherry B. Ortner. Printed at Prabhat Printing Press, Kathmandu, no date.

5. Publications and unpublished work by volunteers at Khunde Hospital

Dawson, Penny, and Jamie Uhrig. "Sherpas and Sickness". *Alpine Journal* 89, no. 333, 1984, 80–83.

——. "Sherpa Health and Kunde Hospital". *Canadian Medical Association Journal* 128, 1983, 1010–12.

Harding, Elizabeth. *You Are A Brave Man: A Kiwi Odyssey in the Himalayas.* Auckland: Random House, 1996.

Heydon, Emma. "A Survey of Iodine Status in a Sherpa Community." B.Med. Sci. thesis, University of Otago, 2006.

Heydon, J., and S. Heydon. "50 Years after the First Ascent of Mt Everest: Progress and Problems". *Travel Medicine and Infectious Disease* 1, 2003, 145–47.

Heydon, Susan. "Sherpa Beliefs and Western Medicine: Providing Health Care at Khunde Hospital, Nepal". In *Soundings in Tibetan Medicine: Historical and Anthropological Perspectives. Proceedings of the Tenth Seminar of the International Association for Tibetan Studies, Oxford, 2003,* ed. Mona Schrempf, 65–87. Boston and Leiden: Brill, 2007.

——. "'High Places': Sir Edmund Hillary, the Sherpa and Health Services in the Mt Everest Area of Nepal." *New Zealand Journal of Asian Studies* 9, no. 1, 2007, 133–55.

——. "Modern Medicine and the Sherpa of Khumbu: Exploring the Histories of Khunde Hospital, Nepal 1966–1998". Ph.D. thesis, University of Otago, 2006.

——. "Kiwis in Khumbu: Negotiating Landscape and Community at Khunde Hospital". In *Landscape/Community: Perspectives from New Zealand History,* ed. Tony Ballantyne and Judith A. Bennett, 133–45. Dunedin: University of Otago Press, 2005.

——. "From Mount Everest to Kunde Hospital". *New Zealand International Review* 28, no. 6, 2003, 20–24.

——. "Change and Continuity: A History of Kunde Hospital, SoluKhumbu, Nepal". *Himalayan Research Bulletin* 17, no. 2, 1997, 27–30.

——. "Parochialism or a Fair Deal? A History of the South Otago Hospital Board". M.A. thesis, University of Otago, 1996.

Lang, Selwyn. "The Highest Schools in the World". *NZ Listener,* 24 May 1971, 10–11.

Lang, S. D. R., and Ann Lang. "The Kunde Hospital and a Demographic Survey of the Upper Khumbu, Nepal". *New Zealand Medical Journal* 74, 1971, 1–8.

Litch, J. A., R. A. Bishop, M. T. Sherpa, G. N. Sherpa and K. T. Sherpa. "Hormonal Contraceptive Use in a Rural District of Nepal". *Journal of Nepal Medical Association* 39, 2000, 199–202.

McKinnon, J. R. "Health Problems of Khumbu in Nepal: The Work at the Kunde Hospital". *New Zealand Medical Journal* 67, 1968, 140–43.

Murdoch, David R. "Symptoms of Infection and Altitude Illness Among Hikers in the Mount Everest Region of Nepal". *Aviation, Space, and Environmental Medicine,* 1995, 148–51.

Murdoch, David, and Lynley Cook. "Altitude Illness in Nepalis". *Journal of Nepal Medical Association* 31, 1993, 288–92.

Murdoch, David R., Elizabeth G. Harding and John T. Dunn. "Persistence of Iodine Deficiency 25 years After Initial Correction Efforts in the Khumbu Region of Nepal". *New Zealand Medical Journal* 112, 1999, 266–68.

6. Interviews

Formal and informal interviews and conversations took place, and were documented, throughout. In many cases this information was gathered on multiple occasions and the date is noted in the footnotes throughout the book. Oral material was also supplemented on occasions by further communication by email, the date of which is also noted in the footnotes. I am very grateful to the following people:

Ang Danu Sherpa, manager of the Khumbu Bijuli Company who trained as a government health assistant in the late 1970s

Ang Pasang Sherpa, hospital assistant in the 1970/79, now lodge owner in Lukla who also helps with hospital matters

Ang Rita Sherpa, chief administrative officer of the Himalayan Trust

Ang Tashi Sherpa, friend and lodgeowner at Kenzuma on the main tourist trail

Dawa Phuti Sherpa, nurse-assistant in 1978/79, now living in Lukla and very active in women's affairs in the area; member of the Himalayan Trust Advisory Committee

Gayse Nuru Sherpa, medical assistant, Khunde Hospital, from 1997

Dr Kami Temba Sherpa, village health worker 1976 and medical assistant at Khunde Hospital from 1977, trained in medicine at the Fiji School of Medicine from 1997, worked at Patan Hospital in Kathmandu and doctor-in-charge at Khunde Hospital from October 2002

Dr Lhakpa Norbu Sherpa, The Mountain Institute, first Sherpa to be awarded a Ph.D., in forest resources, works for conservation and development in mountain areas; formerly warden of the Sagarmatha National Park

Mingma Nuru Sherpa, dental therapist at Namche Dental Clinic and now a trained dentist

Mingma Temba Sherpa, medical assistant, Khunde Hospital, from 1979 and hospital manager from 1997

Nawang Doka Sherpa, dental therapist at Namche Dental Clinic and assists with running the family lodge in Namche Bazar

Nima Yangen Sherpa, first nurse-assistant at Khunde Hospital, 1966/68

Betty Joplin, secretary for Hillary since 1958

Professor David Murdoch and Dr Lynley Cook, volunteers at Khunde Hospital, 1991–93

Sir Edmund Hillary, chairman of the Himalayan Trust until his death in 2008

Elizabeth Hawley, New Zealand's Honorary Consul in Nepal, who has been involved with Hillary's work in Nepal since the 1960s

George Lowe, with Hillary on Everest in 1953; established the Sir Edmund Hillary Himalayan Trust UK in 1989

Professor James Fisher, anthropologist, Peace Corps teacher with Hillary's 1964 Himalayan School Expedition (email interview)

Dr Jim Wilson, member of the Himalayan Trust and friend of Hillary from the early 1960s

Dr John and Diane McKinnon, first volunteers at Khunde Hospital, 1966–68; continued involvement with the Trust, John becoming chairman of the medical sub-committee in 1980; Diane became chairperson of VSA in 1984

Dr John Heydon, volunteer at Khunde Hospital, 1996–98, member of the Himalayan Trust Council

Dr John Reekie, volunteer at Khunde Hospital, 1979/81

Professor John West, Professor of Medicine and Physiology at the University of California, specialising in high-altitude research; he was as a member of the 1960/61 Hillary expedition

Dr John Wilson, volunteer at Solu (Phaphlu) Hospital in 1975/77

June Lady Hillary, has been involved with Trust activities since the 1960s, chairperson of the Himalayan Trust from 2008

Professor H. Kaye Ibbertson, carried out iodine deficiency research in Khumbu in the 1960s and early 1970s

Dr Michael (Mike) Gill, member of the Himalayan Trust and involved with Hillary's activities since 1960

Murray Ellis, member of the Himalayan Trust and long-time family friend of Hillary

Neville Wooderson, plumber during the building of Khunde Hospital in 1966 and continued to be involved with building activities

W. F. (Zeke) O'Connor, founder and president of the Sir Edmund Hillary Foundation of Canada, from 1973

Rex Hillary, brother, builder for many of the Trust projects

Dr Richard and Lesley Evans, volunteers at Khunde Hospital, 1968–69

Drs Selwyn and Ann Lang, volunteers at Khunde Hospital, 1969/71

Shyam Pradhan Krishna, teacher from 1965, then headmaster at Khumjung School

8. Other

Collection of newspaper cuttings, "Sir Edmund Hillary: Everest and Beyond" exhibition, Otago Museum (Dunedin, New Zealand), 16 October 2004–20 March 2005.

The Sherpas of Everest, prod. and dir. by Ned Kelly, 50 min., BBC Bristol, *The World About Us* series, 1971.

Digital Himalaya, Census of Nepal 2001
http://www.digitalhimalaya.com/collections/nepalcensus/form.php

SECONDARY SOURCES

Acharya, S. "Monitoring and Evaluation of an IDD Control Program in Nepal". In Hetzel, Dunn and Stanbury, *The Prevention and Control of Iodine Deficiency Disorders,* 213–16.

Adams, Vincanne. *Tigers of the Snow and Other Virtual Sherpas: An Ethnography of Himalayan Encounters.* Princeton: Princeton University Press, 1996.

——. "The Production of Self and Body in Sherpa-Tibetan Society". In *Anthropological Approaches to the Study of Ethnomedicine,* ed. Mark Nichter, 149–89. New York: Gordon and Breach, 1992.

——. "Healing Buddhas and Mountain Guides: The Production of Self Within Society Through Medication". Ph.D. thesis, University of California, Berkeley, 1989.

——. "Modes of Production and Medicine: An Examination of the Theory in Light of Sherpa Medical Traditionalism". *Social Science & Medicine* 27, no. 5, 1988, 505–13.

Ahern, Brian. "A Hospital for Kunde". *New Zealand Alpine Journal* 22, no. 1, 1967, 13–19.

Ali, Almas. *Status of Health in Nepal.* Resource Centre for Primary Health Care Nepal and South-South Solidarity, India, July 1991.

Allen, N. J. "Approaches to Illness in the Nepalese Hills". In *Social Anthropology and Medicine,* ed. J. B. Loudon, 500–52. London: Academic Press, 1976.

Alter, Joseph S., ed. *Asian Medicine and Globalization.* Philadelphia: University of Pennsylvania Press, 2005.

Amrith, Sunil S. *Decolonizing International Health: India and Southeast Asia, 1930–65.* Houndmills: Palgrave Macmillan, 2006.

——. "In Search of a 'Magic Bullet' for Tuberculosis: South India and Beyond, 1955–1965". *Social History of Medicine* 17, no. 1, 2004, 113–30.

Arnold, David. *Science, Technology and Medicine in Colonial India.* The New Cambridge History of India 3, no. 5. Cambridge: Cambridge University Press, 2000.

Aziz, Barbara Nimri. *Tibetan Frontier Families: Reflecting Three Generations from D'ingri.* Durham, North Carolina: Carolina Academic Press, 1978.

Baker, G. C. (prepared by). "Forestry in Sagarmatha National Park: Nepal. A Collection of Unpublished Reports, 1970–1995". New Zealand Forest Research Institute, PO Box 465 Rangiora, New Zealand, August 1995.

Baker, P. T., ed. *The Biology of High-Altitude Peoples.* Cambridge: Cambridge University Press, 1978.

Bam, Dirgh Singh, and Ian Smith. "Principles of Effective Tuberculosis Control in Nepal". *Journal of Nepal Medical Association* 34, 1996, 3–7.

Bashford, Alison, and Claire Hooker, eds. *Contagion: Historical and Cultural Studies*. London: Routledge, 2001.

Basu, Amitabha, Ranjan Gupta and Sanat K. Bhattacharya. "Altitude and Biology in the Sherpa: An Alternative Approach to the Study of High Altitude Biology in the Context of the Eastern Himalayan Situation". *Journal of the Indian Anthropological Society* (Calcutta) 14, 1979, 139–48.

Belich, James. *Paradise Reforged: A History of New Zealanders from the 1880s to the Year 2000.* Auckland: Allen Lane/Penguin Press, 2001.

Berreman, Gerald D. *Hindus of the Himalayas: Ethnography and Change.* Berkeley: University of California Press, 1972.

Bhattacharya, Sanjoy. *Expunging Variola: The Control and Eradication of Smallpox in India, 1947–1977.* New Delhi: Orient Longman, 2006.

——. "Uncertain Advances: A Review of the Final Phases of the Smallpox Eradication Program in India, 1960-1980". *American Journal of Public Health* 94, no. 11, 2004, 1875–83.

Bhattacharya, Sanjoy, Mark Harrison and Michael Worboys. *Fractured States: Smallpox, Public Health and Vaccination Policy in British India, 1800–1947.* New Delhi: Orient Longman, 2005.

Bista, Dor Bahadur. *People of Nepal.* Kathmandu: Ratna Pustak Bhandar, 1972 [1967].

Bolam, Alison, Dharma S. Manandhar, Purna Shrestha, Matthew Ellis and Anthony M. de L. Costello. "The Effects of Postnatal Health Education for Mothers on Infant Care and Family Planning Practices in Nepal: A Randomised Controlled Trial". *British Medical Journal* 316, 1998, 805–11.

Booth, Pat. *Edmund Hillary: The Life of a Legend.* Auckland: Hodder Moa Beckett, 1993.

Brodhead, Tim. "NGOs: In One Year, Out the Other?" *World Development* 15, Supplement, 1987, 1–6.

Brooking, Tom. *The History of New Zealand.* Westport, Connecticut: Greenwood Press, 2004.

Brower, Barbara. *Sherpa of Khumbu: People, Livestock and Landscape.* Delhi: Oxford University Press, 1992 [1991].

Brown, Diana. "'Stepping-stone to Cretinism': Goitre in New Zealand, 1920–1950". B.A. Hons. diss., University of Otago, 2000.

Bryant, L. V. *New Zealanders and Everest.* Wellington: A. H. & A. W. Reed, 1953.

Bryder, Linda, ed. *A Healthy Country: Essays on the Social History of Medicine in New Zealand.* Wellington: Bridget Williams Books, 1991.

Buckle, Sam. "A Conscience Issue? Attitudes of New Zealand Governments to International Aid, 1967–1975". B.A. Hons. diss., University of Otago, 1996.

Burghart, Richard. "The Formation of the Concept of Nation-State in Nepal". *Journal of Asian Studies* 14, no. 1, 1984, 101–25.

Burnet, Sir Macfarlane. *Natural History of Infectious Disease.* 3rd ed. Cambridge: Cambridge University Press, 1962.

Bynum, W. F. *Science and the Practice of Medicine in the Nineteenth Century.* Cambridge: Cambridge University Press, 1994.

Camelon, Gelaine. *Rising to New Heights.* Toronto: Sir Edmund Hillary Foundation of Canada [1999].

Caplan, Lionel. *Warrior Gentlemen: "Gurkhas" in the Western Imagination.* Providence: Berghahn Books, 1995.

——. "'Bravest of the Brave': Representations of 'The Gurkha' in British Military Writings". *Modern Asian Studies* 25, no. 3, 1991, 571–97.

Central Bureau of Statistics. *Statistical Year Book of Nepal 2001.* Kathmandu: Central Bureau of Statistics, 2001.

Chand, Diwaker. *Development through Non-Government Organisations in Nepal.* Kathmandu: Institute for National Development Research and Social Services, 1991.

Chertow, Jennifer. "Gender, Medicine, and Modernity: Childbirth in Tibet Today—China's Control of Reproductive Choice in Tibet". *Harvard Asia Quarterly* 7, no. 4, 2003. http://www.asiaquarterly.com/content/view/140/40/

Clark, Keren. *The Two-Way Street: A Survey of Volunteer Service Abroad.* Wellington: New Zealand Council for Educational Research, 1978.

Clarke, Graham E. "Blood, Territory and National Identity in Himalayan States". In Tønnesson and Antlöv, *Asian Forms of the Nation,* 205–36.

Clifford, Terry. *Tibetan Buddhist Medicine & Psychiatry: The Diamond Healing.* Delhi: Motilal Banarsidass, 2001.

Connor, Linda H. "Healing Powers in Contemporary Asia". In Connor and Samuel, *Healing Powers and Modernity*, 3–21.

Connor, Linda H., and Geoffrey Samuel, eds. *Healing Powers and Modernity: Traditional Medicine, Shamanism, and Science in Asian Societies.* Westport, Connecticut: Bergin & Garvey, 2001.

Cooper, Frederick, and Randall Packard, eds. *International Development and the Social Sciences: Essays on the History and Politics of Knowledge.* Berkeley: University of California Press, 1997.

——. "Introduction". In Cooper and Packard, *International Development and the Social Sciences*, 1–41.

Cooter, Roger, and John Pickstone, eds. *Medicine in the Twentieth Century.* Amsterdam: Harwood Academic Publishers, 2000.

Cueto, Marcos. "The Origins of Primary Health Care and Selective Primary Health Care". *American Journal of Public Health* 94, no. 11, 2004, 1864–74.

Cunningham, Andrew, and Bridie Andrews, eds. *Western Medicine as Contested Knowledge.* Manchester: Manchester University Press, 1997.

——. "Introduction: Western Medicine as Contested Knowledge". In Cunningham and Andrews, *Western Medicine as Contested Knowledge*, 1–23.

Cunningham, John S. *Kingdom in the Sky.* London: Souvenir Press, 1975.

Das, Veena, ed. *The Oxford India Companion to Sociology and Social Anthropology.* New Delhi: Oxford University Press, 2003.

Dash, Arthur Jules. *Darjeeling.* Alipore: Bengal District Gazetteers, 1947.

Degnbol-Martinussen, John, and Poul Engberg-Pedersen. *Aid: Understanding International Development Cooperation.* Translated by Marie Bille. London: Zed Books/Copenhagen: Mellemfolkeligt Samvirke, Danish Association for International Cooperation, 2003.

De Nebesky-Wojkowitz, Réne. *Oracles and Demons of Tibet.* 's-Gravenhage [The Hague]: Mouton & Co, 1956.

Department of External Affairs. *New Zealand Foreign Affairs Review,* 22, no. 1, 1972.

Desjarlais, Robert R. *Body and Emotion: The Aesthetics of Illness and Healing in the Nepal Himalayas.* Philadelphia: University of Pennsylvania Press, 1992.

Despande, Satish. "Modernization". In Das, *The Oxford India Companion to Sociology and Social Anthropology,* 63–98.

Dixit, Hemang. *The Quest for Health: The Health Services of Nepal.* Kathmandu: Educational Enterprise, 1995 and 1999.

Dodin, Thierry, and Heinz Räther, eds. *Imagining Tibet: Perceptions, Projections & Fantasies.* Boston: Wisdom Publications, 2001.

Douglas, Ed. *Tenzing: Hero of Everest; A Biography of Tenzing Norgay.* Washington DC: National Geographic, 2003.

Drabek, Anne Gordon, ed. "Development Alternatives: The Challenge for NGOs". *World Development,* Supplement, 1987.

Draper, John. "Beyond Medicine: Sickness, Healing, and Order in Sherpa Society". Ph.D. thesis, University of Sydney, [1995].

——. "Lama Knows: Religion and Power in Sherpa Society". In Samuel, Gregor and Stutchbury, *Tantra and Popular Religion in Tibet*, 79–134.

——. "The Sherpas Transformed: Towards A Power-Centred View of Change in the Khumbu". *Contributions to Nepalese Studies* 15, no. 2, 1988, 139–62.

Dunn, Frederick L. "Medical-Geographical Observations in Central Nepal". *Milbank Memorial Fund Quarterly* 40, 1962, 125–48.

Dunn, J. T., and G. A. Medeiros-Neto, eds. *Endemic Goiter and Cretinism: Continuing Threats to World Health.* Pan-American Health Organization Scientific Publication No. 292, 1974.

Ebrahim, Alnoor. *NGOs and Organizational Change: Discourse, Reporting and Learning.* Cambridge: Cambridge University Press, 2003.

——. "NGO Behaviour and Development Discourse: Cases From Western India". *Voluntas* 12, no. 2, 2001, 79–101.

Ehrenreich, John, ed. *The Cultural Crisis of Modern Medicine.* New York: Monthly Review Press, 1978.

Elsner, Jás, and Joan-Pau Rubiés, eds. *Voyages and Visions: Towards a Cultural History of Travel.* London: Reaktion Books, 1999.

Ernst, Waltraud, ed. *Plural Medicine, Tradition and Modernity, 1800–2000.* London: Routledge, 2002.

——. "Plural Medicine, Tradition and Modernity: Historical and Contemporary Perspectives; Views from Below and Above". In Ernst, *Plural Medicine, Tradition and Modernity,* 1–18.

ESCAP. *Population of Nepal.* Country Monograph Series No. 6. Bangkok: United Nations, 1980.

Ferguson, James. "Anthropology and Its Evil Twin: 'Development' in the Constitution of a Discipline." In Cooper and Packard, *International Development and the Social Sciences*, 150–75.

Fisher, James. *Sherpas: Reflections on Change in Himalayan Nepal.* Delhi: Oxford University Press, 1997 [1990].

——. "The Historical Development of Himalayan Anthropology". *Mountain Research and Development* 5, no. 1, 1985, 99–111.

Fisher, Michael H. *Indirect Rule in India: Residents and the Residency System, 1764–1858.* Delhi: Oxford University Press, 1991.

Fletcher, Grace Nies. *The Fabulous Flemings of Kathmandu: The Story of Two Doctors in Nepal.* London: Quality Book Club, 1964.

Funnell, Don, and Romola Parish. *Mountain Environments and Communities.* London: Routledge, 2001.

Gaenszle, Martin. "The Shaman and the Doctor: Conflicting Systems of Interpretation and Diagnosis in East Nepal". In Sich and Gottschalk, *Acculturation and Domination in Traditional Asian Medical Systems,* 53–60.

Gauld, Robin, ed. *Comparative Health Policy in the Asia-Pacific.* Maidenhead: Open University Press, 2005.

Gellner, David N., Joanna Pfaff-Czarnecka and John Whelpton, eds. *Nationalism and Ethnicity in a Hindu Kingdom: The Politics of Culture in Contemporary Nepal.* Amsterdam: Harwood Academic Publishers, 1997.

Gimlette, G. H. D. *Nepal and the Nepalese.* London: H. F. & G. Witherby, 1928.

Gordon, David. "A Sword of Empire? Medicine and Colonialism at King William's Town, Xhosaland, 1856–91". In Sutphen and Andrews, *Medicine and Colonial Identity,* 41–60.

Green, Edward C. *Indigenous Theories of Contagious Disease.* Walnut Creek, London: AltaMira Press, 1999.

Gurung, Harka. *Nepal: Social Demography and Expressions.* Kathmandu: New Era, 2001.

Gutschow, Niels, Axels Michaels, Charles Ramble and Ernst Steinkellner, eds. *Sacred Landscape of the Himalaya: Proceedings of an International Conference at Heidelberg, 25-27 May 1998.* Vienna: Austrian Academy of Sciences Press, 2003.

Hackett, P. H., D. Rennie and H. D. Levine. "The Incidence, Importance, and Prophylaxis of Acute Mountain Sickness". *Lancet,* 1976, 1149–54.

Hagen, Toni. *Nepal: The Kingdom in the Himalayas.* New Delhi: Oxford and IBH, 1980 [1961].

Hamilton, Joyce. "Woman's Eye-View of Trekking with Hillary in Nepal". *New Zealand Woman's Weekly,* 10 February 1969, 6–9.

Hansen, Peter H. "Why Is There No Subaltern Studies for Tibet?" *Tibet Journal* 28, no. 4, 2003, 7–22.

——. "Confetti of Empire: The Conquest of Everest in Nepal, India, Britain and New Zealand". *Comparative Studies in Society and History 42,* 2000, 307–32.

——. "Partners: Guides and Sherpas in the Alps and Himalayas, 1850s–1950s." In Jás Elsner and Joan-Pau Rubiés, *Voyages and Visions,* 210–31.

——. "Debate: Tenzing's Two Wrist-Watches: The Conquest of Everest and Late Imperial Culture in Britain 1921–1953". *Past and Present* 157, 1997, 159–77.

Harrison, Mark. *Disease and the Modern World: 1500 to the Present Day.* Cambridge: Polity, 2004.

——. "Differences of Degree: Representations of India in British Medical Topography, 1820-c.1870". In Rupke, *Medical Geography in Historical Perspective,* 51–69.

——. *Public Health in British India: Anglo-Indian Preventive Medicine, 1859–1914.* Cambridge: Cambridge University Press, 1994.

Haynes, Douglas E. "From Tribute to Philanthropy: The Politics of Gift Giving in a Western Indian City". *Journal of Asian Studies* 46, no. 2, May 1987, 339–60.

Heath, Donald, and David Reid Williams, *High-Altitude Medicine and Pathology.* London: Butterworths, 1989.

Helman, Cecil. *Culture, Health and Illness: An Introduction for Health Professionals.* 3rd ed. Oxford: Butterworth Heinemann, 1994.

Hetzel, Basil S. *The Story of Iodine Deficiency: An International Challenge in Nutrition.* Oxford: Oxford University Press, 1989.

——. "The Prevention and Control of Iodine Deficiency Disorders". Rome: Administrative Committee on Coordination—Sub-Committee on Nutrition (ACC/SCN) State-of-the-Art Series, Nutrition Policy discussion Paper No. 3, March 1988.

——., ed. *Basic Health Care in Developing Countries: An Epidemiological Perspective.* Oxford: Oxford University Press, 1978.

Hetzel, Basil S., John T. Dunn and John B. Stanbury, eds. *The Prevention and Control of Iodine Deficiency Disorders.* Amsterdam: Elsevier, 1987.

Hetzel, B. S., and O. D. Pharoah, eds. *Endemic Cretinism.* Monograph Series No. 2. Papua New Guinea: Institute of Human Biology, 1971.

Hewa, Soma, and Philo Hove, eds. *Philanthropy and Cultural Context: Western Philanthropy in South, East, and Southeast Asia in the Twentieth Century*. New York: University Press of America, 1997.

Hickey, Sam, and Giles Mohan. "Relocating Participation within a Radical Politics of Development". *Development and Change* 36, no. 2, 2005, 237–62.

Hilton, James. *Lost Horizon.* London: Macmillan, 1933.

Hitchcock, John T., and Rex L. Jones, eds. *Spirit Possession in the Nepal Himalayas.* Warminster: Aris and Phillips, 1976.

Hornbein, Thomas F., and Robert B. Schoene, eds. *High Altitude: An Exploration of Human Adaptation*. New York: Marcel Dekker, 2001.

Houston, Charles S. *Going High: The Story of Man and Altitude.* 3rd. ed. Boston: Little, Brown, 1987.

——. *Going High: The Story of Man and Altitude.* Burlington: Charles S. Houston and The American Alpine Club, 1980.

Howell, Joel D. "Hospitals". In Cooter and Pickstone, *Medicine in the Twentieth Century,* 503–18.

Hu, Shu-Tsu. "Hypoxia Research in China: An Overview". In Sutton, Houston and Jones, *Hypoxia, Exercise, and Altitude,* 157–71.

Huang, Yukon. *Nepal: Development Performance and Prospects.* Washington: South Asia Regional Office, World Bank, 1979.

Hunt, John. *The Ascent of Everest.* London: Hodder and Stoughton, 1953.

Hunt, Nancy Rose. *A Colonial Lexicon: Of Birth Ritual, Medicalization and Mobility in the Congo.* Durham: Duke University Press, 1999.

Husain, Asad. *British India's Relations with the Kingdom of Nepal, 1857–1947: A Diplomatic History of Nepal.* London: George Allen and Unwin, 1970.

Hutt, Michael, ed. *Nepal in the Nineties.* New Delhi: Oxford University Press, 1993.

Ibbertson, H. K. "Goitre and Cretinism in the High Himalayas". *New Zealand Medical Journal* 80, no. 529, 1974, 484–88.

——. "Himalayan Goitre". In Richardson, *Abbottempo,* 30–33.

Ibbertson, H. K., P. D. Gluckman, M. S. Croxson and L. J. W. Strang. "Goiter and Cretinism in the Himalayas: A Reassessment". In Dunn and Medeiros-Neto, *Endemic Goiter and Cretinism,* 129–34.

Ibbertson, H. K., J. M. Tait, M. Pearl, T. Lim, J. McKinnon and M. B. Gill. "Endemic Cretinism in Nepal". In Hetzel and Pharoah, *Endemic Cretinism,* 71–88.

Izzard, Ralph. *An Innocent on Everest.* New York: E. P. Dutton, 1954.

Janes, Craig R. "Tibetan Medicine at the Crossroads: Radical Modernity and the Social Organization of Traditional Medicine in the Tibet Autonomous Region". In Connor and Samuel, *Healing Powers and Modernity,* 197–221.

——. "The Health Transition, Global Modernity and the Crisis of Traditional Medicine: The Tibetan Case". *Social Science & Medicine* 48, 1999, 1803–20.

Johnston, Alexa. *Sir Edmund Hillary: An Extraordinary Life.* Auckland: Penguin Viking, 2005.

Jones, Margaret. *Health Policy in Britain's Model Colony: Ceylon, 1900–1948.* New Delhi: Orient Longman, 2004.

Jones, Rex L. "Sanskritization in Eastern Nepal". *Ethnology* 15, no. 1, 1976, 63–75.

Joshi, Rupa, Kedar Sharma and Basanta Thapa, eds. *Twice Blessed: The Art of Giving.* Lalitpur, Nepal: Tewa, 2000.

Justice, Judith. *Policies, Plans, & People: Foreign Aid and Health Development.* Kathmandu: Mandala in association with University of California Press, 1986.

Keiser, Anne B., and Cynthia Russ Ramsay. *Sir Edmund Hillary and The People of Everest.* Kansas City: Andrews McMeel, 2002.

Kennedy, Dane. *The Magic Mountains: Hill Stations and the British Raj.* Berkeley, California: University of California Press, 1996.

Khadka, Narayan. *Foreign Aid and Foreign Policy: Major Powers and Nepal.* New Delhi: Vikas Publishing House, 1997.

King, Michael. *The Penguin History of New Zealand.* Auckland: Penguin Books, 2003.

Kuhn, Alice S. "Ladakh: A Pluralistic Medical System under Acculturation and Domination". In Sich and Gottschalk, *Acculturation and Domination in Traditional Asian Medical Systems,* 61–73.

Kunwar, Ramesh Raj. *Fire of Himal: An Anthropological Study of the Sherpas of the Nepal Himalayan Region.* New Delhi: Nirala, 1989.

Lambert, Helen. "Plural Traditions? Folk Therapeutics and 'English' Medicine in Rajasthan". In Cunningham and Andrews, *Western Medicine as Contested Knowledge*, 191–211.

Landon, Perceval. *Nepal.* 2 vols. New Delhi: Asian Educational Services, 1993 [1928].

Larkin, T. C., ed. *New Zealand's External Relations*. Wellington: New Zealand Institute of Public Administration and London: Oxford University Press, 1962.

Lee, Sung. "WHO and the Developing World: The Contest for Ideology". In Cunningham and Andrews, *Western Medicine as Contested Knowledge,* 24–65.

Leslie, Charles. "Interpretation of Illness: Syncretism in Modern Ayurveda". In Leslie and Young, *Paths to Asian Medical Knowledge,* 177–208.

——. ed. *Asian Medical Systems: A Comparative Study.* Berkeley: University of California Press, 1976.

Leslie, Charles, and Allan Young, eds. *Paths to Asian Medical Knowledge.* Berkeley,: University of California Press, 1992.

Lindell, Jonathan. *Nepal and the Gospel of God.* Kathmandu: United Mission to Nepal, 1979.

Litsios, Socrates. "The Christian Medical Commission and the Development of the World Health Organization's Primary Health Care Approach". *American Journal of Public Health* 94, no. 11, 2004, 1884–93.

Livingstone, David N. "Human Acclimatization: Perspectives on a Contested Field of Inquiry in Science, Medicine and Geography". *History of Science* 25, 1987, 359–94.

Lossio, Jorge. "Altitude Medicine and Physiology". *Wellcome History* 29, summer 2005, 9.

Loudon, Irvine, ed. *Western Medicine*. Oxford: Oxford University Press, 1997.

Loudon, J. B., ed. *Social Anthropology and Medicine.* London: Academic Press, 1976.

Ludden, David. "Introduction: A Brief History of Subalternity". In Ludden, *Reading Subaltern Studies,* 1–39.

——, ed. *Reading Subaltern Studies: Critical History, Contested Meaning and the Globalization of South Asia.* London: Anthem Press, 2002.

Luger, Kurt. *Kids of Khumbu: Sherpa Youth on the Modernity Trail.* Kathmandu: Mandala Book Point, 2000.

McCarrison, R. "Observations on Endemic Cretinism in the Chitral and Gilgit Valleys". *Lancet*, 31 October 1908, 1275–80.

McCullagh, S. F. "The Huon Peninsula Endemic: I. The Effectiveness of an Intramuscular Depot of Iodized Oil in the Control of Endemic Goitre". *Medical Journal of Australia,* 1963, 769–77.

McDonald, Bernadette. *I'll Call You in Kathmandu: The Elizabeth Hawley Story.* Seattle: The Mountaineers Books, 2005.

Macfarlane, Alan. "Fatalism and Development in Nepal". In Hutt, *Nepal in the Nineties,* 106–27.

Macfarlane, Robert. *Mountains of the Mind: A History of a Fascination.* London: Granta, 2003.

McGuiness, Jamie. *Trekking in the Everest Region.* 3rd ed. Hindhead: Trailblazer Publications, 1998.

McKay, Alex. *Their Footprints Remain: Biomedical Beginnings Across the Indo-Tibetan Frontier.* Amsterdam: University of Amsterdam Press, 2007.

——. "'Fit for the Frontier: European Understandings of the Tibetan Environment in the Colonial Era". *New Zealand Journal of Asian Studies* 9, no. 1, 2007, 118–32.

——. "'The Birth of a Clinic'? The IMS Dispensary in Gyantse (Tibet), 1904–1910." *Medical History* 49, 2005, 135–54.

——. "British-Indian Medical Service Officers in Bhutan, 1905–1947: A Historical Outline". In Ura and Kinga, *The Spider and the Piglet,* 137–59.

——. *Tibet and the British Raj: The Frontier Cadre, 1904–1947.* Richmond: Curzon, 1997.

McKay, Alex, with Dorje Wangchuk. "Traditional Medicine in Bhutan". *Asian Medicine Tradition and Modernity* 1, no. 1, 2005, 204–18.

McIntyre, W. David. "From Dual Dependency to Nuclear Free". In Rice, *The Oxford History of New Zealand,* 520–38.

Magill, Frank N., ed. *Survey of Social Science,* Sociology Series Volume 2. Pasadena: Salem Press, 1994.

Mahoney, Michael. *Harry Ayres: Mountain Guide.* Christchurch: Whitcoulls, 1982.

Malcolm, Laurence. "Primary Health Care and the Hospital: Incompatible Organisational Concepts?" *Social Science & Medicine* 39, no. 4, 1994, 455–58.

Mason, Kenneth. *Abode of Snow: A History of Himalayan Exploration and Mountaineering.* London: Rupert Hart-Davis, 1955.

Marasini, B. R. "Health and Hospital Development in Nepal: Past and Present". *Journal of Nepal Medical Association* 42, 2003, 306–11.

Mathema, Padma. *Primary Health Care in Nepal.* Kathmandu: Vijaya Ram Mathema, 1987.

Mauss, Marcel. *The Gift: Forms and Functions of Exchange in Archaic Societies.* London: Cohen & West, 1970 [1925].

Medical Student's Wife. "In Support of Husbands in a Delivery Theatre". *Digest* [University of Otago Medical Students' Association] 6, no. 2, 1965, 29–30.

Mihaly, Eugene Bramer. *Foreign Aid and Politics in Nepal: A Case Study.* 2nd ed. Lalitpur: Himal Books, 2002 [1965].

Miles, M. "Goitre, Cretinism and Iodine in South Asia: Historical Perspectives on a Continuing Scourge". *Medical History* 42, 1998, 47–67.

Miller, Robert. "High Altitude Mountaineering, Cash Economy, and the Sherpa". *Human Organization* 24, no. 3, 1965, reprinted in *Himalayan Research Bulletin* 17, no. 2, 1997, 17–22.

Mills, Anne. "Leopard or Chameleon? The Changing Character of International Health Economics". *Tropical Medicine and International Health* 2, no. 10, 1997, 963–77.

Minderhoud, Jan. "The Christian Presence in Nepal before 1951". *Indian Church History Review,* December 1990, 144–64.

Ministry of Foreign Affairs. "The Flow of Resources from New Zealand to Developing Countries 1972/73". Wellington, 1974.

Moller, David. "Challenge on the Roof of the World". *Reader's Digest.* UK ed. May 1999, 92–104.

Morris, James. *Coronation Everest.* London: Faber and Faber, 1958.

Mosse, David. "Global Governance and the Ethnography of International Aid". In David Mosse and David Lewis, *The Aid Effect,* 1–36.

Mosse, David and David Lewis. *The Aid Effect: Giving and Governing in International Development.* London: Pluto Press, 2005.

Mull, Dorothy S., Jon W. Anderson and J. Dennis Mull. "Cow Dung, Rock Salt, and Medical Innovation in the Hindu Kush of Pakistan: The Cultural Transformation of Neonatal Tetanus and Iodine Deficiency". *Social Science & Medicine* 30, no. 6, 1990, 675–91.

Musa, Ghazali. "An Investigation of Travel Health Experiences in High Altitude destinations: Case Studies of Sagarmatha National Park (Nepal) and Tibet (China)". Ph.D. thesis, University of Otago, 2001.

Musa, Ghazali, C. M. Hall and J. E. S. Higham. "Tourism Sustainability and Health Impacts in High Altitude Adventure, Cultural and Ecotourism Destinations: A Case Study of Nepal's Sagarmatha National Park". *Journal of Sustainable Tourism* 12, no. 4, 2004, 306–31.

New Zealand Department of Internal Affairs. *The Dictionary of New Zealand Biography* 5, 1941–1960. http://www.dnzb.govt.nz/dnzb/default.asp

Niermeyer, Susan, Stacy Zamudio and Lorna G. Moore. "The People". In Hornbein and Schoene, *High Altitude,* 43–100.

NZAID. "The Heights of Development". *Currents* 6, 2007, 8–13.

Obituary. *New Zealand Medical Journal* 92, 1980, 364–65.

Oldfield, Henry Ambrose. *Sketches from Nipal.* 2 vols. London: W. H. Allen, 1880.

Oliver, W. H., and B. R. William, eds. *The Oxford History of New Zealand.* Wellington: Oxford University Press, 1981.

Oppitz, Michael. "Myths and Facts: Reconsidering Some Data Concerning the Clan History of the Sherpa". *Kailash* 2, 1974, 120–31.

Ortner, Sherry B. *Anthropology and Social Theory: Culture, Power, and the Acting Subject.* Durham: Duke University Press, 2006.

——. *Life and Death on Mt. Everest: Sherpas and Himalayan Mountaineering.* New Delhi: Oxford University Press, 2000 [1999].

——. "The Case of Disappearing Shamans, or No Individualism, No Relationalism". *Ethnos* 23 no. 3, 1995, 355–90.

——. *High Religion: A Cultural and Political History of Sherpa Buddhism.* Delhi: Motilal Banarsidass, 1999 [1989].

——. *Sherpas through their Rituals.* Cambridge: Cambridge University Press, 1978.

——. "Sherpa Purity". *American Anthropologist* 75, 1973, 49–63.

Ortner Paul, Sherry. "Food for Thought: A Key Symbol in Sherpa Culture". Ph.D. thesis, University of Chicago, 1970.

Packard, Randall M. "Post-Colonial Medicine". In Cooter and Pickstone, *Medicine in the Twentieth Century,* 97–112.

——. "Visions of Postwar Health and Development and Their Impact on Public Health Interventions in the Developing World". In Cooper and Packard, *International Development and the Social Sciences,* 93–115.

Panday, Devendra Raj. *Nepal's Failed Development: Reflections on the Mission and the Maladies.* Kathmandu: Nepal South Asia Centre, 1999.

Parker, Barbara. "Ritual Coordination of Medical Pluralism in Highland Nepal: Implications for Policy". *Social Science & Medicine* 27, no. 9, 1988, 919–25.

Parkes, Charlotte M. "The Impact of the Medicalisation of New Zealand's Maternity Services on Women's Experience of Childbirth, 1904–1937". In Bryder, *A Healthy Country*, 165–80.

Patterson, George N. *Tibetan Journey.* London: Faber and Faber, 1954.

Paul, Robert. "Some Observations on Sherpa Shamanism". In Hitchcock and Jones, *Spirit Possession in the Nepal Himalayas*, 141–51.

Pawson, Eric. "The Meanings of Mountains". In Pawson and Brooking, *Environmental Histories of New Zealand,* 136–50.

Pawson, Eric, and Tom Brooking, eds. *Environmental Histories of New Zealand.* Auckland: Oxford University Press, 2002.

Pawson, I. G. "Growth and Development in High Altitude Populations: A Review of Ethiopian, Peruvian and Nepalese Studies". *Proceedings of the Royal Society of London* B. 194, 1976, 83–98.

Pawson, Ivan G., Dennyse D. Standford and Vincanne A. Adams. "Effects of Modernization on the Khumbu Region of Nepal: Changes in Population Structure, 1970–1982". *Mountain Research and Development* 4, no. 1, 1984, 73–81.

Peat, Neville. *The VSA Way: 25 years of Volunteering Overseas.* Wellington: Compatriot Press for Volunteer Service Abroad, 1987.

Pelling, Margaret. "The Meaning of Contagion: Reproduction, Medicine and Metaphor". In Bashford and Hooker, *Contagion,* 15–38.

Phillips, Jock. *A Man's Country? The Image of the Pakeha Male – A History.* Rev. ed. Auckland: Penguin Books, 1996.

Pigg, Stacy Leigh. "'Found in Most Traditional Societies': Traditional Medical Practitioners Between Culture and Development". In Cooper and Packard, *International Development and the Social Sciences,* 259–90.

——. "The Social Symbolism of Healing in Nepal". *Ethnology* 34, no. 1, winter 1995, 17–36.

——. "Unintended Consequences: The Ideological Impact of Development in Nepal". *South Asia Bulletin* 18, nos. 1 and 2, 1993, 45–58.

——. "Inventing Social Categories Through Place: Social Representations and Development in Nepal". *Comparative Studies in Society and History* 34, 1992, 491–513.

Poffenberger, Mark. *Patterns of Change in the Nepal Himalaya.* Boulder, Colorado: Westview Press, 1980.

Porter, Roy, ed. *The Cambridge Illustrated History of Medicine.* Cambridge: Cambridge University Press, 1996.

Poudel, Byas Jee. *Canadian Development Assistance to Nepal.* Kathmandu: Sharad Shashi Poudel, [1989] 1991.

Pratt, Mary Louise. *Imperial Eyes: Travel Writing and Transculturation.* London: Routledge, 1992.

Purdey, Alice F., Gyan Bahadur Adhikari, Sheila A. Robinson and Philip W. Cox. "Participatory Health Development in Rural Nepal: Clarifying the Process of Community Empowerment". *Health Education Quarterly* 21, no. 3, fall 1994, 329–43.

Putnam, Robert D. *Making Democracy Work: Civic Traditions in Modern Italy.* Princeton: Princeton University Press, 1993.

Rachbauer, Dieter, ed. *Energy from the Top of the World: Small Hydropower Plant Thame-Namche Bazar, Nepal.* Kathmandu: Eco Himal, 2001.

Raheja, Gloria Goodwin. *The Poison in the Gift: Ritual, Prestation, and the Dominant Caste in a North Indian Village.* Chicago: University of Chicago Press, 1988.

Ramanna, Mridula. *Western Medicine and Public Health in Colonial Bombay 1845–1895.* New Delhi: Orient Longman, 2002.

Ramble, Charles. "Tibetan Pride of Place: Or, Why Nepal's Bhotiyas are not an Ethnic Group". In Gellner, Pfaff-Czarnecka and Whelpton, *Nationalism and Ethnicity in a Hindu Kingdom*, 379–413.

Rawat, Indra Singh. *Indian Explorers of the Nineteenth Century.* New Delhi: Publications Division, Ministry of Information and Broadcasting, Government of India, 1973.

Regmi, Mahesh C. *Landownership in Nepal.* Berkeley: University of California Press, 1976.

——. "Nepal Press Digest". Kathmandu: Regmi Research Project, first published in 1956.

Reissland, Nadja, and Richard Burghart. "Active Patients: The Integration of Modern and Traditional Obstetric Practices in Nepal". *Social Science & Medicine* 29, no. 1, 1989, 43–52.

Rice, Geoffrey W., ed. *The Oxford History of New Zealand.* 2nd ed. Auckland: Oxford University Press, 1992.

Richardson, Robert G., ed. *Abbottempo.* Book 3. Amsterdam: Abbott Universal, 1969.

Rist, Gilbert. *The History of Development: From Western Origins to Global Faith.* London: Zed Books, 2002 [1997].

Roberts, Gilbert. "Health and Medicine". In Ullman, *Americans on Everest,* 343–50.

Robinson, Sheila A. "Development and Philanthropy in the Context of South Asia: Moving toward Transformation". In Hewa and Hove, *Philanthropy and Cultural Context,* 295–314.

Rogers, Paul, and John Aitchison. *Towards Sustainable Tourism in the Everest Region of Nepal.* Kathmandu, Nepal: IUCN—The World Conservation Union and ICPL, 1998.

Rose, Leo E. "The National Political Culture and Institutions in Nepal". In Shastri and Wilson, *The Post-Colonial States of South Asia,* 114–38.

Rose, Leo E. and Margaret W. Fisher. *The Politics of Nepal: Persistence and Change in an Asian Monarchy.* Ithaca: Cornell University Press, 1970.

Rosenberg, Charles E. *The Care of Strangers: The Rise of America's Hospital System.* New York: Basic Books, 1987.

Rupke, Nicholaas A., ed. *Medical Geography in Historical Perspective.* London: *Medical History,* Supplement no. 20, Wellcome Trust Centre for the History of Medicine at UCL, 2000.

Samuel, Geoffrey, Hamish Gregor and Elisabeth Stutchbury, eds. *Tantra and Popular Religion in Tibet.* New Delhi: International Academy of Indian Culture and Aditya Prakashan, 1994.

Schremph, Mona, ed. *Soundings in Tibetan Medicine: Historical and Anthropological Perspectives; Proceedings of the Tenth Seminar of the International Association for Tibetan Studies, 2003.* Leiden: Brill, 2007.

Sharma, Sudhindra. "Half a Century of Foreign Aid". In Mihaly, *Foreign Aid and Politics in Nepal: A Case Study*, xix–lx.

Shastri, Amita, and A. Jeyaratnam Wilson, eds. *The Post-Colonial States of South Asia: Democracy, Development and Identity*. New York: Palgrave, 2001.

Sich, Dorothea, and Waltraud Gottschalk, eds. *Acculturation and Domination in Traditional Asian Medical Systems.* Stuttgart: Franz Steiner Verlag, 1994.

Sidel, Marc. "Recent Research on Philanthropy and the Nonprofit Sector in India and South Asia". *Voluntas,* 12, no. 2, 2001, 171–80.

Sinclair, Keith. *A History of New Zealand.* Auckland: Penguin Books, 2000 [1959].

Skerry, Christa A., Kerry Moran and Kay M. Calavan. *Four Decades of Development: The History of U.S. Assistance to Nepal, 1951–1991.* Kathmandu: United States Agency for International Development (USAID), 1991.

Smith, Brian H. *More Than Altruism: The Politics of Private Foreign Aid.* Princeton, New Jersey: Princeton University Press, 1990.

Smith, Philippa Mein. *A Concise History of New Zealand.* Cambridge: Cambridge University Press, 2005.

Stanbury, John B. "Commentary on Dr. Hetzel's Review of the Global Problem of Iodine Deficiency Disorders". In Hetzel, "The Prevention and Control of Iodine Deficiency Disorders", 116–19.

Stevens, Stanley. *Claiming the High Ground: Sherpas, Subsistence and Environmental Change in the Highest Himalaya.* Delhi: Motilal Banarsidass, 1996 [1993].

Stiller, Ludwig F. *Nepal: Growth of a Nation.* [Kathmandu]: Human Resources Development Research Center, 1999 [1993].

Stiller, Ludwig F., and Ram Prakash Yadav. *Planning For People.* [Kathmandu]: Human Resources Development Research Center, 1993 [1978].

Stone, Linda. "Cultural Crossroads of Community Participation in Development: A Case from Nepal". *Human Organization* 48, no. 3, 1989, 206–13.

——. "Primary Health Care for Whom? Village Perspectives from Nepal". *Social Science & Medicine* 22, no. 3, 1986, 293–302.

Streefland, Pieter. "The Frontier of Modern Western Medicine in Nepal". *Social Science & Medicine* 20, no. 11, 1985, 1151–59.

Stutchbury, Elizabeth. "Remembering John Norman Draper, 1955–1994." *Himalayan Research Bulletin* 17, no. 2, 1997, 4–5.

Survey of India. *Records of the Survey of India* 8, *Exploration in Tibet and Neighbouring Regions.* Part 1: 1865–1879 and Part 2: 1879–1892. Dehra Dun: Survey of India, 1915.

Sutphen, Mary P. and Bridie Andrews. *Medicine and Colonial Identity.* London: Routledge, 2003.

Sutton, John R., Charles S. Houston and Norman L. Jones, eds. *Hypoxia, Exercise, and Altitude: Proceedings of the Third Banff International Hypoxia Symposium.* New York: A. R. Liss, 1983.

Taylor, Carl E. "A Medical Survey of the Kali Gandak and Pokhara Valleys of Central Nepal". *Geographical Review* 41, 1951, 421–37.

Temple, Philip. *The World at Their Feet: The Story of New Zealand Mountaineers in the Great Ranges of the World.* Christchurch: Whitcombe & Tombs, 1969.

Tester, Frank James, and Paule McNicoll. "'Why Don't They Get It?' Talk of Medicine as Science. St Luke's Hospital, Panniqtuuq, Baffin Island". *Social History of Medicine* 19, no. 1, 2006, 87–106.

Thompson, Graeme J. *New Zealand's International Aid.* Wellington: The New Zealand Institute of International Affairs, 1967.

Tilman, H. W. *Nepal Himalaya.* Cambridge: Cambridge University Press, 1952.

Tønnesson, Stein and Hans Antlöv, eds. *Asian Forms of the Nation.* Richmond, Surrey: Curzon, 1996.

Ullman, James Ramsey. *Americans on Everest: The Official Account of the Ascent Led by Norman G. Dyhrenfurth.* Philadelphia: J. B. Lippincott, 1964.

Ulvila, Marko and Farhad Hossain. "Development NGOs and Political Participation of the Poor in Bangladesh and Nepal". *Voluntas* 13, no. 2, 2002, 149–63.

Unschuld, Paul U. *Medicine in China: A History of Ideas.* Berkeley: University of California Press, 1985.

Ura, Karma, and Sonam Kinga, eds. *The Spider and the Piglet: Proceedings of the First International Seminar on Bhutan Studies*. Bhutan: Centre for Bhutan Studies, 2004. www.bhutanstudies.org.bt/publications/spdr-pglt/spdr-pglt.htm

Van der Geest, Sjaak, Johan D. Speckmann and Pieter H. Streefland. "Primary Health Care in a Multi-Level Perspective: Towards a Research Agenda". *Social Science & Medicine* 30, no. 9, 1990, 1025–34.

Van Spengen, Wim. *Tibetan Border Worlds: A Geohistorical Analysis of Trade and Traders.* London: Kegan Paul International, 2000.

Von Fürer-Haimendorf, Christoph. *The Sherpas Transformed: Social Change in a Buddhist Society of Nepal.* New Delhi: Sterling Publishers, 1984.

——. *Himalayan Traders: Life in Highland Nepal.* London: John Murray, 1975.

——. *The Sherpas of Nepal: Buddhist Highlanders.* London: John Murray, 1964.

——. "The Role of the Monastery in Sherpa Society". *Ethnologica* 2, 1960, 12–28.

Wade, R. H. "New Zealand's External Aid Programmes". In Larkin, *New Zealand's External Relations,* 79–109.

Ward, Michael. *In This Short Span: A Mountaineering Memoir.* London: Victor Gollancz, 1972.

——. "In Eastern Nepal". *Lancet* 263, no. 2, 1952, 238–39.

Ward, Michael P., James S. Milledge and John B. West. *High Altitude Medicine and Physiology.* 3rd ed. London: Arnold, 2000.

Weiner, Saul J. "'Source Force' and the Nepal Medical Profession". *Social Science & Medicine* 29, no. 5, 1989, 669–75.

Weitz, Charles A., Ivan G. Pawson, M. Velma Weitz, Selwyn D. R. Lang and Ann Lang. "Cultural Factors Affecting the Demographic Structure of a High Altitude Nepalese Population". *Social Biology* 25, fall 1978, 179–95.

West, John B. *High Life: A History of High-Altitude Physiology and Medicine.* New York: Oxford University Press for the American Physiological Society, 1998.

Whelpton, John. *A History of Nepal.* Cambridge: Cambridge University Press, 2005.

Wiley, Andrea S. *An Ecology of High-Altitude Infancy: A Biocultural Perspective.* Cambridge: Cambridge University Press, 2004.

——. "Increasing Use of Prenatal Care in Ladakh (India): The Roles of Ecological and Cultural Factors". *Social Science & Medicine* 55, 2002, 1089–1102.

Winthrop, Robert H. *Dictionary of Concepts in Cultural Anthropology.* New York: Greenwood Press, 1991.

Worboys, Michael. "The Spread of Western Medicine". In Loudon, *Western Medicine,* 249–63.

Worsley, Peter. "Non-Western Medical Systems". *Annual Review of Anthropology* 11, 1982, 315–48.

Worth, Robert M., and Narayan K. Shah. *Nepal Health Survey, 1965–1966.* Honolulu: University of Hawaii Press, 1969.

Index